Contributions to Psychology and Medicine

Contributions to Psychology and Medicine

J.A. Skelton
Robert T. Croyle

Editors

Mental Representation in Health and Illness

With 20 Illustrations

Springer-Verlag
New York Berlin Heidelberg London
Paris Tokyo Hong Kong Barcelona

J.A. Skelton
Department of Psychology
Benjamin D. James Center
Dickinson College
Carlisle, PA 17013-2896
USA

Robert T. Croyle
Department of Psychology
University of Utah
Salt Lake City, UT 84112
USA

Advisor
J. Richard Eiser
Department of Psychology
Washington Singer Laboratories
University of Exeter
Exeter EX4 4QG
England

Library of Congress Cataloging-in-Publication Data
Mental representation in health and illness / J.A. Skelton, Robert T.
Croyle, editors.
    p. cm.—(Contributions to psychology and medicine)
    Includes bibliographical references.
    Includes index.
    ISBN 0-387-97401-6 (alk. paper).—ISBN 3-540-97401-6 (alk.
paper)
    1. Sick—Psychology. 2. Health behavior. 3. Medical
anthropology. 4. Social medicine.   I. Skelton, J.A. II. Croyle,
Robert T. III. Series.
    [DNLM: 1. Attitude to Health. 2. Disease—psychology. 3. Mental
Processes. 4. Sick Role. WM 90 M549]
R726.5.M46 1991
616′.0019—dc20
DNLM/DLC   90-10132

NWSt
I ADB9502

Printed on acid-free paper.

Typeset by Best-Set Typesetters, Ltd., Chai Wan, Hong Kong.
Printed and bound by Edwards Brothers, Inc., Ann Arbor, Michigan.
Printed in the United States of America.

9 8 7 6 5 4 3 2 1

ISBN 0-387-97401-6 Springer-Verlag New York Berlin Heidelberg
ISBN 3-540-97401-6 Springer-Verlag Berlin Heidelberg New York

Contents

Contributors

GEORGE D. BISHOP, PH.D.
Division of Behavioral and Cultural Sciences, University of Texas at San Antonio, San Antonio, TX 78285-0652, USA

DANIEL J. COX, PH.D.
Behavioral Medicine Center, University of Virginia School of Medicine, Blue Ridge Hospital, Charlottesville, VA 22901, USA

ROBERT T. CROYLE, PH.D.
Department of Psychology, University of Utah, Salt Lake City, UT 84112, USA

MICHAEL DIEFENBACH, M.S.
Institute for Health, Health Care Policy, and Aging Research, Rutgers University, New Brunswick, NJ 08903, USA

PAUL FARMER, PH.D., M.D.
Department of Social Medicine, Harvard Medical School, Boston, MA 02115, USA

LINDA A. GONDER-FREDERICK, PH.D.
Behavioral Medicine Center, University of Virginia School of Medicine, Blue Ridge Hospital, Charlottesville, VA 22901, USA

BYRON J. GOOD, PH.D.
Department of Social Medicine, Harvard Medical School, Boston, MA 02115, USA

John B. Jemmott III, Ph.D.
Department of Psychology, Princeton University, Princeton, NJ 08544, USA

J. Michael Lacroix, Ph.D.
Department of Psychology, Glendon College, York University, Toronto, Ontario M4N 3M6, Canada

K. Mark Leek, M.A.
Cancer Prevention Unit, Fred Hutchinson Research Center, Seattle, WA 98104, USA

Howard Leventhal, Ph.D.
Institute for Health, Health Care Policy, and Aging Research, Rutgers University, New Brunswick, NJ 08903, USA

James W. Pennebaker, Ph.D.
Department of Psychology, Southern Methodist University, Dallas, TX 75275, USA

Renate Schober
Department of Psychology, Glendon College, York University, Toronto, Ontario M4N 3M6, Canada

J. A. Skelton, Ph.D
Department of Psychology, Benjamin D. James Center, Dickinson College, Carlisle, PA 17013-2896, USA

David Watson, Ph.D.
Department of Psychology, Southern Methodist University, Dallas, TX 75275, USA

1
Mental Representation, Health, and Illness: An Introduction

J. A. Skelton and Robert T. Croyle

The role played by psychological, social, and cultural factors in human health and health-related behavior is hardly a new theme in the social and behavioral sciences. It is clear, however, that something new is happening in health-related social research. An important new line of theory and research can be traced, a line of work concerning basic questions of how the individual thinks about health and illness. This is the study of health and illness representation. The investigators who examine the mental representation of health and illness seek to answer such questions as these: How does the average person understand and conceptualize "health"? What rules govern the ways in which people mentally represent their own and others' health status, and what are the implications of such representational processes and structures?

Such questions have long been staples of medical anthropology, a field concerned with the culturally transmitted meanings assigned to disease. Medical anthropology studies have served the valuable function of sensitizing us to the contextual character of people's responses to health threats (Chrisman & Kleinman, 1983). Fieldwork with non-Western peoples has disclosed the degree of variability in the meanings assigned to disease; accustomed to thinking of health problems in a largely biomedical framework, we have benefited from the revelation of alternative explanatory structures used to account for symptoms and disease in other cultural groups. For Western psychologists, an awareness of cross-cultural variation in collective representations of disease and illness raises the possibilities that (1) individual representations of health and illness vary within a culture, and (2) such variations may help to account for variation in health- and illness-related behavior.

The field of medical sociology (Mechanic, 1978) has also helped to stimulate interest in fundamental questions of illness representation. Parsons's (1953) insightful analyses of the character of American institutional medicine helped raise awareness of the sometimes incompatible goals of health-care providers and their clients. Hayes-Bautista's (1976) description of physician–patient encounters as "negotiations" further illustrated differences in the ways that laypersons' mental representations of illness may conflict with those of the medical establishment. Although individuals raised in the Western biomedical tradition may share some of the assumptions of their health-care providers, it is now clear that laypersons may construe health threats and their treatment very differently from those having responsibility for diagnosing and applying up-to-date medical techniques to such threats.

Although medical anthropology and sociology provide a host of insights into representational issues, both the methodologies and levels of analysis employed in these disciplines largely preclude our being able to answer questions about the structure of lay illness representations at the individual level, about the deployment of such structures in everyday illness experience, about the relationship of representational structures and processes in the domain of illness to other cognitive structures, and about how to modify the undesirable effects of inadequate representational structures on health-related behavior. From a psychological perspective, answering such questions is a prerequisite for a comprehensive theory of health and illness behavior; yet the basic research needed to address them has only recently begun to flourish.

Illness Schemata and the Representational Approach

Few social and behavioral scientists would dispute that individuals' understanding of events is a primary determinant of their responses to those events. Indeed, the notion that individuals respond to the world as they view it, not necessarily as it is, has achieved the status of a truism. But clichés become clichés, at least in part, because of their utility. In the history of Western psychology, the Lewinian concept of life-space, Brunswik's distinction between stimuli and percepts, and neo-Jamesian theories of emotion-as-appraisal stand as testimony to the usefulness of the simple idea that individuals' mental representations of events somehow matter.

At this writing, 10 years have passed since the appearance of "The Common Sense Representation of Illness Danger" (Leventhal, Meyer, & Nerenz, 1980). In that groundbreaking article, Howard Leventhal, Daniel Meyer, and David Nerenz offered the view that patients' mental representations of health threats determine how patients respond to those threats. Taking as their domain the problem of patient compliance with treatment regimens, Leventhal et al. presented both reasoned argument and empirical data showing that patients employ *implicit theories of illness* (sometimes termed *illness schemata*) in order to achieve an understanding of health threats and to regulate their health behavior.

This was not the first time that social scientists working in the area of health and illness accorded an important role to patients' beliefs in health-related behavior. The Health Belief Model (HBM) attempted to explain cooperation (or, more often, noncooperation) with prevention and treatment recommendations partly in terms of subjectively perceived seriousness of and vulnerability to health threats (Becker, 1974; Haynes, Taylor, & Sackett, 1979). A critical shortcoming of the HBM and related approaches to understanding health behavior, however, lay in the sheer quantity of nonprioritized variables that could be hypothesized to affect health-related behavior; for example, Becker and Maimon (1983) catalogued over 80 empirical correlates of health-related behaviors discovered in extant studies.

Leventhal et al.'s notion of illness schemata went beyond the HBM in at least two important respects. First, it proposed that patients' health beliefs are *structured*: The core of implicit illness theories consists of subjectively perceived symptoms and attributions concerning the causes of symptoms, the latter being derived in part from information presented in the social environment and in part from patients' past illness experiences. An important characteristic of this proposal is that it prompted recognition that (1) illness schemata operate in the same way as other representational structures, and (2) an understanding of illness representation in particular must be theoretically grounded in an understanding of cognition in general. This was in stark contrast to the essentially ad hoc, atheoretical, and specialized nature of the HBM. The second way in which Leventhal et al.'s conceptualization of illness schemata superseded the HBM was in the proposition that such structures play a specific part in the *process* of health-related behavior: Lay theories guide coping, entry into and use of medical treatment, and evaluations of treatment effects.

Four years after the Leventhal, Meyer, and Nerenz article appeared, Leventhal, Nerenz, and Steele (1984) proposed a more comprehensive self-regulation model of coping with health threats. This work, which is referenced by many of the contributors to this volume, illustrated the tremendous advantages of integrating work on mental representation with basic research in other fields of psychology. The model rests on two important foundations of psychological research, and it is no coincidence that Leventhal has been a major contributor to both. One of these fields, persuasion, has attracted at least cursory attention from many investigators who study health behavior change. The second, emotion, is attended to by theorists who focus on coping processes but has had little impact on public health research. Research and theory from both subfields has much to contribute to our understanding of health and illness behavior. Unfortunately, the efforts by Leventhal and his colleagues to integrate this work into a theory of health psychology are exceptions.

Current Trends in Illness Cognition Research

The generative value of Leventhal et al.'s recasting has been inestimable in furthering our understanding of how laypeople understand illness (to paraphrase Bishop, this volume) and respond to it. It has spawned a theoretically oriented search for the structural components and the processes of lay illness representations. For example, subsequent research by Leventhal and his associates (Baumann, Cameron, Zimmerman, & Leventhal, 1989; Meyer, Leventhal, & Gutmann, 1985) and by others (Lau, Bernard, & Hartman, 1989; Lau & Hartman, 1983) has produced agreement that lay theories of illness include the elements of (1) concrete *symptoms* and a *label* (e.g., a common cold vs. pneumonia) that facilitate identification of the health problem, beliefs about (2) the immediate and long-term *consequences* of the problem and (3) its *temporal course*, and attributions concerning (4) the *cause* of the problem and (5) the means by which a *cure* may be affected. Schober and Lacroix (this volume) demonstrate that implicit illness theories of the 18th century, as inferred from archival material, parallel in a striking way those discovered in contemporary research.

Specific components of the Leventhal et al. representational model have become the object of study by many investigators. For example, Bishop and his associates (Bishop, Briede, Cavazos, Grotzinger, & McMahon, 1987; Bishop & Converse, 1986) have examined how individuals accomplish the task of identifying health problems. They propose that specific symptoms are matched with identifying labels through a *prototype-matching process*. By calling attention to the parallels between illness beliefs and more general concepts from cognitive psychology, the idea of illness schemata also provided a context for integrating a burgeoning literature on the determinants of symptomatic experience and symptom-reporting behavior (Pennebaker, 1982; Pennebaker & Skelton, 1981). The notion that illness representations and symptom experiences are linked in schematic structures has led to studies of how activation of prior illness episodes contributes to immediate symptom-reporting behavior (Skelton, 1987; Skelton & Strohmetz, 1990). The fact that physical symptoms are also linked to emotion episodes has generated studies of how affect influences people's health appraisals (Croyle & Uretsky, 1987; Salovey & Birnbaum, 1989) and of the "interchangeability" of symptom and mood reports (Watson & Pennebaker, 1989).

Processes of illness representation, especially the ways in which people appraise their own health status, have also come under increased scrutiny in recent years. Jemmott, Croyle, and their associates have examined the ways in which individuals react to information about their own health status (Jemmott, Ditto, & Croyle, 1986). In line with the proposition that information-processing strategies in illness cognition are simply special cases of more general strategies, these investigators found that simple heuristics can account for the seriousness with which people regard the news that they have a disease. In addition, they have found that the threat implications of diseases depend in rather surprising ways on perceptions of the population prevalence of the disease (Jemmott, Croyle, & Ditto, 1988).

Studies of illness cognition such as those noted are now sufficiently numerous to merit special mention in recent reviews of the field of health psychology (Rodin & Salovey, 1989; Taylor, 1990). This should indicate the degree to which the mental representational emphasis has become an influential force in the social and behavioral sciences that are concerned with health. Perhaps an even more important indicator, however, is the growing number of applications of the concept of illness schemata. For example, Lacroix (this volume) reports the creation of an instrument for assessing patients' understanding of disabling chronic low back pain and promising results in using this measure to predict return to work. This development holds out the hope of developing interventions to alter patients' illness schemata and thereby facilitate their reintegration into the working world. Gonder-Frederick and her colleagues (Gonder-Frederick & Cox, this volume) have devoted several years' effort to delineating the implicit theories that guide diabetic patients' behavior in response to a life-threatening disease. They have identified patients' erroneous beliefs about the characteristic symptoms of the disease and are implementing an education program aimed at increasing patients' competence in regulating their own treatment. Lacroix's and Gonder-Frederick's work responds effectively to Leventhal et al.'s (1980) criticism of much compliance research of the time, which focused on patients' inherently unalterable dispositions. Their work represents the fulfillment of a prophecy made by Leventhal, Meyer, and Nerenz, who expressed hope that educational interventions would eventually become routine, were the concept of illness schemata embraced in all its implications.

The Present Volume

Rather than previewing each chapter in this book, we offer here an orientation to its structure and central themes. The opening chapter by Schober and Lacroix, noted earlier, presents an overview of the multicomponent model of illness cognition originally proposed by Leventhal et al. (1980) and adduces evidence for its cross-historical generality. The next three chapters focus on illness representation at the individual level. Bishop presents a summary of current knowledge about the process and consequences of illness identification. Watson and Pennebaker reprise their extensive work on the relationship between perceived symptoms and affective temperament and raise important questions about which measures of health status are most appropriate. Croyle and Jemmott examine individuals' reactions to the increasingly common practice of risk factor testing. Skelton provides a transition from the individual to the collective levels of illness representation by considering how third parties react to patients' illness complaints. Then, Farmer and Good present their anthropological analysis of the cultural transformation of illness representations, using AIDS in Haiti as a case in point. Leek continues the examination of how sociocultural factors are implicated in illness representation by focusing on a community's failure to agree on an approach to alcohol education and treatment. Leek argues that the failure was a result of conflicting implicit models of alcohol abuse among those who establish health policy. Lacroix and Gonder-Frederick and Cox then describe their applications of illness schema concepts to patients with chronic diseases. Finally, Leventhal and Diefenbach look back at the forces that led to the genesis of the illness schema concept and look ahead at its future prospects.

Future Directions for Research and Theory in Illness Cognition

We are heartened by the widespread impact of Leventhal et al.'s (1980) seminal theoretical contributions. Indeed, this volume is testimony to the Lewinian dictum that nothing is so practical as a good theory. Nevertheless, there exist numerous gaps in research on illness representations that we hope can be addressed in future work. Rather than repeat those identified by our authors, we have chosen to focus on three areas of overriding importance.

Perhaps the most critical of these as-yet-unaddressed issues concerns the means by which erroneous illness representations might be changed. If we assume that illness schemata carry behavioral and coping implications, then faulty schemata may result in dysfunctional responses (Kelly, 1955). For example, people appear to judge the severity of a disease in inverse proportion to its population prevalence (Croyle & Jemmott, this volume), and this judgment heuristic may cause failures to take appropriate action in the face of potentially life-threatening conditions. To cite another example, both hypertension and diabetes patients regulate self-treatment on the basis of inappropriate symptomatic "pseudo-concomitants" of their disease, thereby undermining the efficacy of treatment (Gonder-Frederick & Cox, this volume; Leventhal et al., 1980). A major priority is to discover how best to overcome such faulty representations, and this is a task for both basic and applied researchers. Illness schemata represent experience-based, over-learned patterns of perception and conceptualization and hence would seem extremely resistant to change (cf. Lacroix, this volume). The lengths to which Gonder-Frederick and her associates have found it necessary to go in order to achieve modest gains in control over diabetes bespeak the difficulty of inducing accommodation in laypersons' representational systems.

Yet change does occur, and it strikes us as exceedingly important to acquire an understanding of how it occurs. To achieve this understanding, basic researchers should utilize theoretical concepts derived from studies of attitude and behavior change. Applied researchers can assist by identifying patients whose implicit models of illness have undergone radical change and by specifying the most appropriate measures of change. Only through such targeted joint efforts can we hope to develop adequate theories and interventions to promote adaptive changes in faulty models—and to do so in a cost-effective manner.

Another priority for the future is a strengthening of bonds between the theoretical and empirical literatures on coping with health threats and those concerning illness representation. The concept of implicit illness models was developed in the context of attempts to understand the coping process, yet much of the research on coping in social and health psychology has proceeded in relative isolation from that on illness representation. For example, recent reviews in the field of health psychology have treated coping and illness representation as separate issues (Rodin & Salovey, 1989; Taylor, 1990). Part of the problem here, we suspect, is that much of the basic research on representational structures and processes has employed healthy participants and/or has used limited or indirect measures of coping behavior (e.g., subjective likelihoods of engaging in certain health-related actions; requests for information about a particular disease). Health-oriented coping research, on the other hand, has tended to focus on populations facing veridical health threats and on "harder" measures of the outcome of coping efforts (Scheier et al., in press; Taylor, Lichtman, & Wood, 1984). For many clinicians, the gap between illness cognition research and clinical practice is too great. Another contributing factor, however, is that illness cognition research—representationally oriented studies, in particular—is pervasively misrepresented as being concerned solely with the problems of illness identification and causal attribution; as the present volume amply demonstrates, such characterizations are wide of the mark. There are signs, however, that the artificial separation of coping from representationally oriented health research is dissolving (Taylor & Schneider, 1989), and we hope for further progress toward such dissolution. When coping is phrased in terms of how individuals mentally represent and respond to threats, it becomes clear that coping is a form of representational activity.

A final suggestion we offer to representationally oriented theorists and researchers concerns the methods used to perform studies of illness cognition. We strongly advocate the use of at-risk populations, individuals who face genuine threats to their health. The study of illness representation structures and processes involves "hot" cognition, and ignoring the heat may seriously constrain the adequacy of our hypothesis tests. As Farmer and Good (this volume) illustrate, many aspects of illness representations manifest themselves as clearly in everyday discourse as in a psychology laboratory. In a similar vein, we urge the conduct of prospective studies (such as those reported by Lacroix and Gonder-Frederick & Cox in this volume) where efforts are made to assess illness schemata in vivo and substantive behavioral outcomes are measured. It would be useful for us to remember that Leventhal et al.'s (1980) formulation of the representational perspective was based on observations of "real" patients.

References

Baumann, L. J., Cameron, L. D., Zimmerman, R. S., & Leventhal, H. (1989). Illness representations and matching labels with symptoms. *Health Psychology*, *8*(4), 449–470.

Becker, M. H. (1974). *The health belief model and personal health behavior*. Thorofare, NJ: Charles B. Slack.

Becker, M. H., & Maimon, L. H. (1983). Models of health-related behavior. In D. Mechanic (Ed.), *Handbook of health, health care, and the health professions* (pp. 539–568). New York: Free Press.

Bishop, G. D., Briede, C., Cavazos, L., Grotzinger, R., & McMahon, S. (1987). Processing illness information: The role of disease prototypes. *Basic and Applied Social Psychology*, *8*, 21–43.

Bishop, G. D., & Converse, S. A. (1986). Illness representations: A prototype approach. *Health Psychology*, *5*, 95–114.

Chrisman, N. J., & Kleinman, A. (1983). Popular health care, social networks, and cultural meanings: The orientation of medical anthropology. In D. Mechanic (Ed.), *Handbook of health, health care, and the health professions* (pp. 569–590). New York: Free Press.

Croyle, R. T., & Uretsky, M. B. (1987). Effects of mood on self-appraisal of health status. *Health Psychology*, *6*(3), 239–253.

Hayes-Bautista, D. E. (1976). Modifying the treatment: Compliance, patient control, and medical care. *Social Science and Medicine*, *10*, 233–238.

Haynes, R. B., Taylor, D. W., & Sackett, D. L. (1979). *Compliance in health care*. Baltimore: Johns Hopkins University Press.

Jemmott, J. B., Croyle, R. T., & Ditto, P. H. (1988). Commonsense epidemiology: Self-based judgments from laypersons and physicians. *Health Psychology*, *7*, 55–73.

Jemmott, J. B., Ditto, P. H., & Croyle, R. T. (1986). Judging health status: Effects of perceived prevalence and personal relevance. *Journal of Personality and Social Psychology*, *50*, 899–905.

Kelly, G. A. (1955). *The psychology of personal constructs*. New York: Norton.

Lau, R. R., Bernard, T. M., & Hartman, K. A. (1989). Further explorations of commonsense representations of common illnesses. *Health Psychology*, *8*(2), 195–220.

Lau, R. R., & Hartman, K. A. (1983). Commonsense representations of common illnesses. *Health Psychology*, *2*, 167–185.

Leventhal, H., Meyer, D., & Nerenz, D. (1980). The common sense representation of illness danger. In S. Rachman (Ed.), *Contributions to medical psychology* (pp. 7–30). New York: Pergamon Press.

Leventhal, H., Nerenz, D., & Steele, D. J. (1984). Illness representations and coping with health threats. In A. Baum, S. E. Taylor, & J. E. Singer (Eds.), *Handbook of psychology and health* (Vol. 4, pp. 219–252). Hillsdale, NJ: Lawrence Erlbaum Associates.

Mechanic, D. (1978). *Medical sociology* (2 ed.). New York: Free Press.

Meyer, D., Leventhal, H., & Gutmann, M. (1985). Commonsense models of illness: The example of hypertension. *Health Psychology, 4,* 115–135.

Parsons, T. (1953). *The social system.* New York: Free Press.

Pennebaker, J. W. (1982). *The psychology of physical symptoms.* New York: Springer-Verlag.

Pennebaker, J. W., & Skelton, J. A. (1981). Selective monitoring of bodily sensations. *Journal of Personality and Social Psychology, 41,* 213–223.

Rodin, J., & Salovey, P. (1989). Health psychology. *Annual Review of Psychology, 40,* 533–579.

Salovey, P., & Birnbaum, D. (1989). Influence of mood on health-relevant cognitions. *Journal of Personality and Social Psychology, 57*(3), 539–551.

Scheier, M. F., Matthews, K. A., Owens, J., Magovern, G. J., Sr., Lefebvre, R. C., Abbott, R. A., & Carver, C. S. (In press). Dispositional optimism and recovery from coronary artery bypass surgery: The beneficial effects on physical and psychological well-being. *Journal of Personality and Social Psychology.*

Skelton, J. A. (1987, June). Symptom suggestibility: Somatic imagery as an underlying process? In J. M. Lacroix (chair), *Illness schemas: Emerging methodological and empirical issues.* Symposium conducted at the meeting of the Canadian Psychological Association, Vancouver, British Columbia, Canada.

Skelton, J. A., & Strohmetz, D. B. (1990). Priming symptom reports with health-related cognitive activity. *Personality and Social Psychology Bulletin, 16,* 449–464.

Taylor, S. E. (1990). Health psychology: The science and the field. *American Psychologist, 45*(1), 40–50.

Taylor, S. E., Lichtman, R. R., & Wood, J. V. (1984). Attributions, beliefs about control, and adjustment to breast cancer. *Journal of Personality and Social Psychology, 46,* 489–502.

Taylor, S. E., & Schneider, S. K. (1989). Coping and the simulation of events. *Social Cognition, 7*(2), 176–196.

Watson, D., & Pennebaker, J. W. (1989). Health complaints, stress, and distress: Exploring the central role of negative affectivity. *Psychological Review, 96,* 234–254.

2
Lay Illness Models in the Enlightenment and the 20th Century: Some Historical Lessons

Renate Schober and J. Michael Lacroix

I lay engrossed in this vision, for an unconscionable time, in a sort of icy, fatalistic despair; groaning, meditating suicide and twiddling my toes. *My toes*! I had forgotten—*my toes were all right*! There they were, pink and lively, twiddling away, as if twiddling in mirth at my absurd train of thought! Grim and gloomy hypochondriac though I might have been, I was not ignorant of elementary neuro-anatomy. A stroke massive enough to have knocked out the rest of the leg would certainly have knocked out the foot as well. As soon as this occurred to me, I burst into a hearty roar of laughter. My brain was all right—I hadn't had a stroke. I didn't know what I did have, but I didn't have a stroke.

Thus, tormented by his subjectively perceived loss of leg, the physician Oliver Sacks (1984, p. 56) lay, longing for his doctor's understanding ear, in a London hospital—with an official diagnosis of torn tendon. The segment captures the fundamental distinction drawn between disease and illness in both the social sciences and medicine (Barondess, 1979; Cott & Pavloski, 1985; Jennings, 1986). Disease is there viewed as a biological event, characterized by pathology in structure and/or function of body organs and systems. Illness, in contrast, is portrayed as comprising the lay perceptions and thoughts as well as behavioral adjustments to disvalued changes in the individual's state of well-being.

The view that disease and illness are not congruent is supported by a recent and popular body of social science research, suggesting that patient dissatisfaction with the nature and quality of health care is in part attributable to the discordance in cognitive models that patient and physician bring

Supported by grant A0659 from the Natural Sciences and Engineering Research Council of Canada. Order of authorship was determined by a coin flip.

to bear on the biomedical encounter (Engel, 1977; Kleinman, Eisenberg, & Good, 1978; Stimson, 1974). However, the possibility that lay illness models may incorporate concepts of disease that predate the advent of 20th-century medicine has not been evaluated in this research and is the focus of the present chapter. Such evaluation is useful in identifying any impact that biomedical science may have on the nature and development of lay medical thought and thereby may suggest clinical strategies for improving patient–physician communication in contemporary medical practice.

This chapter traces the historical development of lay medical thought by comparing contemporary models of illness with those held in the 17th and 18th centuries. In particular, we argue that contemporary illness models differ from those of the Enlightenment period in verbal familiarity with the terminology in modern medicine—verbal familiarity *only*, for the explanatory framework of health and illness in the two eras is fundamentally based in the Hippocratic–Galenic medicine of classic Greek antiquity. The six-component structure of the illness models appears invariant across time, encompassing symptoms, diagnostic labels, cause, cure, estimates of timeline, and consequences of illness. The contents of the cognitive models also appear similar in the two time periods, focusing particularly on protection of the body against environmental influences, dietary intake, rest, stress, and emotional well-being, with respect to both etiology and therapeutics; we argue that these factors can be traced directly back to Hippocratic medicine. Contemporary illness models show some familiarity with the terminology of modern medicine, but this familiarity is at a level of verbal fluency only, as lay explanations of illness remain fundamentally Hippocratic. The influence that medical science thus has on the nature and development of lay medical thought suggests the importance of systematic attention to illness models in contemporary medical practice.

We first consider the structure and contents of contemporary models of illness with particular emphasis on issues of symptomatology, diagnosis, etiology, and therapeutics. This is followed by material on the structure and contents of the cognitive models of the 17th and 18th centuries. We then examine the historical roots of the illness models, an exercise that will take us to the Hippocratic–Galenic medicine of classic Greek antiquity. In a concluding consideration of clinical lessons from historical research, we comment on the impact of medical advances on lay medical thought and its implications for patient–physician encounters in contemporary medical practice.

Contemporary Lay Illness Models

Empirical research examining the nature of lay illness models is of recent origin and forms part of a broader scientific interest in the role of cognition in illness behavior. Researchers in this novel field of inquiry most commonly conceptualize the illness models as generic and organized cognitive representations or schemata that derive from prior experiences in the medical domain and guide the processing of information in a fashion that is consistent with the prior knowledge (e.g., Bishop & Converse, 1986; Lau & Hartman, 1983; Meyer, Leventhal, & Gutmann, 1985). This view has been valuable in stimulating empirical research which enables the preliminary specification of the structural components as well as the contents of the lay illness models. The research is reviewed in this section, which focuses on the contents of the cognitive models.

Structure

Investigations of the structure of lay illness models are few in number but consistent in finding six components according to which experiences of illness are cognitively organized. These components are symptoms, diagnostic label, cause, cure, timeline, and consequences of ill health, as suggested by studies of patient groups as well as subjects free of current medical disorder (e.g., Bishop, Briede, Cavazos, Grotzinger, & McMahon, 1987; Lau & Hartman, 1983; Leventhal, Meyer, & Nerenz, 1980; Meyer et al., 1985). Let us briefly examine this work.

In open-ended unstructured interviews, patients suffering from malignant lymphoma (Leventhal et al., 1980) and hypertension (Leventhal et al., 1980; Meyer et al., 1985) were more than willing to disclose symptom information, to speculate about the duration and consequences of their illness, to reveal their thoughts about causal elements and physiological mechanisms (even though these were commonly discordant with biomedical formulations), and to elaborate on the associated therapeutic regimens in which they engaged (even if these consisted of discontinuing use of prescribed medication). Lau and Hartman (1983) observed that college students, when asked about their most recent illness episode, similarly volunteered symptom information, spontaneously provided a disease label, had no trouble providing an in-depth account of why they had fallen ill, and, logically deriving from this, why they had recovered. Likewise, when asked to free-associate to descriptions of symptom sets, Bishop et al.'s (1987) subjects displayed great ease in recalling representations in memory of diagnostic labels, additional symptoms, cause, cure, timeline, and consequences of ill health. The six components accounted for 91% of all associations made. Collectively, these studies as well as other investigations (e.g., Pennebaker, 1982; Pennebaker, Gonder-Frederick, Cox, & Hoover, 1985) suggest that the individual components of the cognitive models combine to form a generic and organized knowledge structure which is stable, invariant, and impervious to influence by significant experiences in the individual's medical history. This stands in contrast to the *contents* of lay illness models, which have emerged as idiosyncratic by virtue of ties to prevailing circumstances. In the following section, we seek to find some trends in the idiosyncratic data on the contents of the cognitive models. To this end, we examine, in order, (1) conceptions of symptoms in relation to disease labels, (2) perceived etiological contributions to illness, and (3) perceived therapeutic indications.

Content

Symptomatology is a topic with which the contemporary laity has deep familiarity. The existing empirical literature abounds with reports of lay intimacy with symptom experiences indicative of both minor and major disease attacking the various biological systems (e.g., Bishop, 1984; Kutner & Gordon, 1961; Pennebaker, 1982; Safer, Tharps, Jackson, & Leventhal, 1979). Such symptom experience is a tolerated accompaniment of day-to-day living—"tolerated," indeed, for a substantial majority of patients fail to present themselves to the physician for biomedical diagnosis (Hannay & Maddox, 1976; White, Williams, & Greenberg, 1961). It is apparent from the high frequency of self-recognized illness episodes and the correspondingly low frequency of medical consultation that contemporary sufferers tend to perceive their afflictions as private and individualistic occurrences, which are readily managed outside the realms of the formal medical-care system.

The self-management of ill health is very much an active affair that includes lay speculations about symptomatology in reference to diagnostic labels of disease. In this regard, the following segment is instructive:

> No matter what I have got wrong with me, if I go over to the doctor with a terrific headache that I'm getting—"Oh, it's all to do with your chest"— anything, no matter, if I'm worried about something now, and I want to go to the doctor's, see, perhaps I'm getting these headaches or something and I'm getting a bit concerned about them now, no matter what, I can guarantee when I come out of that doctor's, it's to do with my chest. No matter what I get, you're missing a period and he says—"It's to do with your chest." (Stimson, 1974, p. 102)

This quotation reflects the lay sentiment that the sufferer is capable of making informed diagnostic judgments, based on access to symptom information. The validity of this sentiment has only recently begun to be investigated. Bishop and Converse (1986) and Bishop et al. (1987) presented subjects with symptom sets previously judged to reflect diseases both serious (epilepsy, heart attack, ulcer, stomach cancer, stroke, and pneumonia) and nonserious (measles, strep throat, hay fever, flu, mumps, and chicken pox). With access to symptom descriptions only, subjects clearly exhibited diagnostic skills, providing accurate disease labels and showing great confidence in their diagnoses. The diagnostic facilities deteriorated, however, as inconsistent symptoms were introduced in place of the diagnostically consistent symptoms in the original symptom sets. The discovery of diagnostic skills in ordinary people is valuable in more clearly characterizing the nature of lay medical thought.

What is suggested by the findings of lay diagnostic skills is, first, that ordinary people have acquired a distinct verbal fluency with the biomedical taxonomies of our times. Lay linguistic familiarity with biomedical taxonomies has been demonstrated elsewhere, with respect not only to diagnostic labels but also to symptomatic descriptions, human anatomy, and physiological mechanisms (e.g., Blaxter, 1979; Helman, 1978; Kleinman et al., 178; Lau & Hartman, 1983; Leventhal et al., 1980; Tait & Asher, 1955). Second, lay diagnostic abilities clearly indicate that biomedical taxonomies of disease serve as meaningful representations of symptom sets in lay medical thought. This implies that diseases are apperceived as distinct entities, entities that are readily differentiated from one another in reference to symptomatology. However, although it is thus apparent that there exists a degree of lay competence in medical matters, it does not automatically follow that explanatory frameworks of illness are equally informed. Indeed, lay accounts of etiology are interesting in this respect.

What is striking about the lay explanatory framework of illness is the universal perceived relevance of a limited number of causal elements to the whole gamut of disease taxonomies in our times. Exposure to the elements and climate, germs and viruses, food and diet, carelessness, stress and situational factors, nerves, aging, susceptibility, heredity, and God have been claimed to account for a host of disorders from hypertension to colds and flu, arthritis, pneumonia, urinary tract infections, abdominal distress, headaches, allergies, diabetes, and tuberculosis, to name a few (e.g., Blaxter, 1979; Elder, 1973; Helman, 1978; Lau & Hartman, 1983; Leventhal et al., 1980; Marby, 1964). On close examination, patterns are visible in these etiological accounts. Exposure to the elements is a most prominent perceived cause of illness, as seen in this example on arthritis:

> And as a young person I had a very strenuous life on the farm. . . . Wet—wet up to the knees, and in the dew and everything. And getting awful cold . . . after all we weren't well-to-do, . . . and when the feet got wet they stayed wet and cold all day. (Elder, 1973, p. 32)

This claim of exposure as a cause of arthritis is echoed in lay accounts of the etiologies of colds and flu, bronchitis, and even abdominal discomfort, headaches, and racing heart rate (Blaxter, 1979; Helman, 1978; Lau & Hartman, 1983; Marby, 1964). Naturally, the opportunity for exposure is given by the weather or climate, which is invariably described as dangerous when cold and wet (Blaxter, 1979; Elder, 1973; Helman, 1978; Lau & Hartman, 1983). The germs of illness are thus inherent in the individual's relation with the physical environment. This makes our natural habitat a rather dangerous place.

The social environment is equally dangerous, for it too holds the germs of illness in the literal sense of the word. Germs and viruses are elements of risk in any social relation, as is expressed by this patient: "A girl with a strep throat coughed in my face" (Lau & Hartman, 1983). The catching of germs and viruses through social relations need not involve direct contact with a carrier but can be mediated by the physical environment, as is the case when one catches germs from a dirty lavatory seat (Helman, 1978). Germs enter the body via the orifices; travel about the body invading lungs, chest, stomach, and skin; and signal their appearance by the onset of fever, dry coughs, and diarrhea (Helman, 1978). Germs are held responsible for a range of disorders, among them influenza, pneumonia, tuberculosis, measles, chicken pox, and gastroenteritis (e.g., Blaxter, 1979; Helman, 1978; Marby, 1964). What we can gather from such identification of the social and physical environment as primary threats to health is an individualistic vision of bodily integrity. This vision is above all apparent in the importance assigned to self-management of activities by which the individual enters into relations with his or her surroundings.

Elaborating on this theme, our contemporaries commonly blame neglect of temperance in mind and body for a vast number of human afflictions, including cancer, tuberculosis, gastroenteritis, depression, arthritis, headaches, flu, colds, and hypertension (Blaxter, 1979; Elder, 1973; Helman, 1978; Lau & Hartman, 1983; Leventhal et al., 1980; Marby, 1964; Rippiere, 1981). Neglect may be in the form of failure to keep adequate dietary regimens, failure to protect the body against hazardous environmental influences, failure to obtain sufficient rest and sleep, failure to ensure emotional stability through management of stress and situational factors, and even failure to maintain good relations with God. Faulty self-management in respect to these activities assumes importance by virtue of weakening the body's defenses, thereby robbing the individual of allies in the struggle against a naturally hostile environment (Helman, 1978). The importance assigned to self-management in lay etiological accounts of illness extends, as we shall see, to the perception of therapeutic indications.

It is perhaps not entirely surprising to find that lay etiological evaluations entail directives for curative practice. Naturally, cure is a relatively easy undertaking when failure to recruit allies in the struggle against nature underlies the etiology of disease. By way of example, the normalization of hypertension may require stress reduction and an adequate dietary regimen, which may or may not be combined with medication (Leventhal et al., 1980). "I prayed and God healed me"—this may indeed be all that is required to cure a cold (Lau & Hartman, 1983). Colds may also be combated by taking rest, applying warmth, including ample warm food and drink, and consuming, inhaling, and applying sufficient over-the-counter medicines (Helman, 1978). Fortunately, germs can be "washed out" of the body by fluid intake, sweating, reduction in food intake, and ample amounts of antibiotics (see Helman, 1978, for an illuminating account of the logic underlying hot–cold, wet–dry disorders, their symptoms, etiologies, treatment, and agreement with biomedical classifications). Although empirical research on the laity's perceptions of cure is regrettably sparse, the existing evidence combined with the nature of lay etiological accounts point to the individual management of the environment and the self as primary modes of therapeutic thought.

When the lay individual does encounter the physician, explanatory frameworks of illness and opinions on curative practice are bound to conflict. Patients may take issue with physician diagnoses, physician instructions pertaining to medication use, and, more generally, the nature and quality of clinical management and care (Engel, 1977; Kleinman et al., 1978; Meyer et al., 1985; Shorter, 1985). That the growing patient dissatisfaction with professional health care is in part attributable to the nature of cognitive illness models that are brought to bear on the biomedical encounter is suggested by the foregoing pages and is powerfully illustrated in the following example, which we quote at length:

> The patient was a 60-year-old white Protestant grandmother recovering from pulmonary edema secondary to atherosclerotic cardiovascular disease and chronic congestive heart failure on one of the medical wards at the Massachusetts General Hospital. Her behavior in the recovery phase of her illness was described as bizarre by the house staff and nurses. Although her cardiac status greatly improved and she became virtually asymptomatic, she induced vomiting and urinated frequently into her bed. She became angry when told to stop. Psychiatric consultation was requested.
>
> Review of the lengthy medical record showed nothing as to the personal significance of the patient's behavior. When asked to explain why she was engaging in it and what meaning it had for her, the patient's response was most revealing. Describing herself as the wife and daughter of plumbers, the patient noted that she was informed by the medical team responsible for her care that she had "water in the lungs." Her concept of the anatomy of the human body had the chest hooked up to two pipes leading to the mouth and the urethra. The patient explained that she had been trying to remove as much water from her chest as possible through self-induced vomiting and frequent urination. She analogized the latter to the work of the "water pills" she was taking, which she had been told were getting rid of the water on her chest. She concluded: "I can't understand why people are angry at me." After appropriate explanations, along with diagrams, she acknowledged that the "plumbing" of the body is remarkable and quite different from what she had believed. Her unusual behavior ended at that time. (Kleinman et al., 1978, p. 254)

This case, combined with the preceding data, is dramatic in teaching us about the length to which ordinary people are willing to go to secure their recovery through the individual self-management of physical symptoms and to the relative exclusion of professional medical care. It is dramatic in teaching us about the sorts of anatomical configurations and causal physiological mechanisms which people construct, "modern" in some respects but without "true" content from biomedical science entering into the explanatory system. And it is dramatic in teaching us about physician–patient encounters and the extent to which these frequently "strained" relations may be neutralized by both parties agreeing to teach and be taught.

In summary, the foregoing review indicates that contemporary lay illness models comprise six structural components (symptoms, label, cause, cure, timeline, and consequences) that serve as cognitive organizers of prior experiences in the individual's medical history. The contents of the cognitive models suggest a verbal fluency with the terminology of modern medicine. However, the lay explanatory framework of health and illness focuses on the self-management of weather and climatic conditions, diet, emotional well-being, and sleep and activity cycles and as such appears discordant with contemporary biomedical formulations. In considering the influence that progress in medical science may have had on the nature and development of lay medical thought, it is instructive to examine lay illness models in a period prior to the advent of 20th-century medicine.

Lay Illness Models in the Enlightenment

Gathering information on how illness was apperceived by the laity in times past is no easy undertaking. The history of medicine has been written, but it has been written with a focus on the contributions of medical innovators, to the exclusion of the patient. Only recently has a new breed of historians embarked upon the construction of what Porter termed "the sufferers' history—medical history from below" (1985c, p. 182). Of the many sources available to the historian pursuing this goal, the most fruitful sources of data have been the diaries, correspondences, and magazines, probed for medically relevant material from the present point of view. We draw on 17th- and 18th-century British data, focusing on the Enlightenment, for this is a period which precedes the many medical discoveries that have so fundamentally shaped the 20th-century medical views.

Structure

What is striking about lay medical thought which found expression in 17th- and 18th-century writings is that the cognizing about illness appears to have taken place within the bounds of a cognitive structure compatible with that of contemporary lay illness models. Annoying symptoms were spread across many pages of diaries, correspondences, and magazine submissions, and much space was equally devoted to diagnostic labels, the onset and stages of illness episodes, causes and mechanisms of disease, therapeutic evaluations and practices, and unfortunate consequences, ranging from death to inability to perform one's duties (Barry, 1985; Beier, 1985; Hultin, 1975; Lane, 1985; Porter, 1985a, 1985b, 1985c; Rogers, 1986; Smith, 1985; Wear, 1985). The laity's writings, moreover, leave little doubt about the presence of associative links between the six components of the cognitive illness models, as is briefly illustrated in this section.

Crosstalk between cognitive representations of symptoms, labels, cause, cure, timeline, and consequences of ill health is abundantly evident in 17th-

and 18th-century lay illness accounts. By way of example, on August 29, 1775, Samuel Johnson wrote to Mrs. Thrale:

> This sorry foot! and this sorry Doctor Laurence who says it is the gout! But he thinks every thing the gout, so I will try not to believe him. (Rogers, 1986, p. 135)

Almost a year later, on June 3, 1776, Johnson appeared to have accepted his diagnosis and reconciled himself with the debilitating effects of his affliction:

> The lameness, of which I made mention in one of my notes, has improved to a very serious and troublesome fit of the gout. I creep about and hang by both hands. . . . I enjoy all the dignity of lameness. I receive ladies and dismiss them sitting. Painful pre-eminence. (Rogers, 1986, p. 135)

And on to etiology:

> My opinion is that I have drank too little, and therefore have the gout, for it is of my own acquisition, for neither my father had it nor my mother (Rogers, 1986, p. 136)

submitted Johnson in a letter to Dr. John Taylor on June 23, 1776. Time and again we find sufferers like Johnson making sense of their illness by painstakingly reducing the whole experience to its constituent, yet interdependent, parts. To take another example, Richard Baxter, a 17th-century diarist, had the poor fortune of falling prey to an illness episode which relieved him from professional obligations. His account of the experience reads:

> I came to our Major Swallow's quarters at Sir John Cook's house . . . in a cold and snowy season, and the cold, together with other things coincident, set my nose on bleeding. When I had bled about a quart or two, I opened four veins, but it did not good. I used divers of other remedies for several days to little purpose; at last I gave myself a purge which stopt it. This so much weakened me and altered my complexion, that my acquaintance who came to visit me scarce knew me. Coming after so long weakness, and frequent loss of blood before, it made the physicians conclude me deplorate after it was stopped; supposing I would never escape a dropsy. (Wear, 1985, p. 99)

What is revealed by such correspondence is a network of closely interrelated and medically relevant knowledge structures pertaining, specifically, to symptoms, label, cause, cure, timeline, and consequences of ill health. These knowledge structures combine to provide a schematic frame within which the experience of illness is apperceived. The six-component structure of lay illness models is thus revealed as invariant in time, characterizing, as it does, both Enlightenment and contemporary lay medical thought. In light of the ahistorical nature of the structure of the illness models, it is of interest to examine the extent to which the contents of the cognitive models are historically bound. To this end, we repeat the route taken in our review of contemporary lay illness models and focus, in order, on (1) conceptions of symptoms in relation to disease labels, (2) perceived etiological contributions to illness, and (3) perceived therapeutic indications.

Content

It seems that throughout the course of history, the laity has possessed a most intimate familiarity with physical symptoms. To quote Richard Baxter again:

> I have lain in above forty years constant weakness, and almost constant pains: My chief troubles were incredible inflations of stomach, bowels, back, sides, head, thighs as if I had been daily filled with wind. . . . Thirty physicians (at least) all call'd it nothing but hypochondriack flatulency, and somewhat of a scorbutical malady: great bleeding at the nose also did emaciate me, and keep me in a scorbutickal atrophy. (Wear, 1985, p. 94)

Baxter was joined by many others throughout the 17th and 18th centuries, who described in exquisite detail the aches and pains, the colds and fevers, the infections and diarrheas afflicting their own bodies and the bodies of their loved ones (Beier, 1985; Hultin, 1975; Lane, 1985; Porter, 1985c; Rogers, 1986; Wear, 1985). "I die daily, yet remain alive" (Wear, 1985, p. 98)—Baxter's confession so vividly captures the sentiments of his contemporaries. While Baxter's ailments mandated, by his own admission, frequent visits to numerous doctors, other estimates of physician consultation during that century approximate the rates observed today (Porter, 1985c). Let us turn to examine the sorts of diagnostic categories that could serve as meaningful summary descriptors of symptom experiences in the 17th and 18th centuries.

In this historic period, the patient–physician encounter was governed by a relatively unsophisticated system of medical taxonomies, one in which symptomatic descriptions assumed greater importance than the labeling of states of disease (Ackerknecht, 1982; Jewson, 1974). Accordingly, it was not uncommon for lay accounts of illness episodes to fall short of providing a diagnostic label, being instead confined to such qualitative symptom descriptions as vomiting, sore navel, running eyes, leg cramps, the itch, or just plain feeling sick and sore, to name a few. Added to these were the then well-known diagnostic categories of colds, rheume, distemper, agues and fevers, scurvy, gout, asthma, stone, dropsy, convulsions, consumption, apoplexy, smallpox, plague, and cancer (e.g., Beier, 1985; Hultin, 1975; Lane, 1985; Porter, 1985a, 1985b, 1985c; Rogers, 1986; Wear, 1985). When measured against modern standards, the lay vocabulary of illness was not extensive by any means, but it was nevertheless conceptually parallel with the medical taxonomies of the times (e.g., Lane, 1985; Porter, 1985a, 1985b).

What is of particular importance here is that the laity's competence in medical matters went beyond a mere linguistic familiarity with biomedical taxonomies to include the use of diagnostic labels in the differentiation of discrete symptom sets. Diaries and correspondence show without doubt that diagnosing was thought a relatively easy undertaking when the "diagnostic label" constituted no more and no less than a restatement of symptom experience. This was the case for such conditions as fevers, colds, eye and skin irritations, worms, or diarrhea. But in addition, lay individuals displayed considerable skill and confidence in diagnosing, based on symptom information, cases of ague, ill humors, gout, colic, rickets, dropsy, or kidney stones (e.g., Beier, 1985; Hultin, 1975; Lane, 1985; Porter, 1985c; Wear, 1985). While lay individuals thus appeared competent drawing on symptom information for the purpose of self-diagnosis, they appeared equally competent drawing on symptom information for the purpose of evaluating physician diagnoses. In this regard, there are many effusions on medical misdiagnoses to be found in 17th- and 18th-century writings. In their clearest forms, medical misdiagnoses tended to reveal themselves in the failure of prescribed medication to bring about symptom relief or in the premature demise of patients believed to have been victimized by physician incompetence (Lane, 1985; Porter, 1985c). In addition, misdiagnosis could reveal itself in the intensification of symptomatology in a "healthy" subject, as it did in the case of Baxter, a medically certified hypochondriac, who kept diligent records on his pain:

> 1673 it turned to terrible suffocations of my brain and lungs. So that if I slept I was suddenly and painfully awakened: The abatement of urine, and constant pain, which nature almost yielded to as victorious, renewed my suspicions of the stone, And my old exploration: and feeling my lean back, both the kidneys were greatlier indurate than before, that the membrane is sore to the touch, as if nothing but stone were within them. (Wear, 1985, p. 94)

Baxter's words clearly speak for themselves, but we hasten to add that his kidney stone rested in the British Museum at Montague House from 1766 to 1830.

What such correspondence reveals is that the laity at the time took strong interest in diagnostic matters, habitually self-diagnosing based on symptom information and exhibiting in at least one well-documented case substantial accuracy in diagnostic skills. We believe such diagnostic endeavors reflect a lay perception of diseases as entities, entities that can be differentiated from one another in reference to discrete symptom sets and diagnostic labels, to the extent that the latter were available. The vocabulary of illness was, moreover, shared by laymen and physicians alike, and any lay diagnostic speculations thus took place within the confines of the then unsophisticated medical taxonomies. The explanatory framework within which the diagnostic judgments were made is revealed as we turn our attention to lay conceptions of etiology and cure.

When we examine 17th- and 18th-century diaries, correspondence, and magazine submissions, we find that the whole gamut of ill health known to the laity, as with the contemporary laity, was variously traced to behavioral mismanagement with respect to diet, sleep and activity cycles, emotional well-being, and exposure to hostile climatic and social conditions. For example, Samuel Pepys confided to his diary, "Home to bed, with some pain in making water, having taken cold this morning in staying too long bare-legged to pare my cornes" (Porter, 1985c, p. 179). Elaborating upon this theme, Timothy Burrell declared:

> Yesterday having wetted my feet by walking out in the dew and having eaten a small piece of new cheese, I have been today tortured with flatulent spasms. By taking two doses of hiera picra the pains in my stomach abated. Thanks to the great God for his mercy towards me. (Lane, 1985, p. 244)

Obituary columns in the *Gentleman's Magazine* are written in a similar vein:

> Miss Elizabeth Richardson, daughter of Mr Robert R. of the Six Hundreds in Heckington fen, co. Linc. She had been dancing a few evenings before; and the cause of her death is supposed to have originated from drinking cold water or small beer, and going in to the air before she was cool. (Porter, 1985b, p. 162)

Time and again, weather and climatic conditions, particularly the dimensions of cold and wet, were implicated by the laity in the etiologies of diverse physical derangements, including colds, agues, gout, headaches, abdominal pains, colics, vomiting, and convulsions (e.g., Beier, 1985; Lane, 1985; Porter, 1985b, 1985c; Rogers, 1986; Wear, 1985). Dietary neglect or excess likewise reigned as a primary precipitating factor, lying at the root of such disorders as gout, kidney stones, coughs, fevers, and bowel inflammations (e.g., Porter, 1985b; Rogers, 1986; Wear, 1985). What is thus revealed in 17th- and 18th-century writings is a simple cognitive map of etiological contributions to illness, centering on climatic and dietary hazards. This cognitive map received elaboration through various allusions to sleep and activity cycles, excretions, emotional well-being, as well as constitutional factors and sinful temptations (Beier, 1985; Barry, 1985; Lane, 1985; Porter, 1985b, 1985c; Rogers, 1986; Wear, 1985). In other words, etiological evaluations in the Enlightenment, as in the contemporary era, constitute a narrative of the classic themes of individualism and temperance in mind and body. As will be seen in the following section, these themes are rooted in the Hippocratic–Galenic medicine of classic Greek antiquity.

The themes of individualism and temperance in mind and body applied not only to etiological evaluations but also to perceived therapeutic indications. The Hippocratic–Galenic frame is uniquely captured in this excerpt from "Recipe For an Asthma," which appeared for the benefit of fellow sufferers in a 1751 edition of the *Gentleman's Magazine* (Porter, 1985b, p. 145):

> Restless from quack to quack they range,
> When 'tis themselves they ought to change;
> Nature hates violence and force,
> By method led and gentle course,

Rules and restraint you must endure,
What comes by time 'tis time must cure

These lines reflect, of course, the general guiding principles of self-management and temperance in mind and body, which governed therapeutic thought of lay individuals and physicians alike (e.g., Hultin, 1975; Lane, 1985; Porter, 1985b). Translated into action, this principle encouraged the active participation of sufferers in regimens pertaining to diet, excretions, climate, activity, sleep, and mental passions. Indeed, diaries, letters, and magazine submissions of the time reveal an array of curative practices along the lines of Judith Milbanke's report of her husband's treatment in 1780:

> Milbanke has had some return of the complaint in his stomach & was far from well with it yesterday; the People here think it is owing to his Stomach being so greatly relaxed from the Mercurial medicines he took three Years ago, for which I have long been convinced both Turton & Bromfield deserve to be hanged. The Person we consult here [Harrogate] has put him on a bracing Regimen and has forbid Slopping, Salt Meat & much Wine. (Lane, 1985, p. 219)

Elizabeth Montagu likewise opted for temperance, not in body, but in spirit. In 1739 she resolved:

> I have swollowed the weight of an Apothecary in medicine, and what I am better for it, except more patient and less credulous I know not. I have learnt to bear my infirmities and not to trust the skill of Physicians for curing them. I endeavor to drink deeply of Philosophy, and to be wise when I cannot be merry, easy when I cannot be glad, content with what cannot be mended, and patient where there can be no redress. The mighty can do no more, and the wise seldom do as much. (Porter, 1985c, p. 189)

In lay illness accounts, these modes of intervention stand alongside addresses to the therapeutic values of work and exercise, climatic change, sleep and rest, and regulation of excretions in the treatment of such disorders as colds, agues, fevers, gout, asthma, abdominal distress, convulsions, kidney stones, and nervous afflictions (e.g., Barry 1985; Beier, 1985; Bynum, 1980; Hultin, 1975; Lane, 1985; Porter, 1985b, 1985c; Rogers, 1986; Smith, 1985; Wear, 1985).

The therapeutic regulation of excretions enjoyed particular popularity in the 17th and 18th centuries, as is illustrated in the following examples. In 1663, Samuel Pepys, suffering from itching, inflammation, abdominal pain, and fever, received this piece of advice from his apothecary:

> I am to sweat soundly and that will carry all this matter away; which nature would itself eject, but this will assist nature—it being some disorder given the blood; but by what I know not, unless it be my late great Quantitys of Dantzicke-girkins that I have eaten. (Porter, 1985c, p. 178)

Samuel Pepys was not the only patient "sweating it out." He was joined by uncountable others who endured not only sweating, but also bleeding, purging, and vomiting to combat their various afflictions (e.g., Barry, 1985; Beier, 1985; Hultin, 1975; Lane, 1985; Rogers, 1986; Smith, 1985). In December 1646, for instance, Ralph Josselin was fortunate to have nature on his side, reporting with relief that "After above 30 hours illness in my stomach I fell into a great looseness which I conceive did me much good" (Beier, 1985, p. 112). And Josselin, like his contemporaries, was prepared to give nature a helping hand, when this was indicated. During an attack of ague, he was self-physicking with syrup of roses, which, in his opinion, "wrought very kindly with me, gave me 9 stools brought away much choler" (Beier, 1985, p. 117). The laity was intimately familiar with these modes of therapeutic intervention, taking upon themselves the self-monitoring of urine, stools, vomit, sweat, and blood, and showing delight when such evacuations occurred (e.g., Lane, 1985; Porter, 1985b; Wear, 1985). What is thus revealed in the laity's writings is a simple cognitive map of therapeutics, centering on the excretions, and framed by considerations to diet, climate, activity, sleep, and mental passions. This cognitive map reflects an individualistic vision of health and illness and as such is true to the Hippocratic–Galenic medicine in classic Greek antiquity.

In summary, lay illness models in the Enlightenment period appear to be characterized by a six-part structure encompassing symptoms, label, cause, cure, timeline, and consequences of ill health. The contents of the cognitive models reflect a verbal facility with the unsophisticated medical taxonomies of the times as well as an explanatory framework of health and illness which centers on themes of self-management and temperance in mind and body. It is noteworthy here that although the cognitive models of health and illness were shared by Enlightenment patients and physicians alike, conflict was nevertheless a fundamental part of the patient–physician encounter in this frame of time. Thus, and against the background of unprecedented advances in 19th- and 20th-century medicine, Enlightenment lay illness models bear a close resemblance to the illness models in the contemporary era, from which they differ only in a lack of familiarity with the terminology in modern medicine.

A Historical Note on Hippocratic–Galenic Medicine

We have suggested that both contemporary and Enlightenment lay illness models derive from Hippocratic traditions. The roots of modern medicine are often traced to classic Greek antiquity and, specifically, to Hippocrates (about 460–397 B.C.), the acclaimed "father of medicine" (e.g., Ackerknecht, 1982; Elliot-Binns, 1978; Gordon, 1949). We believe that lay illness models may be similarly traced. Hence we outline here features of the Hippocratic approach to disease within which the organizing matrix of contemporary and Enlightenment lay medical thought can be discerned. These features pertain specifically to Hippocratic humoural pathology, etiological analyses, therapeutic directives, and physician approach to the patient and his or her affliction. Let us consider these in turn.

→ In Hippocratic medicine, health and disease were seen as inextricably linked to the person's interaction with the environment. What served as the organizing matrix for this perceived intimate relationship between the microcosm and macrocosm was a humoural pathology of great appeal in logic, flexibility, and explanatory power (Ackerknecht, 1982; Chadwick & Mann, 1950; Gordon, 1949; Neuburger, 1910). In humoural pathology, the world was thought to be constituted by the four basic elements of air, water, fire, and earth. These found a correspondence at the level of the individual human body in the form of four bodily fluids, or humors, those of blood, phlegm, yellow bile, and black bile. Blood was anatomically linked to the heart and it was characterized, like air, by hot and moist qualities. Phlegm arose in the brain and its cold and moist qualities were also characteristic of water. Yellow bile, the anatomical derivative of the liver, was analogous to fire in its hot and dry qualities. Black bile, forming in the spleen, was cold and dry, much like the earth. From this schema followed logically the medical insight that health should constitute a physiological state within which the hot, cold, wet, and dry qualities of humors were harmoniously mixed. Disease, in contrast, should constitute a physiological departure from the hypothetical harmonious mixture of humors within the patient. The beauty of this monistic pathology is appreciated upon considering the etiological analyses and curative endeavors which it inspired.

Hippocratic etiological considerations were marked by a vision of the individual in temperate relationship with the environment (Chadwick & Mann, 1950; Gordon, 1949; Neuburger, 1910). Accordingly, weather and climatic conditions posed serious threats to health, to the extent that humoural "life" was subject to the particular status of air, water, and locality. A cold, wet, hot, or dry environment occasioned analogous humoural changes in the bodily fluids of the so afflicted. Humoural changes could likewise be induced by lack of dietary restraint, for any food and drink consumed would become part of the humoural liquids. While the dangers inherent in climatic and dietary conditions formed the focus of medical discourse in Hippocratic writings, attention was also paid to numerous other causative agents arising within the context of temperate management of mind and body. These causative agents were systematically delineated by Galen of Pergamum (A.D. 130–201), who drew a clear distinction between natural and nonnatural causes of disease (Jarcho, 1970; Niebyl, 1971; Smith, 1985). The naturals were innate factors which, following Hippocrates, related to the patient's peculiar humoural constitution. The nonnaturals, of which there were six, were behavioral self-management factors pertaining to air, sleep, activity, diet, evacuations, and passions of the mind. Any activities involving protection of the self against hostile environmental influences as well as self-restraint in mind and body were thus capable of causing disease in the form of humoural disturbance. The six nonnaturals capture the spirit of individualism which governed medical thought about etiology and curative practice.

The guiding principle in therapeutic endeavors was to restore humoural harmony by applying remedies that opposed the patient's physiological imbalance (Ackerknecht, 1982; Chadwick & Mann, 1950; Gordon, 1949; Neuburger, 1910). In combating, for example, a "wet" and "cold" disorder of the phlegm, a "hot" and "dry" remedy had to be devised. To this end, the Hippocratic physician had observed a natural tendency toward recovery, as was evident in the body ridding itself of ill humors by means of such evacuations as sweating, urinating, purging, vomiting, sneezing, or bleeding. Medical opinion held that nature could be assisted by certain modes of intervention. Such intervention was in the form of prescribed regimens pertaining to the six nonnaturals, which, when adjusted appropriately, had observable physiological effects mimicking the natural course of recovery. The modes of therapeutic practice thus centered on themes of food and fluid intake, maintenance of adequate body temperature, climatic change, sleep and activity cycles, and emotional harmony. When these measures were carefully instituted by the supervising physician, a return to humoural balance and harmony within the patient was ensured. Thus the grand design of humoural pathology inspired a medical theory and practice that focused on humoural input and output in relation to the temperate self-management of mind and body. Within the context of this individualistic vision of health and disease, we can discern the Hippocratic approach to the patient and, therein, features of classic medicine that were so widely acclaimed and proved irreplaceable to future generations of medical practitioners.

In encountering the patient, the Hippocratic physician paid tribute to the ideal of individualism (Ballester, 1981; Chadwick & Mann, 1950; Heidel, 1941). Accordingly, the unit of medical analysis comprised the individual patient and his or her verbal report of global psychosomatic disturbance. Access to this unit of analysis was gained through reliance on one singular available tool of medical investigation, that of physician senses. Physician senses were applied, first and foremost, to the patient's symptomatology, or the verbal descriptions of physical and psychological experiences. Also subject to sensory inspection were the psychophysical signs exhibited by the patient and, moreover, the physical and social environment surrounding the diseased. Physician reliance on the senses combined with a patient-centered approach did not yield a diagosis in the modern sense of the word. Indeed, disease did not possess an existence in its own right, independent and apart from the patient, but was instead equated with the symptomatologies of the afflicted. This is readily ascertained from the many case histories presented in Hippocratic writings, case histories consisting of detailed descriptions of patient symptomatologies, with little effort being directed at the classification and labeling of discrete symptom sets (Chadwick & Mann, 1950). In keeping with the focus on the individual patient, the Hippocratic physician employed empirical and inductive methods in gathering clinical data, and excluded a priori religious and magical considerations. It is to this scientific approach to disease that Hippocratic medicine owes its modern acclaim (Ackerknecht, 1982; Ballester, 1981).

What emerges from this consideration of medicine in classic Greek antiquity is a picture of health and disease that is fundamentally individualistic in nature, marked by ideals of moderation in mind and body, and given structure and cohesion within the grand design of humoural theory. Medical opinion held that the opportunity for health and disease was inherent in the individual management of nature, the self, and the environment. This vision of self-management is forcefully captured by Galen's six nonnaturals, which served as an organizing matrix for medical thought from classic Greek antiquity up to and including the Enlightenment period. In keeping with this vision, the patient was above all the measure of disease, directing the physician's sensory gaze and dictating, by means of verbal description of symptomatologies, a holistic, symptom-based, and patient-focused definition of disease.

Clinical Lessons From Historical Research

Any comparative analysis of lay illness models through history is fraught with difficulties, of which the varying sources of data are by no means unimportant. We have drawn on diaries, correspondences, and magazines to evaluate how illness was apperceived in times past, and it can be argued that the content of these submissions is colored by the sociodemographic background and personal motives of those who placed their thoughts on paper. Contemporary data are equally colored, not only by the sociodemographic background of the subjects, but also by the particular interests of the experimental investigators. Yet in this diversity of data, we have found, perhaps surprisingly, an astonishing degree of consensus in the perception of illness.

One striking finding of the comparison of lay illness models currently and in the Enlightenment is the observed invariance, in time, of the structure of the cognitive models. In both eras, symptomatology, diagnostic labels, cause, cure, timeline, and consequences of ill health have emerged as cognitive frames within which the sufferer's illness experience is apperceived. Existing empirical data indicate that these cognitive frames, which contain organized representations of prior experiences in the medical domain, guide the processing of sensory inputs in a fashion that is consistent with the prior knowledge (e.g., Bishop et al., 1987; Pennebaker et al., 1985). We believe it is to the reduction of the complexity of the stimulus world into parsimonious and manageable units that the six-part structure of lay illness models owes its persistence in time and its resistance to change. While the present data thus point to a universal structure of lay illness models, they also suggest that the contents of the cognitive models are, at least in some respects, historically bound.

The present historical analysis has shown that both contemporary and Enlightenment laity exhibit a distinct verbal fluency with the medical taxonomies of their times. This suggests that taxonomic labels of disease entities are readily integrated into lay medical thought, a finding which is in part attributable to the role served by the verbal labels as cognitive organizers of perceived symptom sets (cf. Bishop & Converse, 1986; Helman, 1978). Such classification and labeling of discrete symptom sets comprise a significant extension and departure from Hippocratic medicine, which conceived of diseased patients rather than disease as an entity, separate and distinct from the individual sufferer. Interestingly, medical science has traced the origin of taxonomies of physical symptoms to the 17th-century physician Thomas Sydenham (Pellegrino, 1979), whose fundamental contributions to medicine have been shown to form an integral part of lay medical thought currently and in times past. However, the impact that medical science has had on the illness models of ordinary people is reflected only in verbal facilities with medical terminology, as lay explanations of illness remain fundamentally Hippocratic.

The corpus of medical knowledge in the scientific community was relatively unchanged from classic antiquity up to the Enlightenment period but made unprecedented advances during the 19th and 20th centuries (Ackerknecht, 1982). When measured against this background, lay explanatory accounts of illness have changed little. This is suggested by the present historical analysis, which has shown that contemporary and Enlightenment laity converge in their insistence on self-management as the key to both health and illness. Such individualistic visions of health and illness are fundamentally based in the medical science of classic Greek antiquity. In keeping with that classic era, lay accounts of etiology and therapy center on the importance of individual management of the six nonnaturals, including climate, diet, excretions, sleep, activity, and emotions. A Hippocratic–Galenic–type matrix thus appears to serve as the basic cognitive frame for organizing lay medical thought on etiology and cure, both in the present and in times past. This classic frame appears both flexible and accommodating, which contributes in part to the readiness with which linguistic material from biomedical science is incorporated into lay medical thought (cf. Helman, 1978).

In contemporary and Enlightenment lay illness accounts, health and illness are clearly apperceived within the fundamentally individualistic framework of classic Greek antiquity. It appears that the long-term influence of classic medicine is in part attributable to the fact that its cognitive frame encourages lay self-evaluation of diagnostic labels, etiologies, and therapeutics through reliance on the available tools of perception and description of symptom experiences. In these respects, the lay individual is applying to the self the art and science of the Hippocratic physician. Schober

(1989) has elsewhere captured the lay individual's spirit with the concept of *implicit medicine*. Implicit medicine encompasses the medically relevant knowledge structures or schemata, the behavioral repertoires, and the affections of the mind which together serve to contextualize the sufferer's illness experience. Its schemata encompass beliefs about illness, perceived anatomy, symptomatology, diagnostic labels, and therapeutics as well as etiologies and physiological mechanisms. Together these schemata constitute a complex network of interrelated knowledge structures, which grant a rich source of data upon which to draw when passing through an illness episode. Our focus here has been a historical comparison of the implicit medicines held by contemporary and Enlightenment laity. We have found differences in familiarity with medical terminology in the two eras examined and have traced these differences to progress in medical science. We have found, on the other hand, comparatively few differences in the explanatory framework of health and illness in the two eras. However, the explanatory framework in each has been traced to medical science, medical science in classic Greek antiquity, but medical science nonetheless.

The findings revealed in the present historical analysis are of considerable importance to contemporary medical practice. The patient's implicit medicine there serves as part of the encoding of abstract medical information which is the focus of communication in the patient–physician encounter. Current thinking in social science disciplines holds that the discordance in cognitive models brought to the biomedical encounter contributes in part to patient dissatisfaction with the nature and quality of clinical management and care (Engel, 1977; Kleinman et al., 1978; Stimson, 1974). This view is supported by the present historical data, which point to the multiplicity of conflicts that may potentially arise in patient–physician encounters. The historical data furthermore suggest an important and necessary role for systematic attention to the nature of lay illness models in contemporary medical practice. In view of the impact that medical science has on the development of lay medical thought, it appears particularly necessary for the physician to encourage the patient's encoding of terminologies in modern medicine in reference to both symptomatologies and central features of the prior cognitive framework of health and illness. This approach to the patient may be valuable in establishing "connective" knowledge between the discordant cognitive models and thereby contribute to improved patient–physician communication in contemporary medical practice.

The fundamental clinical lesson from the present historical research is perhaps to be found in the Hippocratic approach to the patient. The Hippocratic physician's devotion was above all to the individual sufferer and his or her experience of symptomatology. This devotion stands in direct contrast to the focus on disease as an entity, a focus that originated in the Enlightenment period and defines the contemporary patient–physician encounter. Although the concept of disease as an entity will undoubtedly continue to play an essential and necessary role in modern medicine, we believe that the physician's tribute to the individual patient may form an equally necessary and powerful ally. This view of the physician's role in clinical medicine was forcefully stated by Ivy McKenzie: "The physician is concerned [unlike the naturalist] . . . with a single organism, the human subject, striving to preserve its identity in adverse circumstances" (cited in Sacks, 1987). It is the physician's participation in this dynamic, this "striving to preserve identity," which may hold the key to conflict resolution in contemporary medical practice.

References

Ackerknecht, E. H. (1982). *A short history of medicine.* Baltimore: Johns Hopkins University Press.

Ballester, L. G. (1981). Galen as a medical practitioner: Problems in diagnosis. In V. Nutton (Ed.), *Galen: Problems and prospects* (pp. 13–46). London: Wellcome Institute for the History of Medicine.

Barondess, J. A. (1979). Disease and illness: A crucial distinction. *American Journal of Medicine, 66,* 375–376.

Barry, J. (1985). Piety and the patient: Medicine and religion in eighteenth century Bristol. In R. Porter (Ed.), *Patients and practitioners: Lay perceptions of medicine in pre-industrial society* (pp. 145–175). Cambridge: Cambridge University Press.

Beier, L. M. (1985). In sickness and in health: A seventeenth century family's experience. In R. Porter (Ed.), *Patients and practitioners: Lay perceptions of medicine in pre-industrial society* (pp. 101–128). Cambridge: Cambridge University Press.

Bishop, G. D. (1984). Gender, role, and illness behavior in a military population. *Health Psychology, 3,* 519–534.

Bishop, G. D., Briede, C., Cavazos, L., Grotzinger, R., & McMahon, S. (1987). Processing illness information: The role of disease prototypes. *Basic and Applied Social Psychology, 8,* 21–43.

Bishop, G. D., & Converse, S. A. (1986). Illness representations: A prototype approach. *Health Psychology, 5,* 95–114.

Blaxter, M. (1979). Concepts of causality: Lay and medical models. In D. J. Osborne, M. M. Gruenberg, & J. R. Eiser (Eds.), *Research in psychology and medicine* (Vol. 2, pp. 154–161). New York: Academic Press.

Bynum, W. F. (1980). Health, disease and medical care. In G. S. Rousseau & R. Porter (Eds.), *The ferment of knowledge: Studies in the historiography of eighteenth century science* (pp. 211–253). Cambridge: Cambridge University Press.

Chadwick, J., & Mann, W. N. (1950). *The medical works of Hippocrates.* Oxford: Blackwell Scientific.

Cott, A., & Pavloski, R. P. (1985). Behavioral medicine: A process for managing performance problems. *Canadian Psychology, 26,* 160–167.

Elder, R. G. (1973). Social class and lay explanations of the etiology of arthritis. *Journal of Health and Social Behavior, 14,* 28–35.

Elliot-Binns, C. (1978). *Medicine: The forgotten art?* London: Pitman Medical.

Engel, G. L. (1977). The need for a new medical model: A challenge for biomedicine. *Science, 196,* 129–136.

Gordon, B. L. (1949). *Medicine throughout antiquity.* Philadelphia: F. A. Davis.

Hannay, D. R., & Maddox, E. J. (1976). Symptom prevalence and referral behavior in Glasgow. *Social Science and Medicine, 10*, 185–189.

Heidel, W. A. (1941). *Hippocratic medicine: Its spirit and method.* New York: Columbia University Press.

Helman, C. G. (1978). "Feed a cold, starve a fever": Folk models of infection in an English suburban community and their relation to medical treatment. *Culture, Medicine and Psychiatry, 2*, 107–137.

Hultin, N. C. (1975). Medicine and magic in the eighteenth century: The diaries of James Woodforde. *Journal of the History of Medicine and Allied Sciences, 30*, 349–366.

Jarcho, S. (1970). Galen's six non-naturals: A bibliographic note and translation. *Bulletin of the History of Medicine, 44*, 372–377.

Jennings, D. (1986). The confusion between disease and illness in clinical medicine. *Canadian Medical Association Journal, 135*, 865–870.

Jewson, N. (1974). Medical knowledge and the patronage system in eighteenth century England. *Sociology, 8*, 369–385.

Jewson, N. (1976). The disappearance of the sick-man from medical cosmology, 1770–1870. *Sociology, 10*, 225–244.

Kleinman, A., Eisenberg, L., & Good, B. (1978). Culture, illness, and care: Clinical lessons from anthropological and cross-cultural research. *Annals of Internal Medicine, 88*, 251–258.

Kutner, B., & Gordon, G. (1961). Seeking care for cancer. *Journal of Health and Human Behavior, 2*, 171–178.

Lane, J. (1985). "The doctor scolds me": The diaries and correspondence of patients in eighteenth century England. In R. Porter (Ed.), *Patients and practitioners: Lay perceptions of medicine in pre-industrial society* (pp. 205–248). Cambridge: Cambridge University Press.

Lau, R. R., & Hartman, K. A. (1983). Common sense representations of common illnesses. *Health Psychology, 2*, 167–185.

Leventhal, H., Meyer, D., & Nerenz, D. (1980). The common sense representation of illness danger. In S. Rachman (Ed.), *Contributions to medical psychology* (Vol. 2 pp. 7–30). New York: Pergamon Press.

Marby, J. H. (1964). Lay concepts of etiology. *Journal of Chronic Disease, 17*, 371–386.

Meyer, D., Leventhal, H., & Gutmann, M. (1985). Common-sense models of illness: The example of hypertension. *Health Psychology, 4*, 115–135.

Neuburger, M. (1910). *History of medicine* (Vol. 1). London: Oxford University Press.

Niebyl, P. H. (1971). The non-naturals. *Bulletin of the History of Medicine, 45*, 486–492.

Pellegrino, E. D. (1979). The sociocultural impact of twentieth-century therapeutics. In M. J. Vogel & C. E. Rosenberg (Eds.), *The therapeutic revolution: Essays in the social history of American medicine* (pp. 245–266). Philadelphia: University of Pennsylvania Press

Pennebaker, J. W. (1982). *The psychology of physical symptoms.* New York: Springer-Verlag.

Pennebaker, J. W., Gonder-Frederick, L., Cox, D. J., & Hoover, C. W. (1985). The perception of general vs specific visceral activity and the regulation of health-related behavior. In E. S. Katkin and S. B. Manuck (Eds.), *Advances in Behavioral Medicine: A Research Annual* (Vol. 1, pp. 165–198). Greenwich, CT: JAI Press.

Porter, R. (1985a). Laymen, doctors and medical knowledge in the eighteenth century: The evidence of the Gentleman's Magazine. In R. Porter (Ed.), *Patients and practitioners: Lay perceptions of medicine in pre-industrial society* (pp. 283–314). Cambridge: Cambridge University Press.

Porter, R. (1985b). Lay medical knowledge in the eighteenth century: The evidence of the Gentleman's Magazine. *Medical History, 29,* 138–168.

Porter, R. (1985c). The patient's view: Doing medical history from below. *Theory and Society, 14,* 175–198.

Rippiere, V. (1981). The survival of traditional medicine in lay medical views: An empirical approach to the history of medicine. *Medical History, 25,* 411–414.

Rogers, J. P. W. (1986). Samuel Johnson's gout. *Medical History, 30,* 133–144.

Sacks, O. (1984). *A leg to stand on.* London: Duckworth.

Sacks, O. (1987). *The man who mistook his wife for a hat.* New York: Harper & Row.

Safer, M., Tharps, D., Jackson, T., & Leventhal, H. (1979). Determinants of three stages of delay in seeking care at a medical clinic. *Medical Care, 17,* 11–29.

Schober, R. (1989). *Implicit medicine: Schemata of illness, symptomatology, and anatomy.* Unpublished manuscript, York University, Toronto.

Shorter, E. (1985). *Bedside manners: The troubled history of doctors and patients.* New York: Simon and Schuster.

Smith, G. (1985). Prescribing the rules of health: Self-help and advice in the late eighteenth century. In R. Porter (Ed.), *Patients and practitioners: Lay perceptions of medicine in pre-industrial society* (pp. 249–282). Cambridge: Cambridge University Press.

Stimson, G. V. (1974). Obeying doctor's orders: A view from the other side. *Social Science and Medicine, 8,* 97–104.

Tait, C. D., & Asher, R. C. (1955). Inside-of-the-body test. *Psychosomatic Medicine, 17,* 139–148.

Wear, A. (1985). Puritan perceptions of illness in seventeenth century England. In R. Porter (Ed.), *Patients and practitioners: Lay perceptions of medicine in pre-industrial society* (pp. 55–99). Cambridge: Cambridge University Press.

White, K. L., Williams, T. F., & Greenberg, B. G. (1961). The ecology of medical care. *New England Journal of Medicine, 265,* 885–892.

3
Understanding the Understanding of Illness: Lay Disease Representations

George D. Bishop

As health psychologists one of our primary goals is to understand the determinants of health-related behavior. Topics such as preventive health behavior, help seeking and the use of medical services, and compliance with medical recommendations occupy center stage in health psychology (Leventhal, 1983; Matarazzo, Weiss, Herd, Miller, & Weiss 1984; Stone, Cohen, & Adler, 1979). In each of these areas we seek to understand individuals' responses to actual or perceived health threats. Further, we are concerned with developing interventions to promote desirable health-related behavior. In this chapter these issues are addressed through examination of cognitive representations of physical illness and the implications of these representations for specific health-related behaviors.

The traditional approach in studies of health-related behavior has emphasized delineation of the different factors, both internal and external, that influence the behavior in question. In addressing the question of help seeking and the use of medical services, for example, the focus has been on such factors as the demographic characteristics of users and nonusers (McKinlay, 1972; Wolinsky, 1978), sociocultural factors influencing use (Zola, 1973), and the characteristics of symptoms that lead people to seek help (Mechanic, 1978). In the compliance domain, researchers have sought the sources of noncooperation in the characteristics of the patient, the nature of the treatment, and the quality of the patient–practitioner relationship (DiMatteo & DiNicola, 1982). Thus the emphasis in these areas has been on identifying independent variables that have either a direct or an indirect influence on health behavior. The fundamental notion has been that by cataloging factors that can be shown to affect various health-related behaviors it will be possible to design effective interventions for changing undesirable behaviors and promoting desirable ones. Although this approach has certainly had its successes, it suffers from a somewhat simplistic model that conceptualizes health behaviors in terms of uni-directional cause–effect relationships. Health behaviors are viewed as outcome variables determined by conceptually distinct causal factors. Mechanic (1978), for example, describes 10 determinants of help seeking that include such factors as the type of symptoms experienced, the kind of situation the person is engaged in, and how others are likely to respond.

Although this unidirectional cause–effect model has been dominant in work on health-related behavior, a more dynamic model—specifically, a systems theory approach—has been called for (Jasnoski & Schwartz, 1985; Leventhal, 1983; Schwartz, 1980). This model views behavior as the product of a dynamic interaction of multiple factors, which are seen as existing on multiple levels and as having reciprocal causal relationships. Thus, depending on the particular situation and purposes of the theorist, a factor can be a cause, an intervening factor, or an effect. Further, behavior is seen as goal-directed and governed by a feedback process in which the results of the person's behavior are evaluated against the goal, with the results of this evaluation producing feedback affecting the original determinants of the behavior.

In applying this approach specifically to health-related behavior, Howard Leventhal and his colleagues (Leventhal, 1983; Leventhal, Meyer, & Nerenz, 1980; Leventhal, Nerenz, & Steele, 1984; Leventhal, Nerenz, & Straus, 1982) proposed a self-regulation/information processing model of responses to health threats. This model views health-related behavior as the result of an iterative process by which the person integrates both internal and external stimulus information with existing cognitive structures to give meaning to the person's experience. This meaning directs the person's coping, the results of which provide feedback by which both the person's coping behaviors and illness interpretations are evaluated. In dealing with potential health threats people seek out information about the health threat, interpret that information according to internal cognitive representations that they have of relevant health matters, and, on the basis of this interpretation, select a means of coping. The results of coping are then evaluated and that evaluation is used in reassessing the illness interpretation and for planning future coping. Two features of this model are central for our purposes. First, people are seen as being active in seeking out and processing illness information. Rather than passively reacting to external stimuli, people actively create meanings out of their experience which then guide their coping. Second, the critical role in guiding coping behavior is played by the cognitive representations that people have of illness.

The remainder of this chapter is concerned with the nature of these cognitive representations and their implications for understanding health-related behavior. With respect to the nature of the representations, research demonstrating the existence and general nature of disease representations is examined first. Then work exploring the composition of disease representations is considered, followed by research on the cognitive organization of disease information. Implications of disease representations are explored for self-diagnosis and help seeking, compliance with medical recommendations, and responses to disease victims. Finally, suggestions are made about some possible future directions for research on disease representations.

The Nature of Disease Representations

General Characteristics

Given that a person's health-related behavior is guided by internal disease representations, the question arises as to the nature of those representations. How is illness information represented in memory and what are the implications of that representation? The general model for addressing this question comes from work in cognition concerned with the kinds of knowledge structures that people use in processing information about objects and events (Fiske & Taylor, 1984; Neisser, 1976). In responding to objects or events, people do not simply react to stimuli but rather construct meanings by relating those stimuli to preexisting schemata that the person has for the objects or events in question. Although the term "schema" has been defined in different ways (Brewer & Nakamura, 1984; Fiske & Taylor, 1984), it generally refers to the organized knowledge that a person has about given types of stimuli. In applying the schema concept to illness, the argument is that people understand health events through the use of organized and reasonably stable disease schemata.

The idea of a disease schema was first explored by Leventhal and his colleagues in their work with hypertension and cancer patients (Leventhal et al., 1980, 1984). In attempting to explain why hypertension patients dropped out of treatment, as well as how cancer patients coped with chemotherapy, Leventhal and his associates noted that the patients seemed to be responding to the treatment situation in terms of implicit theories about the disease and its treatment. For example, patients with malignant lymphoma seemed to gauge the effectiveness of chemotherapy by monitoring the size of their tumors. Paradoxically, patients who experienced a rapid disappearance of their tumors exhibited much higher levels of distress during therapy than did those showing a more gradual remission. This suggested an implicit model of disease in which symptoms defined illness and illness was understood in terms of the symptoms involved. The heightened distress of patients with the most rapid remission apparently reflected the fact that they no longer had a palpable means of monitoring the effectiveness of treatment. On the basis of a series of investigations, Leventhal and his colleagues argued that disease representations such as these form implicit theories of disease that are used to guide coping with the disease and to evaluate and regulate the use of treatment.

In an effort to further elucidate the nature of disease representations and investigate their use in everyday symptom experience, my students and I have been engaged in a series of studies investigating the cognitive processes involved in interpreting illness information. Based on work from cognitive psychology on categorization processes (Rosch, 1978; Rosch & Mervis, 1975; Rosch, Mervis, Gray, Johnson, & Boyes-Braem, 1976; Smith & Medin, 1981), we proposed a prototype model of disease representations. This model argues that people's schemata of diseases can be thought of as idealized representations of the symptoms and other attributes associated with different diseases. These disease prototypes serve as standards against which people match and evaluate information about experienced symptoms. When people experience physical symptoms, they interpret those symptoms by retrieving from memory prototypes of various diseases. The symptoms are interpreted as representing the disease whose prototypical symptoms are most like the ones currently experienced. In line with work on the prototype notion as it applies in other domains, the disease categories involved are not rigidly defined but, rather, "fuzzy" (i.e., people accept some flexibility in the definitions of the categories). Hence a perfect fit between the prototype and the symptoms experienced is not required. The selection of a disease prototype to interpret the symptoms is made on the basis of the "family resemblance" (Rosch & Mervis, 1975; Smith & Medin, 1981) between the symptoms and available prototypes. When interpreting a set of symptoms as being, say, strep throat, people don't require that the symptoms experienced fit their prototype of strep throat exactly. They simply require that there be enough resemblance to the symptoms of strep throat so as to make that a plausible interpretation. Also, the symptoms should fit the prototype for strep throat better than they do other disease prototypes considered.

Evidence for this model of disease representation comes from a series of studies performed in our laboratory (Bishop, Briede, Cavazos, Grotzinger, & McMahon, 1987; Bishop & Converse, 1986; Bishop, Sikes, Schroeder, McGregor, & Holub, 1985). This work has focused on several aspects of disease prototypes and their implications. The first issue explored was the recognition of disease states as a function of the prototypicality of presented symptoms. Specifically, we tested the hypothesis that subjects would be more likely to rate a set of symptoms as indicating a disease and correctly identify the disease involved, and to feel more confident about their disease identifications, when the symptoms in the set more closely resembled the consensual prototype for a given disease. To test this hypothesis, Sharolyn Converse and I (Bishop & Converse, 1986) obtained pilot subjects' ratings of the perceived association between various symptoms and diseases. Based on these ratings, symptom sets were then assembled that varied in the extent of perceived association between the symptoms and specified diseases. High-prototype sets contained six symptoms, all of which were rated by pilot subjects as

Table 3-1. Sample Stimulus Sets Used in Prototype Studies

High prototype (hay fever): This afternoon your friend Bob mentions that for the last
few days he has been (C) sneezing quite a bit, his (C) sinuses have been inflamed
and he has had an (C) itchy nose. Also, he has had (C) nasal congestion with (C)
teary eyes and (C) nasal discharge.

Medium prototype (stroke): Recently Sally has been complaining that she has been
experiencing some (C) sensations of numbness along with (C) dizziness. Also, she
has had a (I) swollen ankle and states that she has a (I) sore throat and her (C)
vision is blurred. You notice that her (C) speech seems to be slurred.

Low prototype (strep throat): Yesterday when you were talking, your friend Bill
mentioned that recently he has had (I) trouble remembering things. He also
mentioned that he has had a (C) sore throat and some (C) difficulty in swallowing
along with some (I) pain over his heart. He has also noticed a (I) swollen wrist and
(I) burning in his eyes.

Random: In talking with Alice today she mentioned that recently she has been
experiencing quite a bit of (I) insomnia. Also, she has noticed that she has (I) lost
weight recently, has had (I) difficulty urinating and has noticed a (I) change in the
color of two warts. This morning she noticed a (I) rash on her skin and currently
feels (I) dizzy.

Key: (C) indicates that the symptom that follows is consistent with the disease prototype. (I)
indicates that the symptom that follows is irrelevant to the disease prototype.
Source: From Bishop and Converse, 1986. Reprinted by permission.

being closely associated with the specified disease entity, whereas medium-
and low-prototype sets contained four related and two unrelated symptoms
or two related and four unrelated symptoms, respectively. In addition,
random symptom sets were assembled in which no two symptoms were
related to any particular disease. Examples of symptom sets used are shown
in Table 3.1. When presented with these symptoms, subjects were indeed
more likely to state that high-prototype symptom sets indicated a disease
than they were with medium- or low-prototype or random sets. Also, as
predicted, when asked to identify the disease entity involved, subjects were
more likely to correctly identify the disease for high-prototype sets and
indicated greater confidence in their disease identification.

With these initial findings in place, we set out to test predictions of the
prototype model for the recall and for the speed of processing illness
information. In particular, we hypothesized that if people use prototypes in
conceptualizing diseases and interpreting symptoms, people should find it
easier to recall symptoms that are consistent with available disease
prototypes. Further, we predicted that prototype-consistent information
would be processed more rapidly than would information not relevant to
available prototypes.

The implications of prototypes for recall were tested in a second study with
Sharolyn Converse (Bishop & Converse, 1986). In this study we presented

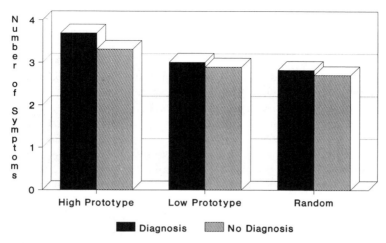

Figure 3-1. Differences in correct symptom recall by prototype level. (Data from Bishop & Converse, 1986.)

subjects with symptom sets varying in prototypicality and later asked them to recall the symptoms. We found, as predicted, that subjects correctly recalled more symptoms from high- than low-prototype or random sets (see Figures 3-1 and 3-2). Further, with low-prototype sets, there was a slight tendency for subjects to recall a greater proportion of symptoms consistent with their prototype for the disease in question than symptoms unrelated to the prototype. This effect was significantly enhanced by giving subjects an

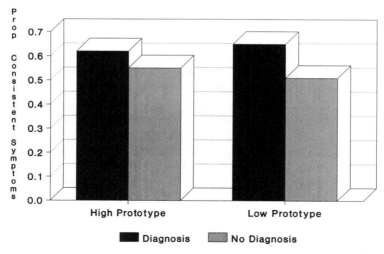

Figure 3-2. Differences in proportion of prototype-consistent symptoms recalled. (Data from Bishop & Converse, 1986.)

explicit diagnosis for the disease involved. Thus, when given a diagnosis for a set of symptoms, subjects were even more likely to recall prototype-consistent symptoms and to neglect irrelevant ones.

The prototype model also implies that closeness of fit between symptom information and available prototypes should affect the speed with which people process that information. If people use prototypes as templates against which to match symptom information, a closer fit between a set of symptoms and an available disease prototype should lead to more rapid processing of symptom information. This hypothesis was tested by presenting symptom sets, varying in prototypicality, on a computer screen. Subjects were asked to read the symptoms and then to indicate, by pressing a key on the keyboard, whether the symptoms represented a specific disease. The latency between presentation of the symptoms and the subjects' response was measured and recorded by the computer. The results showed that, as predicted, subjects required less time to make decisions about high-prototype sets (mean = 14.84 sec) than they did for medium (mean = 18.64 sec) or low-prototype (mean = 18.34 sec) or for random sets (mean = 17.57 sec).

Overall, the results of our studies supported the hypothesis that disease representations can be thought of in terms of prototypes that people have for specific physical diseases. The existence and content of these prototypes appear to influence the process of identifying disease states from symptoms as well as the processing and recall of information about illness episodes. Implications of these findings for self-diagnosis and help seeking are discussed in greater detail later.

Additional studies probing the nature of disease representations have been conducted by Lau and his colleagues (Lau, Bernard, & Hartman, 1989; Lau & Hartman, 1983) and by Croyle and Williams (in press). Lau and his colleagues have been concerned with how laypeople conceptualize everyday illnesses and have confirmed the existence of illness schemata using methods quite different from those used either in our studies or in those by Leventhal. Lau and his colleagues asked subjects to describe recent illness episodes in their own words. These descriptions were then content analyzed for the presence and content of illness schemata. These studies have verified the existence of schemata for common illnesses that are both coherently organized and relatively stable over time.

The work by Croyle and Williams has been concerned with what they term illness stereotypes, that is, the personal characteristics that people associate with individuals who have been diagnosed with different diseases. In their studies they examined stereotypes that their subjects have of hypertensives, noting that these stereotypes are related to the perceived seriousness of this disease. This line of work is very interesting in that it raises the possibility that the disease representations that people have include not only information about the disease per se but also perceptions of persons who have the disease.

Makeup of Disease Representations

The work described thus far concerns the general nature of disease representations, arguing that laypeople have well-organized and stable cognitive representations of diseases that have important implications for interpreting illness information and guiding coping. A second critical question deals with the specific makeup of these representations. There have been two approaches to this question, one examining the components of disease schemata, the other exploring the dimensions or factors that are involved.

In their interviews with hypertension and cancer patients, Leventhal and his associates (1980, 1982, 1984) identified four basic components in their representations of their diseases: identity, cause, timeline, and consequences. *Identity* consists of the label placed on the disease and the symptoms associated with it. As indicated by its name, *cause* refers to the person's ideas about how one gets the disease. *Timeline* is concerned with the expectations the person has about how long the disease is likely to last and its characteristic course. Finally, the component of *consequences* has to do with the expected outcome and sequelae of the disease.

These components are viewed as being the basic building blocks of disease representations and as having important implications for how patients conceptualize and cope with their condition. For example, with regard to the identity component, Leventhal notes that patients have a great deal of difficulty conceptualizing a disease like hypertension, which is said to have no symptoms. Despite medical statements to the contrary, 88% of the hypertension patients interviewed stated that there were symptoms they could monitor to tell when their blood pressure was up (Leventhal et al., 1984). Further, patients appeared to be conceptualizing the timeline component in terms of three different models, acute, cyclic, and chronic. Patients with an acute model viewed hypertension as a disease that when treated goes away, much like an infection or other acute illness. Those holding a cyclic view thought of hypertension as a disease that comes and goes, requiring treatment on a periodic basis. Those utilizing a chronic model correctly regarded hypertension as a condition requiring long-term treatment.

Because the components identified by Leventhal were derived from studies of seriously and/or chronically ill patients, Lau and Hartman (1983) wondered if the same components would be found when relatively healthy individuals were asked to describe their experiences with everyday illnesses such as colds or the flu. Content analysis of descriptions of common illnesses obtained from college students found support for the four components proposed by Leventhal and identified a fifth component, *cure*, which relates to beliefs about how one recovers from an illness. Lau and Hartman suggested that this component is one that is more likely to be detected in descriptions of acute illnesses where recovery is expected than it is in the case of chronic conditions. These five components were confirmed in a second study that examined illness experience over time (Lau et al., 1989). Moreover, these components appear to be stable over time and to have implications for illness behavior. For example, people with strong identity and cure components in their illness cognitions were particularly likely to visit a doctor both for specific illness episodes and for asymptomatic checkups (Lau et al., 1989).

In our work with disease prototypes, my students and I have explored the components of disease representations by examining the kinds of associations that people make to symptom descriptions. Our goals have been to test for the existence of the five components of disease representations, using a somewhat different methodology, and to explore the cognitive processes involved in recalling illness information. We presented subjects with symptom sets varying in the prototypicality of the symptoms and the seriousness of the disease entity involved and asked them to write down their thoughts about what else might be associated with the person's symptom experience. Our data confirmed the existence of the five components in that 90% of the associations fell into the categories of identity (including both labels and other symptoms), cause, timeline, consequences, and cure (Bishop et al., 1987).

Beyond this, our data also allowed us to explore some of the processes involved in evoking these components from the person's store of disease information. One of the prime functions of prototypes is to make disease information readily available to the person, so people's ability to match symptoms to a specific disease prototype can be expected to considerably influence what they feel they know about the condition. In the study just described we predicted that the number and type of associations evoked by a set of symptoms would be a function of its prototypicality. In considering the associations that people might make to symptom sets, we thought it important to distinguish between associations made to individual symptoms as opposed to those made to the symptom set as a whole. This distinction is in line with recent work in social cognition exploring the differences between "category-based" and "piecemeal" processing (Fiske & Pavalchak, 1986). With respect to the processing of disease information, category-based processing occurs when the person responds to an overall disease entity. In this case the person responds to the disease prototype activated in the attempt to identify the source of the symptoms. On the other hand, piecemeal processing occurs when the person responds to individual symptoms without relating them to a larger whole. In our study, we hypothesized that subjects would make more associations to symptom sets *as a whole* as the prototypicality of those sets increased, but we expected that as the prototypicality of symptom sets decreased the overall number of associations might not necessarily decrease but there would be a greater tendency to make associations to individual symptoms. Our reasoning here was that in order to make sense of what was happening to them, people would have a bias toward relating symptom information to specific disease prototypes, thus making additional information about the identified disease entity accessible. Another way of saying this is that they would attempt to engage in "category-based" processing. However, when the symptoms experienced do not fit a disease prototype, a person is likely to be forced back into a more "piecemeal" mode of processing in which inferences are made on the basis of individual symptoms and not a central disease entity. In support of these hypotheses, we (Bishop et al., 1987, Exp. 2) found that subjects made significantly more category-based associations to symptom sets high in prototypicality than to those lower in prototypicality. On the other hand, more associations were made to individual symptoms as the prototypicality of the symptom sets decreased. In processing illness information, then, people do their best to relate symptoms to a given disease entity and, when successful, make associations to the overall set of symptoms. When unsuccessful at relating symptoms to a specific disease, attempts at understanding the symptoms in a holistic fashion are thwarted. People will continue attempts to understand their symptom experience but will do so on the basis of individual symptoms.

It is also instructive to consider how this affects the particular associations made. To examine this issue we made counts of the different categories of associations made to the different symptom sets and analyzed them according to the seriousness and prototypicality of the sets. The largest differences were found for label and cause associations (see Figures 3-3 and 3-4). In a nutshell, we found that for nonserious symptom sets, as the prototypicality of the symptoms decreased the number of label associations decreased while the number of cause associations increased. When faced

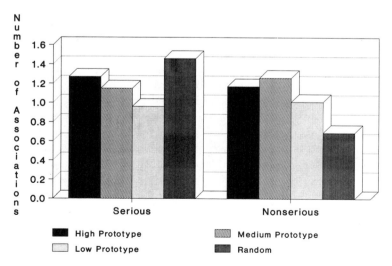

Figure 3-3. Number of label associations made by prototype level and seriousness of symptoms. (Data from Bishop et al., 1987.)

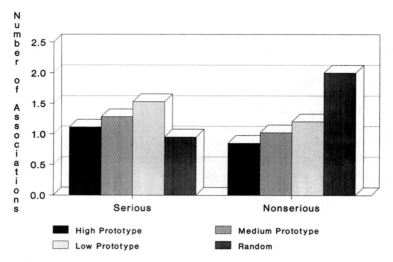

Figure 3-4. Number of cause associations made by prototype level and seriousness of symptoms. (Data from Bishop et al., 1987.)

with nonserious symptoms that could not be related to a prototype, our subjects had trouble coming up with labels but no problem coming up with causes. One possibility is that they identified a separate cause for each symptom. For serious symptoms, however, a different pattern was found. While the pattern for high-, medium-, and low-prototype sets was similar to that for nonserious symptoms (decreasing prototypicality led to decreasing label and increasing cause associations), subjects' responses to random serious symptoms were quite different. Random serious symptoms produced the greatest number of label associations for any cell and the second smallest number of cause associations. This suggests that when faced with serious symptoms that do not fit a known pattern people may well go into overdrive in producing labels for the condition but be at a real loss to figure out what is causing them. This state of affairs is likely to be an anxiety-provoking one for individuals as they attempt to grapple with what is going on. When subjects in another experiment were asked how concerned they would be if they were experiencing the symptoms in each of the sets, they indicated their greatest degree of concern when faced with serious random sets (Bishop et al., 1987, Exp. 1).

Although the data in our laboratory as well as those from Leventhal and Lau provide strong support for the five components of disease representations mentioned here (also see Lacroix & Schober, this volume, for a discussion of historical data relating to this question), a second set of findings has addressed the makeup of disease representations from a somewhat different point of view, by seeking to identify the underlying dimensions used in thinking about diseases. The assumption is that there are certain cognitive dimensions that characterize disease representations. Further, it is often assumed that these dimensions can be deduced through statistical techniques such as factor analysis.

Among the earliest attempts to identify the dimensions of disease representations are the factor analytic studies of Jenkins (1966; Jenkins & Zyzanski, 1968). Using a semantic differential technique (Osgood, Suci, & Tannenbaum, 1957), Jenkins obtained ratings of four different diseases (tuberculosis, cancer, poliomyelitis, and mental illness) from a sample of adults in Florida and then submitted them to factor analysis. Although there was some variance in the factor structures obtained from the different diseases, the results suggested the presence of at least three interpretable factors that appeared to be common to the different diseases. These factors were labeled personal involvement, human mastery, and social desirability. Personal involvement referred to the extent to which respondents saw the disease as salient and felt susceptible to it. Human mastery concerned the degree to which people felt the disease could be understood and controlled. Social desirability was the amount of shame or embarrassment associated with the disease. Ben-Sira (1977a, 1977b) later used these factors to define what he referred to as the "image" of diseases and presented data showing at least a modest relationship between this image and preventive health behavior.

A somewhat different approach was used by Lau and Hartman (1983) in exploring the dimensionality underlying the cause and cure components. When obtaining descriptions of recent illnesses, Lau and Hartman asked subjects to describe in their own words why they had gotten sick and also why they had gotten better. After each set of reasons was given, subjects were asked to rate these reasons on eight attribution scales. Factor analysis of these scales indicated a three-factor structure for both cause and cure attributions. The factors obtained—locus (internal vs. external), stability, and controllability—had also been obtained in a variety of studies examining attributions in other domains (Weiner, 1971). These results are, of course, limited to the cause and cure components but do establish the relevance of common attributional dimensions for lay disease representations.

In an effort to reconcile some of the differences in previous findings relating to the dimensions of disease representations, Turk, Rudy, and Salovey (1986) devised the Implicit Models of Illness Questionnaire (IMIQ). The 38 items of this questionnaire were selected on the basis of the studies by Leventhal, Lau, Jenkins, and others. Included were questions pertaining to the five components of disease representations described earlier and to such disease characteristics as disruptiveness, personal responsibility, and seriousness. The IMIQ was then administered to different subject populations including diabetics, diabetes educators, and college students. Subjects rated two diseases, one with which they were directly familiar (diabetes or flu) and one with which they had no direct personal experience (cancer). Exploratory, followed by confirmatory, factor analyses suggested four factors, which were labeled seriousness, personal responsibility, controllability, and changeability. While these results are suggestive and certainly seem to confirm the relevance of attributional dimensions for disease representations, questions remain about the interpretation of these factors. Examination of loadings for the seriousness factor, for example, reveals that the highest loading for this factor was for contagiousness, suggesting that this factor may in reality be a combination of seriousness and contagion. Turk et al. argue that their data contradict the notion of the five components described by Leventhal and Lau and confirmed in our prototype studies.

On the surface, the results of these studies might be construed as being at odds with those examining components. However, studies exploring the dimensionality of disease representations start with a different set of assumptions and utilize different methods than do those examining components. Studies examining the components of disease representations have used content analysis of respondents' free descriptions of illness experience, whereas the work done on dimensions has generally relied on scale ratings. Also, as Lau et al. (1989) point out, a factor analytic approach examines differences in how people conceptualize objects (in this case diseases) rather than focusing on the common features of disease representations, as does the components approach. These differences in assumptions and methods may well account for many of the differences in outcome. Further, it seems quite likely that these two different approaches simply examine different, but complementary, aspects of the same phenomena. While the components approach looks at the specific content of disease representations, the dimensional approach examines different ways in which people evaluate that content. Indeed, Lau and colleagues (Lau & Hartman, 1983; Lau et al., 1989) explicitly discuss the dimensions used in evaluating the cause and cure components.

Organization of Disease Representations in Memory

Thus far our discussion has been concerned with how people conceptualize individual diseases. A largely unexplored question is how representations of different diseases relate to one another. This is a question that has a number of potential implications and that we have recently begun to explore in our laboratory.

Our approach has been to examine individuals' responses to different diseases in an attempt to identify the categories and/or dimensions that people use in organizing disease information. Note that in this work we have been looking at how people perceive the *relationships between diseases* as opposed to examining the internal structure of disease representations, as was the case for studies discussed in the previous section. Researchers have often overlooked this distinction when examining disease representations.

Initial evidence on the organization of disease information in memory has been obtained in a study examining perceived relationships between different diseases and the implications of this organization for how people respond to disease victims. In this study we obtained ratings for a broad spectrum of 22 diseases on a series of 18 scales (Bishop, in press). The rating scales, which we had found useful in previous studies of illness perception (Bishop, 1987), included such characteristics as contagiousness, seriousness, easiness to get, painfulness, and commonness. In addition, we asked the subjects in a second questionnaire to indicate how willing they would be to engage in six different types of interaction (e.g., meet, work, go to school, spend several hours) with a person having one of these diseases. To assess the perceived relationships between diseases, means were computed across subjects for each rating scale for each disease. These means were used to compute distances between diseases that were submitted to both multidimensional scaling (MDS) (Schiffman, Reynolds, & Young, 1981) and cluster analysis (Anderberg, 1972). The results of these analyses suggested a two-dimensional MDS solution in which diseases were organized according to perceived contagiousness and the extent to which diseases were viewed as serious or life threatening. As expected, the cluster analyses confirmed the MDS results in finding four clusters of diseases that were labeled contagious/life threatening, contagious/non–life threatening, noncontagious/life threatening, and noncontagious/non–life threatening. This MDS solution and the clusterings are seen in Figure 3-5.

Subjects' willingness to interact with disease victims was primarily a function of the perceived contagiousness of the disease in question. On the measure of interaction willingness, the diseases tended to cluster into two groups with contagious diseases in one group and noncontagious diseases in the other. Not surprisingly, subjects indicated a willingness to interact with persons having noncontagious diseases but were quite unwilling to interact with those having contagious conditions.

Although on the surface these results may not seem particularly surprising, what struck us was our subjects' willingness to draw a distinction between contagious and noncontagious diseases without considering differences between the ways in which the diseases are actually spread. For example, even though flu and AIDS are very different and are spread in different ways, subjects did not seem to differentiate between them in their willingness to interact with a person having one of them. Rather, it appeared that our subjects were responding primarily to a general category of contagious disease.

In light of these results, we conducted a second study to obtain a more complete picture of people's understanding of the concept of contagious disease and to explore the possibility that there are specific diseases that people consider to be prototypical of this category. Subjects in this study were asked to give their own definitions of contagious disease, list possible modes of transmission, and rate diseases in terms of how typical they were of

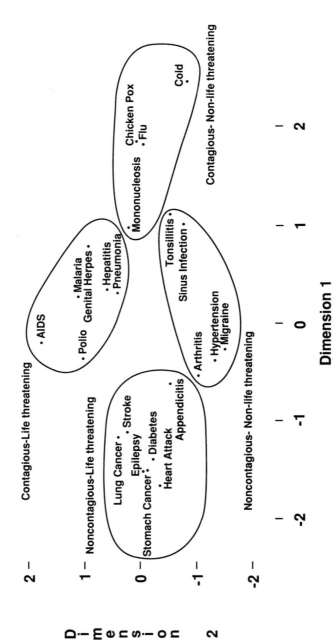

Figure 3-5. Plot of MDS dimensions and disease clusters. (From Bishop, in press. Used by permission.)

the person's concept of a contagious disease. As we suspected, our subjects had a rather undifferentiated concept of contagious disease and tended to identify contagious diseases with some form of "casual" contact (e.g., through the air, via contaminated objects). Content analysis of the definitions indicated that they were relatively simple and straightforward. On the average, each definition contained 2.77 elements. Generally, these included a statement that a contagious disease is one that can be passed from person to person along with one or two possible modes of transmission, most often some form of "casual" contact. Interestingly, 9 of our 53 subjects specifically stated that a contagious disease is one that can be easily transmitted. When asked to state how one gets a contagious disease, subjects listed an average of 3.85 different modes of transmission. Again, casual contact figured most prominently in these responses, with 92% of the subjects mentioning one or more types of casual contact as compared with 69% mentioning one or more types of intimate or blood contact (e.g., sexual intercourse, sharing of needles, blood transfusions, or "exchange of body fluids"). This identification of contagious diseases with casual contact was also obtained when subjects were asked to rate diseases in terms of their typicality as contagious diseases. The three diseases rated most typical (on a seven-point scale with 7 indicating "very typical") were flu (6.20), cold (6.13), and chicken pox (5.83).

These data suggest that laypeople organize diseases into categories based on perceptions of contagiousness and the degree to which diseases are life threatening. Further, with regard to contagiousness, it appears that there is a relatively straightforward consensual definition of contagious disease and that certain diseases are seen as being particularly representative of that category. Another study (Bishop, Brandt, Lawrence, & Leighton, 1988), using a methodology similar to that used in the study of contagious disease, examined perceptions of life-threatening and contagious life-threatening diseases. Preliminary results from this study suggest that AIDS, lung cancer, and heart attack are perceived to be the most typical life-threatening diseases, whereas, among the conditions examined, AIDS stands alone in being perceived as the typical contagious life-threatening disease.

The existence and use of general disease categories in organizing disease information appear to have some important implications. One possibility that we are currently exploring is that designating certain diseases as being prototypical of a disease category provides the person with "default values" when responding to unfamiliar diseases. Suppose, for example, that a person encounters a disease that is known to be contagious but about which the person knows little. How is the person likely to respond to this new disease? The use of cold or flu as a prototypical contagious disease may furnish the person with hypotheses about the characteristics of the new disease, including specific ways in which it might be spread. One situation where this may well have occurred is AIDS hysteria. The implications of general disease categories for AIDS hysteria are discussed later.

Implications of Disease Representations

Thus far I have been concerned with the basic aspects of disease representations, their nature, composition, organization, and source. I now turn to a consideration of the implications of disease representations for health-related behavior. In the sections that follow I discuss the role of disease representations in self-diagnosis and help seeking, adherence to medical recommendations, and people's responses to disease victims.

Self-Diagnosis and Help Seeking

One of the common observations in studies of illness and illness behavior is that there is a great deal of variability in how people respond to physical symptoms (Mechanic, 1978; Pennebaker, 1982). Although people experience symptoms on a fairly regular basis (Bishop, 1984; Pennebaker, 1982; Roghman & Haggerty, 1972), it is often the case that many of these symptoms are ignored or at least go untreated. For example, in a recent health diary study of illness behavior in a military population, respondents reported at least one symptom on about 20% of all diary days. Help seeking was observed, however, for less than 8% of all symptoms (Bishop, 1984). It has also been noted in studies of help seeking for symptoms of cancer and heart attack that victims often delay for significant amounts of time before seeking help (Antonovsky & Hartman, 1974; Matthews, Seigel, Kuller, Thompson & Varat, 1983). Many factors affect treatment delays, but one central issue is the understanding that people have of the symptoms involved and their relationship to various disease entities. For example, the greatest proportion of delay in seeking medical attention for myocardial infarction appears to be attributable to time required for the person to decide that a heart attack is occurring and medical attention is needed (Doehrman, 1977; see also King & Colen, 1989, for a first-person account).

Work on disease representations furthers our understanding of the process of help seeking by laying out the cognitive processes involved in deciding whether one is ill. In our work on disease prototypes we have conceptualized this as a process of self-diagnosis in which the person attempts to understand experienced symptoms by relating them to available disease prototypes. A person who experiences physical symptoms sets in motion a cognitive search aimed at labeling the symptoms and gaining other information about his or her condition. The prototype model argues that the person will attempt to match the symptoms experienced against available prototypes, selecting the best fitting prototype to interpret the symptoms.

This process has several implications both for the person's behavior in response to symptoms and for the symptom experience itself. First, the person's behavior is likely to be a function of the disease prototypes that the person has available as well as the medical appropriateness of those prototypes. One problem that heart attack victims encounter when they first begin experiencing symptoms is that the symptoms may not fit their conception of a heart attack. Often the symptoms are interpreted as gastric distress or simple fatigue (King & Colen, 1989). A particularly interesting situation arises when the person is faced with symptoms that are perceived as serious but do not fit an available prototype. As noted earlier, when subjects were presented with serious random symptoms they seemed to be at a loss to identify the source of the symptoms but proved quite adept at coming up with potential labels (Bishop et al., 1987, Exp. 2). This also seemed to be a very anxiety-provoking situation. When asked to indicate how concerned they would be if they were experiencing these symptoms and how confident they were about what they would do about them, subjects indicated the greatest concern about serious random symptoms (Bishop et al., 1987, Exp. 1) and expressed the greatest confidence in their behavior choices (Bishop et al., 1985). Subjects were very certain that they would immediately seek medical attention.

The prototypes used to interpret somatic experience may also have an impact on the symptom experience itself. Pennebaker (1982, 1984) has pointed out that somatic experience is frequently ambiguous and that symptom perception is often inaccurate. Further, Pennebaker and Skelton (1981) have shown that the perception of symptoms can be influenced significantly by the hypotheses that individuals have about what they should be experiencing. For example, when led to expect an increase in skin temperature in response to an experimental manipulation, subjects reported the expected increase in the absence of any overall objective changes. Disease prototypes used to interpret symptom experience can be expected to have effects similar to the hypotheses that Pennebaker and Skelton examined. Once a particular disease prototype has been selected for interpreting the person's experience, this prototype provides the person with hypotheses about other symptoms that might be present. When our subjects were asked to make associations to symptom sets varying in prototypicality, 14% of those associations were additional symptoms (Bishop et al., 1987, Exp. 2). In line with the results of Pennebaker and Skelton, we can anticipate that expecting these additional symptoms would make it likely that the person would begin to feel these in addition to the symptoms already experienced.

The disease prototypes that the person utilizes in interpreting symptoms are also likely to affect presentation of those symptoms to a health-care provider or, for that matter, anyone else to whom the person describes the symptoms. Specifically, our findings that symptom recall is a function of the relationship of those symptoms to available disease prototypes (Bishop & Converse, 1986) point to likely biases in reporting symptoms to others. People may bias their reports toward consistency with the selected prototype and neglect symptoms they perceive to be irrelevant. There was also evidence in this same experiment that false symptom recall (remembering symptoms not in the original set) tended to be consistent with the prototype in use. Hence, once a self-diagnosis has been made, the person may report symptoms not originally experienced but consistent with the prototype selected.

Adherence to Medical Recommendations

It has long been recognized that patients often do not follow medical recommendations. Although estimates of noncooperation with medical regimens vary widely, depending on the disorder and type of recommendation, it is estimated that roughly one-third of patients do not follow recommendations for short-term treatments, and half or more fail to follow recommendations for long-term treatments (Baekeland & Lundwall, 1975; Sackett & Snow, 1979). Lay disease representations have a number of important implications for this problem as they point out the specific models that patients develop of their illnesses, models that often diverge significantly from the medical understanding of the disease in question. Health professionals think of treatment decisions in terms of a biomedical understanding of disease, but the actual adherence to those treatment recommendations has been shown to be a function of the "common sense" lay models.

To date the most extensive work relating disease representations to treatment behavior is that of Leventhal and his associates (Leventhal et al., 1980, 1982, 1984; Meyer, Leventhal, & Gutmann, 1985). As noted earlier, people tend to define diseases in terms of symptoms, making it difficult to conceptualize asymptomatic diseases such as hypertension. Without symptoms to define the disease and monitor the effectiveness of treatment, people lack familiar guides for their behavior. Leventhal and his colleagues have found that, in order to deal with this situation, hypertension patients almost universally develop a representation of hypertension that includes symptoms that can be monitored to tell when one's blood pressure is elevated. Even though they often state that in general hypertension has no symptoms, 71% of the newly treated hypertensives along with 92% of those continuing and 94% of those reentering treatment state there are symptoms they can monitor to tell when their own blood pressure is up. These beliefs, in turn, exert a strong effect on treatment behavior. Of a group of actively treated hypertensives, 37% believed the treatment affected their symptoms. Among these patients, 70% were judged to be complying with their treatment regimen. For patients who did not perceive a relationship between symptoms and treatment, only 31% were taking their medications as prescribed. As would be expected, patients perceiving a relationship between treatment and symptoms were more likely to be judged by their physicians as being in good control of their blood pressure (Meyer et al., 1985).

Although these findings suggest that symptom monitoring is an adaptive strategy for hypertensives, other data point to important pitfalls. Recent studies have shown that although hypertensives believe strongly in symptoms that indicate heightened blood pressure, the symptoms involved are often highly idiosyncratic and the beliefs largely erroneous. Baumann and Leventhal (1985) examined both actual and perceived symptom–blood pressure relationships and found that symptoms were related to *perceived* blood pressure, but the relationship between predicted and actual blood pressure was quite weak, as was the relationship between actual blood pressure and symptoms. Further, feedback about this lack of relationship appeared to have little effect on subjects' beliefs about their ability to detect heightened blood pressure. Substantially similar results were obtained by Pennebaker and Watson (1988), who found that although 68% of their subjects had at least one symptom that correlated significantly with systolic blood pressure, these symptoms varied considerably between subjects, and subjects' beliefs about symptom–blood pressure relationships were generally inaccurate. In addition, although medicated hypertensives displayed greater confidence in their ability to detect blood pressure changes than did normotensives, hypotensives, and nonmedicated hypertensives, in fact they were no more accurate than the other groups and had fewer symptoms and emotions that were empirically related to blood pressure. These results argue that attempts by hypertensives to use changes in symptoms to monitor the effectiveness of treatment are likely to lead to treatment behavior based on false assumptions. Whether hypertensives can be trained to detect blood pressure accurately via symptoms, as suggested by Pennebaker and Watson, is unknown.

The specific components of disease representations also have important implications for treatment cooperation. In this respect the timeline component appears to be particularly important. The Leventhal group has identified three models, acute, cyclic, and chronic, that people have of the course of a disease. These models reflect the person's expectations about the likely duration of treatment and have been shown to have a significant effect on whether patients stay in treatment. Leventhal et al. (1984) note that hypertensives new to treatment tend to conceptualize their disease in acute rather than chronic terms, whereas hypertensives who have been in treatment for a while see it in chronic terms. Further, among the newly treated hypertensives, those utilizing an acute model are much more likely to drop out of treatment within six months (58%) than are those holding the more accurate chronic model (17%).

Responses to Disease Victims

In addition to influencing help-seeking behavior and cooperation with medical recommendations, lay disease representations also have important implications for people's responses to individuals who are the victims of disease (see also Skelton, this volume). At one time or another, and probably more frequently than we realize, we come in contact with individuals who have different diseases. Work on disease representations argues that an important determinant of our responses to those individuals will be our schemata of the diseases in question. Disease representations include the beliefs that people have about how a disease is contracted and its consequences, so we can certainly anticipate that the contents of the cognitive representation for a given disease will profoundly affect how a person reacts to someone who has the disease.

A good case in point is the fearful reaction that many people have shown toward those with AIDS. We are by now all too familiar with reports of highly fearful reactions when a child with the AIDS virus attends school or when a co-worker or acquaintance develops AIDS, reactions that have included ostracism, dismissal from employment, boycotting of schools, and, in one case, the burning of a family out of their home. Given what we know about AIDS, these responses to persons with the AIDS virus are highly irrational. To date not one person is known to have contracted the AIDS virus through the kind of casual contact involved in school or work settings. As Surgeon General Koop pointed out, AIDS is difficult to get, with transmission of the virus limited to such high-risk behaviors as the sharing of infected needles and sexual relations with an infected person. How, then, can we understand fearful reactions by the public? On the one hand, the stigma associated with homosexuality in our society is certainly a very potent factor (O'Donnell, O'Donnell, & Pleck, 1987; Shilts, 1987). A second major factor is misinformation about the virus and how it is spread. Surveys have shown that although the majority of those responding gave correct answers about the nature of AIDS and how it is contracted, a significant number of people still believe that AIDS can be transmitted through casual contact. For example, in the September 1987 National Health Interview Survey, 18% of those interviewed believed that it was somewhat or very likely that a person could get AIDS by working near someone with AIDS and 36% believed that it was somewhat or very likely that a person could get the AIDS virus from eating in a restaurant where the cook has AIDS (Dawson, Cynamon, & Fitti, 1988).

These factors are undoubtedly important in understanding AIDS hysteria, but our studies of disease representations suggest another significant source of AIDS fear. Even though there has been, and still is, much ignorance among laypeople as to the nature of AIDS and how it is spread, people are acting on the beliefs that they hold about AIDS, regardless of how appropriate or inappropriate these beliefs may be. Our work on the organization of disease representations (Bishop, in press) suggests that one source of these beliefs can be found in the basic categories used to organize diseases. As noted earlier, the category of contagious disease appears to be a fundamental one. Perception of contagiousness was one of the two organizing principles that subjects seemed to be using in thinking about diseases. Willingness to interact with a disease victim was shown to be largely a function of perceived contagiousness. Further, people seem to have a relatively undifferentiated concept of contagious disease, defining it as being simply a disease that can be passed from one person to another and most frequently identifying transmission as occurring through casual contact. Finally, the diseases seen as being most prototypical of contagious disease as a category (flu, cold, and chicken pox) are transmitted relatively easily by casual means.

The implications of these findings for people's responses to AIDS and persons with AIDS are straightforward. When presented with a new disease that is deadly and either thought or known to be transmitted by a virus, people are likely to respond by applying to that disease their overall conception of a contagious disease. The concept of contagious disease is so closely associated with casual contact and prototypical contagious diseases are those that are spread by such means, so it is not surprising that people assume there is at least a strong likelihood this new virus is passed in the same way. This can be expected even when there are no explicit statements that it is spread through casual contact. This argues that hysteria over the possibility of contracting AIDS through everyday contact was quite likely inevitable. Even in the absence of the now infamous "household contact" theory (Shilts, 1987), it is likely that the mere identification of AIDS as a contagious disease, caused by a virus, would have been sufficient to engender fear. These same considerations also point to reasons why the household contact theory was so readily believed by many and why such intensive efforts have been needed to counter public fear over AIDS and its spread.

Future Directions

The work done to date barely scratches the surface of the phenomena associated with disease representations. The studies discussed here lay the groundwork in demonstrating the importance of lay disease representations and exploring their basic characteristics, but much remains to be learned. Future research should build on these initial findings as well as incorporate what has been learned about cognitive structures in other domains (Brewer & Nakamura, 1984; Markus & Zajonc, 1985; Rumelhart, 1984). The following paragraphs describe some possible future directions for the study of disease representations.

The work discussed earlier primarily examines the verbal representations that people have of disease. Although such verbal representations are obviously important and form the foundation for communicating illness information, there is certainly no reason to limit disease representations to this level. One of the critical features of our illness experience is that it is usually (although not always) based on perceptions of physiological sensations. Clearly disease representations exist on the sensory as well as the verbal level. Future research on disease representations needs to explore this sensory level of disease representations more fully. One line of work that has explored aspects of the sensory level of illness schemata is Pennebaker's (1982, 1984) work on symptom perception. This work has explored several aspects of symptom experience, including its environmental determinants and accuracy as well as the relationship of symptoms to emotions. Particularly germane is the work by Pennebaker and his colleagues on accuracy of symptom perception in hypertensives and diabetics (Gonder-Frederick, Cox, Bobbitt, & Pennebaker, 1986; Pennebaker & Watson, 1988). This work has certainly contributed to our understanding of how people perceive symptoms and can serve as a model for further exploration of the sensory aspects of disease representations. Among the topics that might be examined are the sensations associated with specific disease entities, variations between individuals in their sensory representations of different diseases, and sources of inaccuracy in people's disease interpretations.

A second question that has received little attention concerns the activation of disease representations. The implicit assumption in the work thus far is that disease representations exist in memory and are activated under appropriate circumstances. In applying disease representations to self-diagnosis, I argued above that the experience of symptoms sets off a cognitive search resulting in the activation in memory of the disease prototype that is believed to best fit the symptoms. This is certainly only one path to activation. Work in social cognition has pointed out that schemata are activated under a variety of conditions with various implications (Markus & Zajonc, 1985). It seems highly likely that this is the case in illness cognition as well. On the one hand, disease representations can be activated by internal physiological events or by internally generated memories. On the other hand, they might be activated by stimuli in the social environment, such as another person pointing out a potential abnormality (e.g., a lump on the skin), social conversation about health, or media discussion of particular diseases. As yet we know very little of the details of the processes involved or the implications for illness interpretation or behavior.

The social context of disease representations is a third area that has yet to be explored. Our experience of illness, even though often based on internal sensations, commonly occurs in a social context. People describe their symptoms and discuss possible interpretations with others, both lay and professional. The symptoms that people report and the interpretation of those symptoms can have important social implications, such as release from work or school or sanctions for presumed undesirable behavior, as with drunkenness or illicit drug use. Work on person schemata has shown that the goals that a person has when processing information about others as well as whether a person is communicating or interpreting information can have significant effects on how that information is organized and what is remembered (Markus & Zajonc, 1985). Might it be the case that the processing of disease information is also significantly affected by these types of social context considerations? For example, what are the differences in the way in which people process disease information on weekends as opposed to workdays? In addition to perhaps a greater tendency to perceive symptoms as indicating disease on workdays, might there also be a difference in the schemata used and in the symptom information recalled? A particularly important illness-related social context is the interaction of doctor and patient. Work in social cognition has pointed out that transmitters of information tend to organize information more tightly than do receivers of that information (Markus & Zajonc, 1985). In the realm of illness cognition this suggests that there may be significant differences between how people organize disease information for presentation to others (such as a doctor) and how they organize information when listening to another's symptom complaints. Skelton (this volume) has begun examining issues related to perceived symptom legitimacy, but clearly more work is needed.

Another important area that has generated much speculation but few hard data concerns the source of lay disease representations. Currently we know very little about where disease representations come from and how they develop. In their work with medical patients, Leventhal et al. (1980, 1984) suggest three basic sources of disease representations. First, people's schemata for diseases derive from cultural factors, such as semantics (e.g., the common confusion between hypertension and heightened emotional tension), and the organization of medical care to deal with acute symptomatic disease. Second, disease representations are formed on the basis of information from other people, both health care professionals and laypersons (see Sanders, 1982, for a discussion of "lay conferral"). Third, disease representations derive from the person's illness experience. To this list I would add the cognitive organization of disease information. The disease categories described earlier appear to be a potent source of information about diseases when the person has little a priori information about a disease other than a general idea of the category into which it falls.

These suggestions provide a logical starting point for understanding the sources of disease representations, but there is as yet little empirical evidence to either confirm or elaborate on these possibilities. This needs to be corrected in future research. In my laboratory we are examining the influence of general disease categories on perceptions of unfamiliar diseases. If people do, in fact, view certain diseases as being prototypical of a category, we can expect that the characteristics of the prototypical diseases will strongly influence the perceived characteristics of the new disease. We are testing this possibility by presenting subjects with a fictitious disease ("Meyer–Zweig disease") that is described as falling into one of the following four categories: contagious/life threatening, contagious/non–life threatening, noncontagious/life threatening, and noncontagious/non–life threatening. We expect that subjects will respond to Meyer–Zweig disease in ways that are similar to how they respond to the prototypes identified for the different disease categories.

Conclusion

This chapter has explored laypeople cognitive representations of disease. These disease representations are the critical feature in a self-regulation model of responses to health-related events. Knowledge of how laypeople conceptualize diseases is essential for understanding their health-related behavior. The work to date on disease representations indicates that people possess well-structured and stable schemata for diseases, which guide their coping with health threats. These schemata include at least five components: identity, cause, timeline, consequences, and cure. In addition, there appear to be several dimensions that people use in evaluating these components. Work in our laboratory suggests these schemata can be thought of as prototypes of different diseases that the person compares with experienced symptoms in an effort to interpret the illness experience. The use of these prototypes influences both the process of identifying disease states and later symptom recall. In addition, there is reason to believe that the prototypes in use may also influence the symptom experience itself.

Less well researched are questions concerning the organization and source of disease representations. Available evidence suggests that disease representations are organized into categories based on perceived contagiousness and the extent to which the disease is seen as serious/life threatening. In addition, it appears likely that people have in mind diseases that they see as being particularly representative or prototypical of the different categories. As noted, this type of organization appears to have important implications for how people respond to diseases that are unfamiliar but are identified as falling into a given category. Studies are currently under way to examine further the organization of disease representations and to test the implications of this organization.

The implications of disease representations for health-related behavior were explored with a focus on help seeking, adherence to medical recommendations, and responses to disease victims. Even though these three areas are concerned with different aspects of people's responses to health events, they are all closely related to lay disease representations. In each case people's behavior can be understood as being guided by their schemata of diseases.

Finally, a number of suggestions were made about possible future directions for research on disease representations. Although much has been learned about the nature of disease representations and their implications, many issues have yet to be explored. The suggestions made by no means cover all or even a substantial part of the possibilities. However, they point out important areas for consideration and, I hope, provide a taste of the kinds of questions remaining to be addressed.

References

Anderberg, M. R. (1972). *Cluster analysis for applications*. New York: Academic Press.

Antonovsky, A., & Hartman, H. (1974). Delay in detection of cancer: A review of the literature. *Health Education Monographs*, *2*(2), 98–127.

Baekeland, F., & Lundwall, L. (1975). Dropping out of treatment: A critical review. *Psychological Bulletin*, *82*, 738–783.

Baumann, L. J., & Leventhal, H. (1985). "I can tell when my blood pressure is up, can't I?" *Health Psychology*, *4*, 203–218.

Ben-Sira, Z. (1977a). Involvement with a disease and health-promoting behavior. *Social Science and Medicine*, *11*, 165–173.

Ben-Sira, Z. (1977b). The structure and dynamics of the image of diseases. *Journal of Chronic Diseases*, *30*, 831–842.

Bishop, G. D. (1984). Gender, role and illness behavior in a military population. *Health Psychology*, *3*, 519–534.

Bishop, G. D. (1987). Lay conceptions of physical symptoms. *Journal of Applied Social Psychology*, *17*, 127–146.

Bishop, G. D. (in press). Lay disease representations and responses to victims of disease. *Basic and Applied Social Psychology*.

Bishop, G. D., Brandt, M., Lawrence, K., & Leighton, K. (1988). Unpublished data.

Bishop, G. D., Briede, C., Cavazos, L., Grotzinger, R., & McMahon, S. (1987). Processing illness information: The role of disease prototypes. *Basic and Applied Social Psychology*, *8*, 21–43.

Bishop, G. D., & Converse, S. A. (1986). Illness representations: A prototype approach. *Health Psychology*, *5*, 95–114.

Bishop, G. D., Sikes, L., Schroeder, D., McGregor, U. K., & Holub, D. (1985, August). *Behavior in response to physical symptoms*. Paper presented at the meeting of the American Psychological Association, Los Angeles.

Brewer, W. F., & Nakamura, G. V. (1984). The nature and functions of schemas. In R. S. Wyer & T. K. Srull (Eds.), *Handbook of social cognition* (Vol. 1, pp. 119–160). Hillsdale, NJ: Lawrence Erlbaum Associates.

Croyle, R. T., & Williams, K. D. (in press). Reactions to medical diagnosis: The role of illness stereotypes. *Basic and Applied Social Psychology*.

Dawson, D. A., Cynamon, M., & Fitti, J. E. (1988, January 18). AIDS knowledge and attitudes for September 1987: Provisional data from the National Health Interview Survey. *NCHS Advance Data from Vital and Health Statistics*, No. 148, 1–12.

DiMatteo, M. R., & DiNicola, D. D. (1982). *Achieving patient compliance*. New York: Pergamon Press.

Doehrman, S. R. (1977). Psychosocial aspects of recovery from coronary heart disease: A critical review. *Social Science and Medicine*, *11*, 199–218.

Fiske, S. T., & Pavalchak, M. A. (1986). Category-based versus piecemeal-based affective responses: Developments in schema-triggered affect. In R. M. Sorrentino & E. T. Higgins (Eds.), *The handbook of motivation and cognition: Foundations of social behavior* (pp. 167–203). New York: Guilford Press.

Fiske, S. T., & Taylor, S. E. (1984). *Social cognition*. Reading, MA: Addison-Wesley.

Gonder-Frederick, L. A., Cox, D. J., Bobbitt, S. A., & Pennebaker, J. W. (1986). Blood glucose symptom beliefs of diabetic patients: Accuracy and implications. *Health Psychology*, *5*, 327–341.

Jasnoski, M. L., & Schwartz, G. E. (1985). A synchronous systems model for health. *American Behavioral Scientist, 28*, 468–485.

Jenkins, C. D. (1966). Group differences in perception: A study of community beliefs and feelings about tuberculosis. *American Journal of Sociology, 71*, 417–429.

Jenkins, C. D., & Zyzanski, S. J. (1968). Dimension of belief and feeling concerning three diseases, poliomyelitis, cancer, and mental illness: A factor analytic study. *Behavioral Science, 13*, 372–381.

King, L., & Colen, B. D. (1989). *"Mr. King, you're having a heart attack": How a heart attack and bypass surgery changed my life.* New York: Delacorte Press.

Lau, R. R., Bernard, T. M., & Hartman, K. A. (1989). Further explorations of common sense representations of common illnesses. *Health Psychology, 8*, 195–219.

Lau, R. R., & Hartman, K. A. (1983). Common sense representations of common illnesses. *Health Psychology, 2*, 167–185.

Leventhal, H. (1983). Behavioral medicine: Psychology in health care. In D. Mechanic (Ed.), *Handbook of health, health care, and the health professions* (pp. 709–743). New York: Free Press.

Leventhal, H., Meyer, D., & Nerenz, D. (1980). The common sense representation of illness danger. In S. Rachman (Ed.), *Contributions to medical psychology* (Vol. 2, pp. 7–30). Oxford: Pergamon Press.

Leventhal, H., Nerenz, D. R., & Steele, D. J. (1984). Illness representations and coping with health threats. In A. Baum, S. E. Taylor & J. E. Singer (Eds.), *Handbook of psychology and health: Vol. IV. Social psychological aspects of health* (pp. 219–252). Hillsdale, NJ: Lawrence Erlbaum Associates.

Leventhal, H., Nerenz, D., & Straus, A. (1982). Self-regulation and the mechanisms of symptom appraisal. In D. Mechanic (Ed.), *Symptoms, illness behavior, and help-seeking* (pp. 55–86). New York: Prodist.

Markus, H., & Zajonc, R. B. (1985). The cognitive perspective in social psychology. In G. Lindzey & E. Aronson (Eds.), *Handbook of social psychology* (3rd ed., Vol. 1, pp. 137–230). Reading, MA: Addison-Wesley.

Matarazzo, J. D., Weiss, S. M., Herd, S. A., Miller, N. E., & Weiss, S. M. (Eds.) (1984). *Behavioral health: A handbook of health enhancement and disease prevention.* New York: Wiley.

Matthews, K. A., Seigel, J. M., Kuller, L. H., Thompson, M., & Varat, M. (1983). Determinants of decisions to seek medical treatment by patients with acute myocardial infarction symptoms. *Journal of Personality and Social Psychology, 44*, 1144–1156.

McKinlay, J. B. (1972). Some approaches and problems in the study of the use of services: An overview. *Journal of Health and Social Behavior, 13*, 115–152.

Mechanic, D. (1978). *Medical sociology* (2nd ed.). New York: Free Press.

Meyer, D., Leventhal, H., & Gutmann, M. (1985). Common-sense models of illness: The example of hypertension. *Health Psychology, 4*, 115–135.

Neisser, U. (1976). *Cognition and reality.* San Francisco: Freeman.

O'Donnell, L., O'Donnell, C. R., & Pleck, J. H. (1987). Psychosocial responses of hospital workers to acquired immune deficiency syndrome (AIDS). *Journal of Applied Social Psychology, 17*, 269–285.

Osgood, C. E., Suci, G., & Tannenbaum, P. (1957). *The measurement of meaning.* Urbana: University of Illinois Press.

Pennebaker, J. W. (1982). *The psychology of physical symptoms.* New York: Springer-Verlag.

Pennebaker, J. W. (1984). Accuracy of symptom perception. In A. Baum, S. E. Taylor, & J. E. Singer (Eds.), *Handbook of psychology and health: Vol. IV. Social psychological aspects of health* (pp. 189–212). Hillsdale, NJ: Lawrence Erlbaum Associates.

Pennebaker, J. W., & Skelton, J. A. (1981). Selective monitoring of bodily sensations. *Journal of Personality and Social Psychology, 41,* 213–223.

Pennebaker, J. W., & Watson, D. (1988). Blood pressure estimation and beliefs among normotensives and hypertensives. *Health Psychology, 7,* 309–328.

Roghman, K. J., & Haggerty, R. J. (1972). The diary as a research instrument in the study of health and illness behavior. *Medical Care, 10,* 143–163.

Rosch, E. (1978). Principles of categorization. In E. Rosch & B. B. Lloyd (Eds.), *Cognition and categorization* (pp. 27–48). Hillsdale, NJ: Lawrence Erlbaum Associates.

Rosch, E., & Mervis, C. (1975). Family resemblances: Studies in the internal structure of categories. *Cognitive Psychology, 7,* 573–605.

Rosch, E., Mervis, C., Gray, W., Johnson, D., & Boyes-Braem, P. (1976). Basic objects in natural categories. *Cognitive Psychology, 8,* 382–439.

Rumelhart, D. E. (1984). Schemata and the cognitive system. In R. S. Dwyer & T. K. Srull (Eds.), *Handbook of social cognition* (Vol. 1, pp. 161–188). Hillsdale, NJ: Lawrence Erlbaum Associates.

Sackett, D. L., & Snow, J. C. (1979). The magnitude of compliance and noncompliance. In R. B. Haynes, D. W. Taylor, & D. L. Sackett (Eds.), *Compliance in health care* (pp. 11–22). Baltimore: Johns Hopkins University Press.

Sanders, G. S. (1982). Social comparison and perceptions of health and illness. In G. S. Sanders & J. Suls (Eds.), *Social psychology of health and illness* (pp. 129–157). Hillsdale, NJ: Lawrence, Erlbaum Associates.

Schiffman, S. S., Reynolds, M. L., & Young, F. W. (1981). *Introduction to multidimensional scaling.* New York: Academic Press.

Schwartz, G. E. (1980, winter). Behavioral medicine and systems theory: A new synthesis. *National Forum,* 25–30.

Shilts, R. (1987). *And the band played on: Politics, people, and the AIDS epidemic.* New York: St. Martin's Press.

Smith, E. E., & Medin, D. L. (1981). *Categories and concepts.* Cambridge, MA: Harvard University Press.

Stone, G. C., Cohen, F., & Adler, N. E. (Eds.) (1979). *Health psychology—A handbook.* San Francisco: Jossey-Bass.

Turk, D. C., Rudy, T. E., & Salovey, P. (1986). Implicit models of illness. *Journal of Behavioral Medicine, 9,* 453–474.

Weiner, B. (1971). *Achievement motivation and attribution theory.* Morristown, NJ: General Learning Press.

Wolinsky, F. D. (1978). Assessing the effects of predisposing, enabling, and illness-morbidity characteristics on health service utilization. *Journal of Health and Social Behavior, 19,* 384–396.

Zola, I. K. (1973). Pathways to the doctor—From person to patient. *Social Science and Medicine, 7,* 677–689.

4
Situational, Dispositional, and Genetic Bases of Symptom Reporting

David Watson and James W. Pennebaker

Self-report health measures are widely used in health psychology research, but they are as yet poorly understood. In this chapter, we argue that physical symptom reporting—in addition to reflecting the respondent's current physiological state—is affected by numerous psychological factors. We summarize extensive evidence demonstrating that phasic situational factors, enduring dispositions of personality and temperament, and genetic determinants all influence symptom reporting. Whereas our earlier work focused on how perceptual and cognitive factors influence the reporting of internal states, more recent research strongly implicates the pervasive personality trait of negative affectivity (NA) as a central determinant in the reporting of physical symptoms, stress, subjective distress, and psychopathology. Further, recent NA research suggests that trait NA—and, by extension, the proclivity to perceive and report symptoms—is highly heritable. After discussing the situational, dispositional, and genetic bases of symptom reporting, we raise several questions about the nature of self-reports in the area of health psychology.

The Prevailing View of Health Complaints: Naive Realism

In recent years there has been an explosion of research examining psychosocial factors that may play an etiological role in death and disease. Hypothesized precursors of organic pathology have included major life changes, chronic stresses and role strains, daily microstressors, depression,

Preparation of this manuscript was funded, in part, by grants HL32547 from the National Institutes of Health and BNS 8606764 from the National Science Foundation.

helplessness, hopelessness, and personality traits such as pessimism, cynicism, (lack of) hardiness, and the Type A behavior pattern (e.g., Friedman & Booth-Kewley, 1987; Holmes & Rahe, 1967; Kobasa, Maddi, & Kahn, 1982; Matthews, 1982; Pearlin, Lieberman, Menaghan, & Mullan, 1981; Shekelle et al., 1981).

An enormous range of health criteria has been used in these studies, from objective biological markers (e.g., physiological levels, immune system functioning, serum risk factors) and medical evidence of dysfunction or pathology (including long-term mortality rates) to criteria that more clearly involve overt psychological factors, such as physician or health-center visits or illness-related absences from work or school (Costa & McCrae, 1985, 1987; Watson & Pennebaker, 1989). However, the most commonly used criteria are self-reports, especially health complaint measures in which subjects indicate the presence, frequency, or intensity of various physical symptoms (e.g., DeLongis, Coyne, Dakof, Folkman, & Lazarus, 1982; Eckenrode, 1984; Rhodewalt & Zone, 1989; Scheier & Carver, 1985).

Some investigators have been interested in the perception and reporting of physical symptoms per se (e.g., Pennebaker, 1982, and the various contributors to this volume). For the most part, however, health complaints have been used as surrogates for hard health criteria (e.g., mortality, objective evidence of pathology) that are more difficult and time-consuming to obtain. This reliance on self-report assessment is readily understandable: Health complaint scales are quick to administer, easy to obtain, simple and objective to score, and generally reliable (see Pennebaker, 1982; Watson & Pennebaker, 1989). The assumptions underlying their use are that physical symptom reports are veridical, that they can be taken more-or-less at face value, and that they therefore provide a valid index of the respondent's current health status. This view—which Costa and McCrae (1985) call *naive realism*—is the prevailing conceptual model of symptom reporting.

The assumptions underlying the naive realism view are not entirely unfounded. In fact, considerable evidence indicates that somatic complaints are significantly related to other types of health measures. Pennebaker (1982), for example, presents data indicating that high scorers on his Pennebaker Inventory of Limbic Languidness (PILL) make more physician and health-center visits, take more aspirin, and have more illness-related work absences than low PILL responders. Other research has demonstrated that physical symptom scales correlate significantly with physicians' health ratings, medical records, and documented health visits (e.g., LaRue, Bank, Jarvik, & Hetland, 1979; Linn & Linn, 1980; Maddox & Douglas, 1973; Meltzer & Hochstim, 1970; Pennebaker, 1982). Furthermore, prospective studies have shown that self-report health measures are significant predictors of mortality from ischemic heart disease and other causes (Kaplan & Camacho, 1983; Kaplan & Kotler, 1985). These findings indicate that physical symptom scales can play a valid and useful role in the study of disease states.

However, although statistically significant, the correlations between symptom reports and other types of health measures are typically low to moderate in magnitude. For example, correlations between self-reported and physician-rated health typically range from .30 to .40 (e.g., Maddox & Douglas 1973; Tessler and Mechanic, 1978). However, coefficients as low as .14 have also been reported (McCrae, Bartone, & Costa, 1976); correlations such as these clearly reflect a very weak level of convergence between these supposedly interchangeable measures.

A related line of evidence that undermines the naive realism view has evolved from work in visceral perception wherein researchers assess the correspondence between perceived and actual physiological activity. Numerous laboratory studies have clearly demonstrated that the ability to perceive accurately normal fluctuations in heart rate, blood pressure, blood glucose, and stomach contraction is extremely limited. Indeed, across experiments employing a variety of paradigms, the mean within-subject correlations between actual and perceived physiological activity range between .15 and .42, averaging around .28 (Cox et al., 1985; Katkin, 1985; Pennebaker & Watson, 1988a; Whitehead & Drescher, 1980).

Overall, then, the accumulated data do not support a strong version of the prevailing naive realism model. That is, the available evidence indicates that self-report scales are not strongly related to other health indicators and that they should not be used as surrogates for these other measures. Rather, it is increasingly clear that symptom reporting reflects several distinct factors, some of which are organically based and obviously health-relevant, whereas others are more subjective and psychological (Costa & McCrae, 1985, 1987; Leventhal, 1975; Mechanic, 1979, 1980; Pennebaker, 1982; Watson & Pennebaker, 1989).

These data are consistent with the theoretical distinction that has been made between *disease* and *illness* (Barondess, 1979; Jennings, 1986). According to Barondess (1979), a disease reflects actual pathologic changes in the body, whereas an illness represents the experienced suffering of the patient. In terms of this model, self-report measures are best viewed as measures of illness that directly assess the subjective experience of the individual. Their relation to actual physical pathology is more indirect and problematic, although they are also likely to contain a significant disease component. In light of this situation, health research needs to adopt a more sophisticated conceptual model that acknowledges the influence of psychological variables on the perception, interpretation, and reporting of physical symptoms.

Situational Factors That Influence Health Complaints

Over the years, Pennebaker and his colleagues have developed a general model of symptom perception that incorporates the influence of several social psychological variables on the perception and reporting of physical symptoms. A detailed examination of this model is beyond the scope of our chapter. Instead, we focus on two aspects that are especially relevant to the present discussion.

Based on the assumption that people can process only a finite amount of information at any given time, Pennebaker (1982) proposed that internal and external stimuli compete for attention. That is, as the number and salience of external cues increase, attention to internal stimuli will necessarily decrease, and vice versa. When the environment lacks meaningful external stimuli (e.g., when subjects are engaged in tedious, repetitive tasks), attention will tend to focus more internally, and symptom reporting will consequently increase. Thus, people should perceive and report more symptoms such as headaches and fatigue in an unstimulating environment than in an interesting one.

Considerable research has supported this competition-of-cues model. For example, studies have demonstrated that subjects report higher levels of fatigue (Pennebaker & Lightner, 1980) and cough more (Pennebaker, 1980) in unstimulating settings. Further, manipulations inducing heightened self-attention (e.g., through the use of a mirror, attending to one's own heart and breathing rate) also increase physical symptom reporting (Duval & Wicklund, 1972; Fillingim & Fine, 1986; Wegner & Giuliano, 1980; see also Mechanic, 1983, 1986).

Another line of research is based on the assumption that organisms actively search their environment for information that will enable them to behave more adaptively (e.g., Gibson, 1979). This scanning is typically not random or unselective but is instead guided by organizational frameworks (beliefs, schema, etc.) that direct the ways in which information is sought and ultimately found. This general principle is also relevant to the formation of health complaints: Subjects' health-related beliefs and schema influence how they attend to—and interpret—bodily sensations (Pennebaker, 1982; Pennebaker & Watson, 1988b).

Pennebaker and Skelton (1981) demonstrated this principle in a series of experiments. In one study, for example, subjects were led to believe that bogus ultrasonic noise caused either vasodilation or vasoconstriction. Consistent with their experimentally induced schema, subjects selectively attended to sensations indicating either an increase (vasodilation) or a decrease (vasoconstriction) in skin temperature. This, in turn, led to corresponding changes in estimated skin temperature—when, in fact, skin temperature was not systematically affected by any external stimuli.

Schemas and selective search also seem to play an important role in cases of mass psychogenic illness (Colligan, Pennebaker, & Murphy, 1982), in which many individuals report a related set of physical symptoms that have no demonstrable organic basis. Mass illness of this sort develops when one person in a setting becomes overtly sick and displays externally observable symptoms such as nausea and fainting. These symptoms affect the belief processes of others in the setting, who consequently experience and report similar physical problems (Colligan et al., 1982; Pennebaker, 1982).

Dispositional Bases of Symptom Reporting:
The Central Role of Negative Affectivity

Recently, investigators have begun to examine the role that personality variables play in the formation of health complaints (Costa & McCrae, 1985, 1987; Watson & Pennebaker, 1989). Most of this research has focused on a mood-based disposition we call "negative affectivity," or trait NA. In our research we have also examined the role of a second, complementary mood disposition, which we call "positive affectivity," or trait PA. Trait NA is more or less synonymous with several other dispositional constructs such as neuroticism, trait anxiety, pessimism (vs. optimism), and general maladjustment. Trait PA, on the other hand, is strongly associated with extraversion (see Tellegen, 1985; Watson & Clark, 1984, in press).

Our research in this area has been guided by extensive data indicating that subjective emotional experience is dominated by two broad and largely independent factors: negative affect (NA) and positive affect (PA) (Diener & Emmons, 1984; Mayer & Gaschke, 1988; Watson, 1988b; Watson, Clark, & Tellegen, 1984, 1988; Watson & Tellegen, 1985). Both factors can be measured either as a state (i.e., short-term mood fluctuations) or as a trait (i.e., consistent and enduring differences in general affective level). It is important to note that both trait NA and trait PA are highly stable over time (e.g., Costa & McCrae, 1988; Watson & Clark, 1984; Watson & Slack, in press). Furthermore, both dispositions have been shown to have a strong genetic basis (e.g., Tellegen et al., 1988), a point we develop later.

Trait NA is a dimension that reflects pervasive individual differences in negative mood and self-concept (Watson & Clark, 1984). High-NA individuals are more likely to experience significant levels of distress and dissatisfaction in any given situation. High-NA subjects are also more introspective, and they differentially dwell on their failures and shortcomings. They tend to be negativistic and to focus on the negative side of themselves, others, and the world in general (a cognitive style that is highly reminiscent of Beck's notion of the depressogenic "negative triad"; see Beck, 1967). Consequently, they have a less favorable self-view and are less satisfied with their lives (see also Watson, 1988a; Watson, Clark, & Carey, 1988).

Trait PA reflects general levels of energy and enthusiasm. High–trait PA individuals lead a full, enjoyable, and interesting life and maintain a generally high activity level (Costa & McCrae, 1980a; Tellegen, 1985; Watson, 1988a). Tellegen (1985) further suggests that trait PA levels may reflect individual differences in sensitivity to pleasurable stimuli—that is, high-PA individuals are able to derive more pleasure and enjoyment from ongoing life experiences. Because of this, high-PA subjects engage in more active, pleasure-seeking behavior (e.g., greater social activity; see also Depue, Krauss, & Spoont, 1987; Watson, 1988a).

Watson and Pennebaker (1989) provide a comprehensive review of the relations among trait NA, trait PA, and symptom reporting. We summarize and extend these findings here, presenting personality and health complaint data collected from four large subject samples. Two of these data sets were included in the Watson and Pennebaker (1989) review: The current student-1 sample ($N = 193$) corresponds to their student-1 group, whereas the adult sample ($N = 212$; M age = 40.7 years) combines their wellness-1, wellness-2, and adult groups (see Watson & Pennebaker, 1989, for more details regarding these data sets). We also include two new samples of undergraduate psychology students (student-2, $N = 245$; student-3, $N = 568$) that have not previously been reported. After examining these data, we discuss possible explanations for the observed relations.

In the adult, student-1, and student-2 samples, trait NA and PA were assessed using the 14-item Negative Emotionality (Nem) and 11-item Positive Emotionality (Pem) scales from the Multidimensional Personality Questionnaire (MPQ; Tellegen, in press), a general true–false personality inventory. The Nem and Pem scales have been extensively validated as measures of trait NA and PA (see Watson, 1988a; Watson, Clark, & Carey, 1988; Watson & Pennebaker, 1989). Both scales are homogeneous and highly stable over time (Watson & Slack, in press; Watson & Pennebaker, 1989).

In the student-3 sample, trait emotionality was assessed using the NA and PA scales from the Positive and Negative Affect Schedule (PANAS; Watson, Clark, & Tellegen, 1988). Each scale consists of 10 items that are good factor markers of either high NA (e.g., *scared, guilty, irritable, distressed*) or high PA (e.g., *excited, enthusiastic, interested, alert*). The PANAS scales have been shown to be highly reliable and valid measures of the underlying NA and PA dimensions (Watson, Clark, & Tellegen, 1988). These scales can be used with various temporal instructions; in this sample we used the trait form, in which subjects rated the extent to which they generally experienced these mood states.

In all four samples, health complaints were assessed using the PILL (Pennebaker, 1982). The PILL consists of 54 physical symptoms and complaints (e.g., racing heart, chest pain, diarrhea); subjects rate how frequently they have experienced each of these problems during the past year. In addition, subjects in the student-1 and student-2 samples completed the SMU Health Questionnaire (SMU-HQ) Symptom Scale (Watson & Pennebaker, 1989). On this scale, subjects check any of 13 commonly reported health complaints (e.g., headaches, cramps) they have experienced during the past year. Finally, the student-1 and student-2 subjects were also assessed using the Somatization Scale of the Hopkins Symptom Checklist (HSCL; Derogatis, Lipman, Rickels, Uhlenhuth, & Covi, 1974). The HSCL Somatization Scale is composed of 12 items describing various physical problems (e.g., trouble getting your breath; faintness or dizziness); subjects rate how intensely they have experienced each of these problems during the preceding week.

Table 4-1. Correlations Between Trait NA, Trait PA, and Health Complaints

| Symptom Measure/Sample | N | Correlations With | |
		Trait NA	Trait PA
PILL			
Adult	211	.42**	−.10
Student-1	192	.42**	−.02
Student-2	245	.40**	−.03
Student-3	568	.43**	−.19**
SMU-HQ Symptom Scale			
Student-1	192	.42**	−.02
Student-2	120	.41**	−.05
HSCL Somatization Scale			
Student-1	190	.40**	−.08
Student-2	120	.53**	−.28**

Note: A subsample of the student-2 group ($N = 120$) completed the SMU-HQ Symptom Scale and the HSCL Somatization Scale. Nem and Pem are the trait NA and trait PA measures, respectively, in the adult, student-1, and student-2 samples. The general form of the PANAS NA and PA scales are the trait NA and trait PA measures, respectively, in the student-3 sample. *$p < .05$ (two−tailed); **$p < .01$ (two−tailed).

Table 4−1 presents correlations between the trait emotionality scales and health complaints in the four data sets. Several aspects of the table are noteworthy. First, consistent with previous research (Watson, 1988a; Watson & Pennebaker, 1989), trait PA scales are largely unrelated to symptom reporting. The PA–health complaint correlations are invariably low, and only two of them reach significance ($r = −.28$ with the HSCL Somatization Scale in the student-2 sample, and $r = −.19$ with the PILL in the student-3 sample). Although now well established, this finding is nevertheless striking, because it indicates that subjects can report leading an active, happy, and interesting life while simultaneously complaining of numerous physical problems.

In contrast, trait NA is moderately correlated with health complaints, with coefficients ranging from .40 to .53. Moreover, health complaint scales correlate about as highly with trait NA as they do with each other. In the student-1 sample, for example, the correlations among the individual health complaint scales range from .41 to .55. These results indicate that there is no clear psychometric distinction between physical and psychological complaining and further suggest that NA and physical symptom measures all tap a common, underlying factor of somatopsychic distress (see also Watson, 1988a; Watson & Pennebaker, 1989). We consider this issue in more detail later.

Furthermore, the NA–health complaint correlations are remarkably consistent across samples and measures. For example, the PILL's correlations with trait NA range only from .40 to .43 across the four data sets. The coefficients are also largely consistent within a given data set: In the student-1 sample, for instance, trait NA correlates .42, .42, and .40 with the PILL, SMU-HQ Symptom Scale, and the HSCL Somatization Scale, respectively. Thus, the NA–symptom relationship is highly robust and is unaffected by the particular population (adult vs. student), trait NA scale (Nem vs. PANAS NA), or health complaint measure that is examined.

This last finding is especially noteworthy when one considers that the symptom scales differ in the number and content of the problems assessed, the time frame involved, and the type of response format used (checklist, frequency or intensity of the problem). This consistency across measures suggests that the association between trait NA and health complaints is quite general and that NA is related to a very broad range of physical symptoms. To test this idea further, we correlated trait NA scores with the individual PILL items in each of the four samples. Of the 54 PILL items, 27 (50%) were significantly correlated ($p < .05$, two-tailed) with trait NA in all four samples. Moreover, an additional 24 PILL items were significantly correlated with trait NA in at least one of the data sets. Thus, only 3 of the 54 PILL items (hemorrhoids, boils, and nonfacial acne) had nonsignificant coefficients in all four samples. These data replicate the results of Costa and McCrae (1980b), who reported that high-NA subjects scored significantly higher on all 12 somatic sections of the Cornell Medical Index (Brodman, Erdmann, & Wolff, 1949). Taken together, these findings clearly indicate that trait NA has a general, nonspecific relationship with physical symptom reporting.

Heritable Bases of Symptom Reporting

Thus far we have presented data indicating that symptom reporting is influenced by various situational cues and also by broad dispositional differences in distress and complaining. Closely allied with this dispositional evidence is the idea that the tendency to report physical symptoms/negative affect is genetically based. The heritability argument reflects common assumptions about the phenotypical bases of physiological functioning and more recent discoveries concerning the inheritance of perceptual and emotional styles.

The awareness and reporting of physical symptoms depend in large part on the way information is processed in different parts of the brain. Lesions in the somatosensory cerebral cortex, for example, fundamentally affect how individuals perceive sensations in their bodies (Luria, 1980). Beyond basic perception, the ability to report symptoms is dependent on the proper functioning of the language centers in the temporal lobes. Furthermore, it is well documented that central nervous system structure and function are, in turn, highly influenced by genetic factors. Monozygotic twins, for example, have remarkably similar (although not identical) cortical structures, neurotransmitter activity, EEG patterns, and autonomic nervous system activation compared with dizygotic twins (see, for example, Lykken, 1982). In short, the corticoneurological hardware that enables us to perceive symptoms and sensations clearly has a heritable basis.

More striking is a series of discoveries pointing to the genetic bases of personality dispositions and their associated cognitive–perceptual–behavioral styles. Of greatest relevance here are the findings of Tellegen and his associates (Tellegen et al., 1988), who recently conducted a large-scale examination of the heritability of trait NA and trait PA. Tellegen et al. investigated over 400 pairs of identical and fraternal twins, reared either together or apart. Trait NA and PA were assessed using higher order factor scales from the MPQ (Tellegen, in press). Overall, an estimated 55% of the variance on trait NA could be attributed to genetic factors, whereas only 2% was due to the shared familial environment. For trait PA, the genetic component was smaller but nevertheless substantial: Specifically, 40% of the variance was estimated to be heritable, compared with 22% attributable to shared family experiences. Several other studies have reported similar findings regarding the heritability of trait NA .and trait PA (e.g., Floderus-Myrhed, Pedersen, & Rasmuson, 1980; Fulker, 1981; Pedersen, Plomin, McClearn, & Friberg, 1988; Rose, Koskenvuo, Kaprio, Sarna, & Langin-vainio, 1988).

Other research has explored the biological substrate of trait NA and trait PA. We focus here on trait NA, which is more directly relevant to our earlier examination of symptom reporting. Gray (1982,1985) has linked trait NA to the operation of the Behavioral Inhibition System (BIS), which he locates in the septal and hippocampal areas of the limbic system. Cloninger (1987a, 1987b) places the BIS similarly and further links it to the serotonergic neurotransmitter system. In the Gray–Cloninger model, the BIS regulates extinction and passive avoidance behavior in response to signals of punishment. Thus, through the operation of the BIS, trait NA may be related to a biologically based sensitivity to conditioned signals of punishment (see Cloninger, 1987a, 1987b; Gray, 1985; Tellegen, 1985).

The cognitive–perceptual organization of physical symptoms and affective states is therefore strongly linked to genetic and biological processes. It is true that psychological factors influence physical symptom reporting, but these same factors themselves ultimately reflect neurogenetic processes. The research relating trait NA and symptom reporting indicates that it is not sufficient to examine how psychological variables influence somatic processes, or vice versa; rather, the data force us to confront the fact that physical and psychological variables are inextricably intertwined.

Integrating the Situational, Dispositional, and Heritability Approaches

Thus far we examined several of the factors underlying symptom reporting and negative affect. However, we have not yet addressed the possible causal links between these variables. Most importantly, why do high-NA individuals report more health problems? As we discussed earlier, in the naive realism view of symptom reporting, health complaints are assumed to be veridical. Therefore, this model presumes that high-NA individuals actually have more health problems than do those low in NA.

The direction of causality underlying this relationship therefore remains the major unresolved theoretical issue in the naive realism view. There are two obvious (and not mutually exclusive) possibilities. One explanation is a variant of the classic *psychosomatic hypothesis:* High trait NA—which is associated with persistently high levels of anxiety, tension, anger, and depression—produces health problems. Psychosomatic models of disease have long played an influential role in health psychology and currently remain an integral part of psychiatric classification (American Psychiatric Association, 1987). At one time or another, chronic negative affect has been causally implicated in a wide array of disorders, including headaches, ulcers, heart disease, arthritis, asthma, and diabetes (Anderson, Bradley, Young, McDaniel, & Wise, 1985; Diamond, 1982; Friedman & Booth-Kewley, 1987; Harrell, 1980).

A second possibility is what we call the *disability hypothesis:* Health problems cause high NA. According to this model, health difficulties can have important personality and emotional sequelae, including the development of higher trait NA. Health problems may be associated with a number of stressful and aversive consequences, including pain and discomfort, physical disability, and an impairment of social and/or occupational functioning. Given these adverse effects, it is easily understandable why health difficulties might produce a general increase in subjective distress and dissatisfaction, and thus higher trait NA.

As has been discussed elsewhere, the existing evidence fails to support both the psychosomatic and the disability models (Costa & McCrae, 1985, 1987; Watson & Pennebaker, 1989). For example, trait NA is not consistently associated with various risk factors for heart disease, such as elevated blood pressure and serum cholesterol; nor is it related to the occurrence of coronary heart disease (Brozek, Keys, & Blackburn, 1966; Costa, Fleg, McCrae, & Lakatta, 1982), myocardial infarction (Ostfeld, Lebovitz, Shekelle, & Paul, 1964), or heart-related mortality (Keehn, Goldberg, & Beebe, 1974; Shekelle et al., 1981).

Similarly, high NA is not consistently associated with either cancer or immune system dysfunction (e.g., Dattore, Shontz, & Coyne, 1980; Kaplan & Reynolds, 1988; Keehn et al., 1974; Kiecolt-Glaser et al., 1984; Kissen,

1964; Kissen & Eysenck, 1962; Levy, Herberman, Maluish, Schlien, & Lippman, 1985; Shekelle et al., 1981; C. G. Watson & Schuld, 1977). More generally, trait NA is unrelated to overall mortality rates (Costa and McCrae, 1987; Kaplan & Reynolds, 1988; Keehn et al., 1974; Shekelle et al., 1981).

In addition, trait NA is generally uncorrelated with various illness-related behavioral measures, such as number of physician and health-center visits, days hospitalized, and days of work or school missed because of illness during the past year (Mechanic, 1980; Tessler, Mechanic, & Dimond, 1976; Watson & Pennebaker, 1989). Finally, trait NA is not significantly associated with indicators of physical fitness and health-related lifestyle (e.g., frequency of smoking; hours of sleep per night; alcohol, caffeine, and aspirin consumption; see Watson & Pennebaker, 1989).

The Symptom Perception Model

The available evidence indicates that trait NA is not clearly or consistently related to objective indicators of risk, dysfunction, or pathology. This does not necessarily mean, however, that trait NA is completely unrelated to actual health status. First, NA scores have not been correlated with every available health measure or every kind of health problem. In particular, most of the reviewed studies have examined major health problems, and so it remains possible that trait NA may be related to minor, low-level dysfunction (as has been suggested by Depue & Monroe, 1986).

Moreover, in some instances the data are inconsistent or unclear rather than entirely negative, suggesting that additional factors may be involved (see Watson & Pennebaker, 1989). Several studies have, in fact, reported significant but low correlations between trait NA and objective health measures. For example, Booth-Kewley and Friedman's (1987) meta-analysis indicated that various types of negative affect were modestly but significantly related to the subsequent development of heart disease (for anxiety, $r = .14$; for depression, $r = .17$; for anger/hostility, $r = .07$; see Booth-Kewley & Friedman, 1987, Table 7).

Nevertheless, the data demonstrate that trait NA is much more strongly and consistently related to health complaints (as in Table 4-1) than it is to objective indicators of health per se. This, in turn, indicates that neither the psychosomatic nor the disability model can fully explain the correlation between NA and physical symptom reporting. Instead, the data support what we call the *symptom perception hypothesis*. Various explanatory models have been proposed, but they all share the basic idea that individuals differ systematically in how they perceive, respond to, and/or complain about body sensations. A strong form of the symptom perception model argues that the association between trait NA and health complaints is completely spurious and simply reflects the fact that high-NA subjects are more likely to attend to or complain about their internal physical sensations. A weaker form of the model posits that high-NA individuals exaggerate or magnify their actual health problems. There are not yet sufficient data to choose between the various forms of this model, but the available research clearly indicates that high-NA individuals overreport physical problems, thus supporting at least a weak form of the symptom perception view.

Why is trait NA associated with symptom magnification? The specific mechanisms involved are as yet unknown, but we can note some promising areas for future research. First, Watson and Clark's (1984) review indicated that high-NA individuals tend to be more introspective and ruminative than those low in trait NA. Similarly, Watson, Clark, and Carey (1988) reported that high trait NA was associated with clinically significant manifestations of obsessive–compulsive symptomatology. Taken together, these findings suggest that high-NA subjects report more physical problems because they are more internally focused and are therefore especially likely to attend to normal body sensations and minor discomforts. In support of this contention, several studies have found that subjects who are generally more introspective and internally focused also report higher levels of somatic complaints (Mechanic, 1983, 1986; Pennebaker, 1982). Moreover, as was discussed earlier, intraindividual analyses indicate that symptom reporting generally increases when subjects are internally focused (e.g., Pennebaker, 1982).

Recent research also suggests that trait NA is related to an unsettled and vigilant cognitive mode in which the individual scans the environment with uncertainty and apprehension (Gray, 1982, 1985; Tellegen, 1985). Gray (1982, 1985) links this vigilant style to the operation of the Behavioral Inhibition System (BIS), which was described earlier. According to Gray, the BIS checks incoming stimuli to see if they match an expected pattern. Furthermore, the BIS identifies certain stimuli as particularly important and requiring especially careful checking. Gray further theorizes that high-NA subjects (whom he calls trait anxious) have an overactive BIS, one that identifies all incoming stimuli as important and as requiring careful inspection. Because of this, high-NA individuals are hypervigilant, constantly scanning their world for signs of impending trouble (Cloninger, 1987a; Pennebaker, 1989).

The hypervigilance of high-NA subjects may affect their health complaints in two ways. First, consistent with our earlier discussion, they may be more likely to notice normal body sensations and minor aches and pains. Second, because their scanning is fraught with anxiety and uncertainty (Tellegen, 1985), high-NA subjects may be more likely to interpret minor symptoms and sensations as painful or pathological (Barsky & Klerman, 1983; Costa & McCrae, 1985). In this regard, it is noteworthy that several studies have found that high-NA individuals are more likely to interpret ambiguous stimuli in a negative or threatening manner (for a review, see Watson & Clark, 1984).

Interestingly, Barsky, Goodson, Lane, and Cleary (1988) similarly argue that hypervigilance, selective attention, and the tendency to view normal somatic sensations as ominous or problematic are all important elements in the amplification of somatic symptoms. Thus the perceptual/attentional style of high-NA individuals—introspective, obsessive, apprehensive, negativistic, and vigilant—may be largely responsible for their enhanced somatic complaining.

Beyond these perceptual/attentional factors, we must again emphasize the intimate connection between psychological and somatic forms of distress. Strong emotional states are inherently characterized not only by their affective, hedonic component, but also by notable physiological symptoms (e.g., Pennebaker, 1982). Indeed, several writers have noted that the subjective and physiological components of emotional distress have been clearly distinguished from one another in thought and language only during the last 200 years (e.g., Kleinman & Kleinman, 1985; Leff, 1977). Leff (1977), for example, has noted that the modern words "anxiety," "anger," and "angina" all ultimately derive from the same Greek root, which means "to press tight"; originally, this group of words was used nonspecifically to refer to the unpleasant chest sensations that accompany many states of strong negative affect. Thus, the strong covariation of negative affect and physical symptoms is not surprising but reflects in part their common origin.

Along these same lines, research has consistently demonstrated strong cultural and class differences in the somatization of emotion. Specifically, individuals in culturally traditional non-Western societies tend to express distress more somatically, and less in purely cognitive/affective terms. Increased somatization of emotion is also reliably observed among poorer, more rural, and less educated individuals in the West (e.g., Kleinman & Kleinman, 1985; Leff, 1977; Mezzich & Raab, 1980; Westermeyer, 1985). These data again illustrate the tenuousness of the split between "somatic" and "psychological" forms of distress. Moreover, because our own data are based on relatively affluent and well-educated Westerners, we should expect to find even stronger connections between NA and symptom reporting in lower class and non-Western samples.

Implications of the Findings

The data we have reviewed have important implications for research in health psychology. As we have seen, the processes that govern the perception and reporting of physical symptoms are influenced by situational, dispositional, and genetic factors. In the following section we consider how and when symptom reports can be used as indicators of physical pathology. We then explore trait NA's role as a general nuisance factor in health research.

Finally, we conclude with some general recommendations concerning efficient health psychology research designs that can best control for unwanted individual differences in trait NA.

The Use of Symptom Scales as Health Criteria

Although somatic complaint scales have low to moderate correlations with objectively assessed health, we have presented extensive evidence demonstrating that symptom reporting is also strongly influenced by various psychological factors that have no direct connection with the individual's actual health status (i.e., the current level of disease or dysfunction). Thus, health complaint scales assess both somatic and psychological sources of variance. Because of this subjective psychological component, use of symptom scales as general surrogate or proxy measures of an individual's current health status is problematic. Self-report and objective health indicators are not interchangeable and in fact can be expected to yield widely discrepant results in many instances (Costa & McCrae, 1985, 1987; Watson & Pennebaker, 1989). Ultimately, as we noted earlier, physical symptom scores are best viewed as measures of subjectively perceived illness rather than objectively defined disease per se.

We are not arguing that physical symptom scales be eliminated as health criteria. These measures are indispensable for many types of health research. They are quick and easy to administer and, moreover, clearly contain a valid somatically based component. Furthermore, because individuals may act on their illness perceptions (whether they are veridical or not), symptom scores are likely to have important implications for various aspects of the health-care system (Bishop & Converse, 1986; Jemmott, Croyle, & Ditto, 1988; Lau & Hartman, 1983). Finally, the individual's subjective experience of pain and discomfort is an interesting and important variable in its own right.

Nevertheless, it is increasingly clear that self-report measures should not be used as the sole criteria in health research. Given the data, we strongly recommend that physical symptom scales be used in conjunction with other health indicators, such as biological markers (immune system functioning, serum risk factors, etc.), outcome variables (objective evidence of pathology, disease incidence and mortality, etc.), and illness-related behaviors (physician visits, absences, etc.). More generally, we advocate a multimodal approach to health status assessment in which a wide range of health indicators are examined. None of these different types of health measures is interchangeable with another; instead, each can be expected to provide unique information that is not readily obtainable through any other modality. Of course, the specific health criteria chosen for any given study will necessarily depend on the underlying variables of interest and the goals of the research.

Trait NA as a Nuisance Factor

The influence of trait NA on symptom reporting has more troubling implications, because it forces a reevaluation of much of the existing research in health psychology. As we have seen, trait NA is more strongly correlated with health complaints than with the respondent's actual health status. Thus, trait NA can be expected to act as a general nuisance factor in health research. We must be skeptical of any study that uses a health complaint scale as its sole criterion for health and that includes, as a psychological predictor, a measure with an NA-related component. The problem, of course, is that significant predictor–criterion correlations may reflect— either partly or completely—individual differences in subjective distress rather than in health per se.

Consider, for example, the frequently reported finding that measures of perceived stress (e.g., major life changes, chronic stresses or strains, daily hassles) correlate significantly with health complaints (e.g., Cohen, Kamarck, & Mermelstein, 1983; DeLongis et al., 1982; Eckenrode, 1984; Rhodewalt & Zone, 1989). Such results are usually taken to indicate that elevated stress levels cause illness and other health problems. This interpretation is complicated, however, by the fact that perceived stress measures have been found to have a substantial subjective distress component and therefore to correlate significantly with NA scales (e.g., Dohrenwend & Shrout, 1985; Schroeder & Costa, 1984; Watson, 1988a; Watson & Pennebaker, 1989). It thus seems likely that stress–symptom correlations partly or largely reflect their overlapping NA component.

We examined this issue by assessing perceived stress levels in several of our samples. Subjects in the student-1, student-2, and student-3 samples completed the Hassles Scale (Kanner, Coyne, Schaefer, & Lazarus, 1981), which assesses both chronic concerns (financial problems, unsatisfactory relationships, etc.) and minor irritants (e.g., traffic, the weather). Subjects check any hassles that have occurred during the past month and then rate the severity of each problem on a three-point scale. We summed these responses to yield an overall stress score. Subjects in the student-1 and student-2 samples completed the original 117-item form of the Hassles Scale, whereas the student-3 subjects completed a revised 55-item version (DeLongis, Folkman, & Lazarus, 1988).

A subset of the student-2 sample was also assessed on the Perceived Stress Scale (PSS; Cohen et al., 1983), a 14-item scale that measures the extent to which individuals appraise current situations in their lives as stressful. Subjects rate, on a five-point scale, how often they have experienced various thoughts and feelings (e.g., feeling upset, stressed) during the past month.

Consistent with previous research, these stress measures were substantially related to trait NA. The Hassles Scale was significantly correlated with trait NA in all three samples (for student-1, $r = .45$; for student-2, $r = .47$; for student-3, $r = .39$); the PSS had a corresponding

Table 4-2. Simple and Partial Correlations (Controlling for Trait NA) Between Perceived Stress and Health Complaints

Sample/Measure	Hassles Scale		Perceived Stress Scale	
	Simple	Partial	Simple	Partial
Student-1				
PILL	.32**	.16*	—	—
SMU-HQ	.31**	.12	—	—
HSCL Somatization	.42**	.28**	—	—
Student-2				
PILL	.29**	.09	.40**	.13
SMU-HQ	.33**	.16	.35**	.09
HSCL Somatization	.38**	.18	.56**	.32**
Student-3				
PILL	.41**	.30**	—	—

Note: N's are 164 (student-1), 117 (student-2), and 564 (student-3). Trait NA is assessed using the Nem scale in the student-1 and student-2 samples, and using the general form of the PANAS NA scale in the student-3 sample. See text for more details.
*$p<.05$ (two-tailed); **$p<.01$ (two-tailed).

correlation of .67 in the student-2 data. And, as expected, perceived stress and symptom reporting were also consistently related. Table 4–2 presents these correlations, which range from .29 to .56, with a median coefficient of .39. This general pattern of relationships suggests that trait NA is common to (and likely accounts for much of the observed correlation between) perceived stress and health complaints.

To test this possibility, we computed partial correlations between stress and symptoms that removed the influence of trait NA. As can be seen in Table 4-2, partialling out trait NA substantially reduces the magnitude of the association between stress and health complaints. The partial coefficients range from .09 to .32, with a median value of .16; moreover, only 4 of the 10 correlations are now significant. These results clearly demonstrate that trait NA is largely responsible for the observed correlations between perceived stress and health complaints. Furthermore, these findings suggest that stress–symptom correlations are subject to the same interpretive problems we observed in connection with trait NA.

To examine this issue further, we performed a principal components analysis on the emotionality (Nem and Pem), mood (state versions of the PANAS scales in which subjects rated how they had felt during the past week), perceived stress (PSS and Hassles), and health complaint measures (PILL, SMU-HQ Symptom Scale, HSCL Somatization Scale) in a subset of the student-2 sample for whom complete data were available ($n = 115$). We

Table 4-3. Varimax-Rotated Factor Loadings of the Personality, Mood, Stress, and Health Measures in the Student-2 Subsample

Measure	Varimax Loading on		
	Factor 1	Factor 2	Factor 3
Nem	**.78**	−.21	−.01
HSCL Somatization	**.77**	−.15	.18
PILL	**.75**	.09	.24
PSS	**.74**	−.40	.02
Hassles	**.74**	−.01	−.03
PANAS NA	**.65**	−.41	.00
SMU-HQ Symptom	**.64**	.06	.36
Pem	−.16	**.84**	.04
PANAS PA	−.05	**.79**	−.27
Health-related absences	.09	−.16	**.77**
Illness visits	.10	−.02	**.76**

Note: $N = 115$. The highest loading for each variable is shown in boldface.

also included two behavioral health measures (physician visits for illness, illness-caused absences during the past year) in this analysis.

Three large dimensions emerged, together accounting for 63.5% of the total variance. These were then rotated using Varimax. The rotated factor loadings are shown in Table 4-3. The first factor is a large, NA-based dimension, which again indicates that the NA, stress, and symptom measures all tap a common underlying construct. It is also noteworthy that the loadings on this dimension do not show any obvious or clear separation among the various types of measures. This pattern suggests that the conceptual/semantic distinctions that are customarily made in health research (i.e., emotional distress vs. stress vs. physical symptoms) are somewhat arbitrary and inadequate. Rather, it appears that there is a single pervasive trait of subjective distress that is nonspecifically expressed through diverse modalities, including negative affective states, perceived stressors, and somatic complaints.

As expected, the PA scales essentially define a separate factor, although the PSS and PANAS NA scales also have significant secondary (negative) loadings on this dimension; these results again demonstrate that the positive emotions are largely independent of negative affect, stress, and health complaints (see also Watson, 1988a; Watson & Pennebaker, 1989). Finally, the behavioral measures comprise an independent third dimension, indicating that the general distress factor defined by the NA, stress, and symptom scales was essentially unrelated to illness-related visits and absences.

Although the sample size in this analysis is relatively small, the findings in Table 4-3 closely replicate those reported by Watson and Pennebaker (1989) using similar measures and a somewhat larger number of subjects ($n = 164$). Given these results, it seems likely that perceived stress scales show an overall pattern similar to that seen with trait NA; that is, such scales are probably much more highly correlated with health complaints than with health per se. Self-report stress measures may well prove to be significantly correlated with objectively defined disease status, but physical symptom scales probably overestimate this relationship to a considerable extent.

Between-Subjects Versus Within-Subject Designs in Health Psychology

A final issue concerns the research designs that health psychologists employ. Many health investigators continue to use strict between-subjects designs, wherein large numbers of respondents are assessed on a single occasion. Because they are based solely on interindividual variability, such designs allow individual differences variables such as trait NA to confound the results, thus producing data that may be virtually uninterpretable.

Given that trait NA invariably influences overall levels of health complaints, perceived stress, and many other variables, health researchers would be wise to make more use of within-subjects designs that focus on *changes* in symptom reporting over time and across different situations. People typically visit physicians, for example, when they note a significant increase or other change in physical symptoms. Medication use, restriction of daily activities, and other self-initiated health behaviors are similarly based on perceived changes in body state (e.g., Bishop & Converse, 1986; Lau & Hartman, 1983).

This may help to explain one of the remaining puzzles in our data, namely, why trait NA is unrelated to illness visits. Because trait NA is virtually synonymous with subjective distress, our data are superficially inconsistent with the sizable literature showing that highly distressed individuals make more extensive use of medical facilities and that a surprisingly high percentage of patient visits to primary care physicians are for psychological rather than physical reasons (e.g., Katon, 1984; Katon, Ries, & Kleinman, 1984; Locke & Gardner, 1969; Regier, Goldberg, & Taube, 1978). However, trait NA is related to *chronic, stable individual differences* in symptom level; and, as noted, illness-related behaviors are likely to be more affected by perceived changes in symptoms than by the absolute level of symptomatology per se.

The problem of self-reports and dispositions is nicely illustrated by two female undergraduates who assisted in our research. In the year that they worked for us, one student always reported aches, pains, fatigue, and assorted symptoms, whereas the other never noted any symptoms or sensations. During the year, both women had a single illness episode (associated with high fever and vomiting) for which they visited a physician. During this illness, both students reported symptoms that were far above their baseline level of complaining. Interestingly, however, several months after the illness episode the students had each returned to their preillness symptom reporting rates.

The point of this story is to demonstrate that symptom reports can be useful. Indeed, they can be predictive of both internal physiological activity and behavior change. We again emphasize, however, that symptom reports will prove most valuable when viewed from the context of within-subject designs, wherein researchers can detect symptom change rather than simply symptom level. Having said this, we should also note that between- and within-subjects designs are in no way incompatible or mutually exclusive of one another; in fact, combining the two in a single study can produce heuristically powerful results (e.g., Epstein, 1983; Watson, 1988a) in which both intraindividual symptom change and interindividual symptom levels can be examined. The point we wish to stress is that failing to consider the central role of trait NA in between-subjects research will produce studies that add little to our understanding of health.

Acknowledgments. We wish to thank Marilyn Barr, director of the SMU Wellness Program, for her assistance in collecting the data reported in this chapter. Thanks also to Lee Anna Clark for her helpful comments on an earlier version of the manuscript.

References

American Psychiatric Association. (1987). *Diagnostic and statistical manual of mental disorders* (3rd ed., rev.). Washington, DC: Author.

Anderson, K. O., Bradley, L. A., Young, L. D., McDaniel, L. K., & Wise, C. M. (1985). Rheumatoid arthritis: Review of psychological factors related to etiology, effects, and treatment. *Psychological Bulletin, 98,* 358–387.

Barondess, J. A. (1979). Disease and illness: A crucial distinction. *American Journal of Medicine, 66,* 375–376.

Barsky, A. J., Goodson, J. D., Lane, R. S., & Cleary, P. D. (1988). The amplification of somatic symptoms. *Psychosomatic Medicine, 50,* 510–519.

Barsky, A. J., & Klerman, G. L. (1983). Overview: Hypochondriasis, bodily complaints, and somatic styles. *American Journal of Psychiatry, 140,* 273–283.

Beck, A. T. (1967). *Depression: Clinical, experimental, and theoretical aspects.* New York: Harper & Row.

Bishop, G. D., & Converse, S. A. (1986). Illness representations: A prototype approach. *Health Psychology, 5,* 95–114.

Booth-Kewley, S., & Friedman, H. S. (1987). Psychological predictors of heart disease: A quantitative review. *Psychological Bulletin, 101,* 343–362.

Brodman, K., Erdmann, A. J., & Wolff, H. G. (1949). *Cornell Medical Index: Health Questionnaire.* New York: Cornell University Medical College.

Brozek, J., Keys, A., & Blackburn, H. (1966). Personality differences between potential coronary and non-coronary subjects. *Annals of the New York Academy of Sciences, 134,* 1057–1064.

Cloninger, C. R. (1987a). Neurogenetic adaptive mechanisms in alcoholism. *Science*, *236*, 410–416.

Cloninger, C. R. (1987b). A systematic method for clinical description and classification of personality variants. *Archives of General Psychiatry*, *44*, 573–588.

Cohen, S., Kamarck, T., & Mermelstein, R. (1983). A global measure of perceived stress. *Journal of Health and Social Behavior*, *24*, 385–396.

Colligan, M. J., Pennebaker, J. W., & Murphy, L. (Eds.). (1982). *Mass psychogenic illness: A social psychological analysis*. Hillsdale, NJ: Lawrence Erlbaum Associates.

Costa, P. T., Jr., Fleg, J. L., McCrae, R. R., & Lakatta, E. G. (1982). Neuroticism, coronary heart disease, and chest pain complaints: Cross-sectional and longitudinal studies. *Experimental Aging Research*, *8*, 37–44.

Costa, P. T., Jr., & McCrae, R. R. (1980a). Influence of extraversion and neuroticism on subjective well-being: Happy and unhappy people. *Journal of Personality and Social Psychology*, *38*, 668–678.

Costa, P. T., Jr., & McCrae, R. R. (1980b). Somatic complaints in males as a function of age and neuroticism: A longitudinal analysis. *Journal of Behavioral Medicine*, *3*, 245–257.

Costa, P. T., Jr., & McCrae, R. R. (1985). Hypochondriasis, neuroticism, and aging: When are somatic complaints unfounded? *American Psychologist*, *40*, 19–28.

Costa, P. T., Jr., & McCrae, R. R. (1987). Neuroticism, somatic complaints, and disease: Is the bark worse than the bite? *Journal of Personality*, *55*, 299–316.

Costa, P. T., Jr., & McCrae, R. R. (1988). Personality and adulthood: A six-year longitudinal study of self-reports and spouse ratings on the NEO Personality Inventory. *Journal of Personality and Social Psychology*, *54*, 853–863.

Cox, D. J., Clarke, W. L., Gonder-Frederick, L. A., Pohl, S., Hoover, C. W., Snyder, A., Zimbelman, L., Carter, W. R., Bobbitt, S., & Pennebaker, J. W. (1985). Accuracy of perceiving blood glucose in IDDM. *Diabetes Care*, *8*, 529–535.

Dattore, P. J., Shontz, F. C., & Coyne, L. (1980). Premorbid personality differentiation of cancer and noncancer groups: A test of the hypothesis of cancer proneness. *Journal of Consulting and Clinical Psychology*, *48*, 388–394.

DeLongis, A., Coyne, J. C., Dakof, G., Folkman, S., & Lazarus, R. S. (1982). Relationship of daily hassles, uplifts, and major life events to health status. *Health Psychology*, *1*, 119–136.

DeLongis, A., Folkman, S., & Lazarus, R. S. (1988). The impact of daily stress on health and mood: Psychological and social resources as mediators. *Journal of Personality and Social Psychology*, *54*, 486–495.

Depue, R. A., Krauss, S. P., & Spoont, M. R. (1987). A two-dimensional threshold model of seasonal bipolar affective disorder. In D. Magnusson & A. Öhman (Eds.), *Psychopathology: An interactional perspective* (pp. 95–123). Orlando, FL: Academic Press.

Depue, R. A., & Monroe, S. M. (1986). Conceptualization and measurement of human disorder in life stress research: The problem of chronic disturbance. *Psychological Bulletin*, *99*, 36–51.

Derogatis, L. R., Lipman, R. S., Rickels, K., Uhlenhuth, E. H., & Covi, L. (1974). The Hopkins Symptom Checklist (HSCL): A self-report symptom inventory. *Behavioral Science*, *19*, 1–15.

Diamond, E. L. (1982). The role of anger and hostility in essential hypertension and coronary heart disease. *Psychological Bulletin*, *92*, 410–433.

Diener, E., & Emmons, R. A. (1984). The independence of positive and negative affect. *Journal of Personality and Social Psychology, 47,* 1105–1117.

Dohrenwend, B. P., & Shrout, P. E. (1985). "Hassles" in the conceptualization and measurement of life stress variables. *American Psychologist, 40,* 780–785.

Duval, S., & Wicklund, R. A. (1972). *A theory of objective self-awareness.* New York: Academic Press.

Eckenrode, J. (1984). Impact of chronic and acute stressors on daily reports of mood. *Journal of Personality and Social Psychology, 46,* 907–918.

Epstein, S. (1983). A research paradigm for the study of personality and emotions. In M. M. Page (Ed.), *Personality—Current theory and research: 1982 Nebraska Symposium on Motivation* (pp. 91–154). Lincoln: University of Nebraska Press.

Fillingim, R. B., & Fine, M. A. (1986). The effects of internal versus external information processing on symptom perception in an exercise setting. *Health Psychology, 5,* 115–123.

Floderus-Myrhed, B., Pedersen, N., & Rasmuson, I. (1980). Assessment of heritability for personality based on a short-form of the Eysenck Personality Inventory: A study of 12,898 twin pairs. *Behavior Genetics, 10,* 153–161.

Friedman, H. S., & Booth-Kewley, S. (1987). The "disease-prone personality": A meta-analytic view of the construct. *American Psychologist, 42,* 539–555.

Fulker, D. W. (1981). The genetic and environmental architecture of psychoticism, extraversion, and neuroticism. In H. J. Eysenck (Ed.), *A model for personality* (pp. 88–122). New York: Springer-Verlag.

Gibson, J. J. (1979). *The ecological approach to visual perception.* Boston: Houghton Mifflin.

Gray, J. A. (1982). *The neuropsychology of anxiety: An enquiry into the functions of the septo-hippocampal system.* New York: Oxford University Press.

Gray, J. A. (1985). Issues in the neuropsychology of anxiety. In A. H. Tuma & J. D. Maser (Eds.), *Anxiety and the anxiety disorders* (pp. 5–25). Hillsdale, NJ: Lawrence Erlbaum Associates.

Harrell, J. P. (1980). Psychological factors and hypertension: A status report. *Psychological Bulletin, 87,* 482–501.

Holmes, T. H., & Rahe, R. H. (1967). The Social Readjustment Rating Scale. *Journal of Psychosomatic Research, 11,* 213–218.

Jemmott, J. B., III, Croyle, R. T., & Ditto, P. H. (1988). Commonsense epidemiology: Self-based judgments from laypersons and physicians. *Health Psychology, 7,* 55–73.

Jennings, D. (1986). The confusion between disease and illness in clinical medicine. *Canadian Medical Association Journal, 135,* 865–870.

Kanner, A. D., Coyne, J. C., Schaefer, C., & Lazarus, R. S. (1981). Comparison of two modes of life stress measurement: Daily hassles and uplifts versus major life events. *Journal of Behavioral Medicine, 1,* 1–39.

Kaplan, G. A., & Camacho, T. (1983). Perceived health and mortality: A nine-year follow-up of the Human Population Laboratory cohort. *American Journal of Epidemiology, 117,* 292–304.

Kaplan, G. A., & Kotler, P. L. (1985). Self-reports predictive of mortality from ischemic heart disease: A nine-year follow-up of the Human Population Laboratory cohort. *Journal of Chronic Diseases, 38,* 195–201.

Kaplan, G. A., & Reynolds, P. (1988). Depression and cancer mortality and morbidity: Prospective evidence from the Alameda County Study. *Journal of Behavioral Medicine, 11,* 1–13.

Katkin, E. S. (1985). Blood, sweat, and tears: Individual differences in autonomic self-perception. *Psychophysiology, 22,* 125–137.

Katon, W. (1984). Depression: Relationship to somatization and chronic medical illness. *Journal of Clinical Psychiatry, 45,* 4–12.

Katon, W., Ries, R., & Kleinman, A. (1984). The prevalance of somatization in primary care. *Comprehensive Psychiatry, 25,* 208–215.

Keehn, R. J., Goldberg, I. D., & Beebe, G. W. (1974). Twenty-four year mortality follow-up of army veterans with disability separations for psychoneurosis in 1944. *Psychosomatic Medicine, 36,* 27–46.

Kiecolt-Glaser, J. K., Ricker, D., George, J., Messick, G., Speicher, C. E., Garner, W., & Glaser, R. (1984). Urinary cortisol levels, cellular immunocompetency, and loneliness in psychiatric inpatients. *Psychosomatic Medicine, 46,* 15–23.

Kissen, D. M. (1964). Relationship between lung cancer, cigarette smoking, inhalation, and personality. *British Journal of Medical Psychology, 37,* 203–216.

Kissen, D. M., & Eysenck, H. J. (1962). Personality in male lung cancer patients. *Journal of Psychosomatic Research, 6,* 123–127.

Kleinman, A., & Kleinman, J. (1985). Somatization: The interconnections in Chinese society among culture, depressive experiences, and the meanings of pain. In A. Kleinman & B. Good (Eds.), *Culture and depression: Studies in the anthropology and cross-cultural psychiatry of affect and disorder* (pp. 429–490). Berkeley: University of California Press.

Kobasa, S. C., Maddi, S. R., & Kahn, S. (1982). Hardiness and health: A prospective study. *Journal of Personality and Social Psychology, 42,* 168–177.

LaRue, A., Bank, L., Jarvik, L., & Hetland, M. (1979). Health in old age: How do physicians' ratings and self-ratings compare? *Journal of Gerontology, 34,* 687–691.

Lau, R. R., & Hartman, K. A. (1983). Common sense representations of common illnesses. *Health Psychology, 2,* 167–185.

Leff, J. (1977). The cross-cultural study of emotions. *Culture, Medicine, and Psychiatry, 1,* 317–350.

Leventhal, H. (1975). The consequences of depersonalization during illness and treatment. In J. Howard & A. Strauss (Eds.), *Humanizing health care* (pp. 119–161). New York: Wiley.

Levy, S. M., Herberman, R. B., Maluish, A. M., Schlien, B., & Lippman, M. (1985). Prognostic risk assessment in primary breast cancer by behavioral and immunological parameters. *Health Psychology, 4,* 99–113.

Linn, B. S., & Linn, M. W. (1980). Objective and self-assessed health in the old and very old. *Social Science and Medicine, 14,* 311-315.

Locke, B. Z., & Gardner, E. A. (1969). Psychiatric disorders among the patients of general practitioners and internists. *Public Health Reports, 84,* 167–173.

Luria, A. R. (1980). *Higher cortical functions in man.* New York: Basic Books.

Lykken, D. T. (1982). Research with twins: The concept of emergenesis. *Psychophysiology, 19,* 361–373.

Maddox, G. L., & Douglas, E. B. (1973). Self-assessment of health: A longitudinal study of elderly subjects. *Journal of Health and Social Behavior, 14,* 87–93.

Matthews, K. A. (1982). Psychological perspectives on the Type A behavior pattern. *Psychological Bulletin, 91,* 293–323.

Mayer, J. D., & Gaschke, Y. N. (1988). The experience and meta-experience of mood. *Journal of Personality and Social Psychology, 55,* 102–111.

McCrae, R. R., Bartone, P. T., & Costa, P. T., Jr. (1976). Age, anxiety, and self-reported health. *Aging and Human Development, 7,* 49–58.

Mechanic, D. (1979). Correlates of physician utilization: Why do major multivariate studies of physician utilization find trivial psychosocial and organizational effects? *Journal of Health and Social Behavior, 20,* 387–396.

Mechanic, D. (1980). The experience and reporting of common physical complaints. *Journal of Health and Social Behavior, 21,* 146–155.

Mechanic, D. (1983). Adolescent health and illness behaviour: Hypotheses for the study of distress in youth. *Journal of Human Stress, 9,* 4–13.

Mechanic, D. (1986). The concept of illness behaviour: Culture, situation and personal predisposition [Editorial]. *Psychological Medicine, 16,* 1–7.

Meltzer, J., & Hochstim, J. (1970). Reliability and validity of survey data on physical health. *Public Health Reports, 85,* 1075–1086.

Mezzich, J., & Raab, E. (1980). Depressive symptomatology across the Americas. *Archives of General Psychiatry, 37,* 818–823.

Ostfeld, A. M., Lebovitz, B. Z., Shekelle, R. B., & Paul, O. (1964). A prospective study of the relationship between personality and coronary heart disease. *Journal of Chronic Diseases, 17,* 265–276.

Pearlin, L. I., Lieberman, M. A., Menaghan, E. G., & Mullan, J. T. (1981). The stress process. *Journal of Health and Social Behavior, 22,* 337–356.

Pedersen, N. L., Plomin, R., McClearn, G. E., & Friberg, L. (1988). Neuroticism, extraversion, and related traits in adult twins reared apart and reared together. *Journal of Personality and Social Psychology, 55,* 950–957.

Pennebaker, J. W. (1980). Perceptual and environmental determinants of coughing. *Basic and Applied Social Psychology, 1,* 83–91.

Pennebaker, J. W. (1982). *The psychology of physical symptoms.* New York: Springer-Verlag.

Pennebaker, J. W. (1989). Confession, inhibition, and disease. In L. Berkowitz (Ed.), *Advances in experimental social psychology* (Vol. 22, pp. 211–244). Orlando, FL: Academic Press.

Pennebaker, J. W., & Lightner, J. M. (1980). Competition of internal and external information in an exercise setting. *Journal of Personality and Social Psychology, 39,* 165–174.

Pennebaker, J. W., & Skelton, J. A. (1981). Selective monitoring of bodily sensations. *Journal of Personality and Social Psychology, 41,* 213–223.

Pennebaker, J. W., & Watson, D. (1988a). Blood pressure estimation and beliefs among normotensives and hypertensives. *Health Psychology, 7,* 309–328.

Pennebaker, J. W., & Watson, D. (1988b). Self-reports and physiological measures in the workplace. In J. J. Hurrell, Jr., L. R. Murphy, S. L. Sauter, & C. L. Cooper (Eds.), *Occupational stress: Issues and developments in research* (pp. 184–199). New York: Taylor & Francis.

Regier, D., Goldberg, I. D., & Taube, C. H. (1978). The de facto U. S. mental health service system. *Archives of General Psychiatry, 35,* 685–693.

Rhodewalt, F., & Zone, J. B. (1989). Appraisal of life change, depression, and illness in hardy and nonhardy women. *Journal of Personality and Social Psychology, 56,* 81–88.

Rose, R. J., Koskenvuo, M., Kaprio, J., Sarna, S., & Langinvainio, H. (1988). Shared genes, shared experiences, and similarity of personality: Data from 14,288 adult Finnish co-twins. *Journal of Personality and Social Psychology, 54,* 161–171.

Scheier, M. F., & Carver, C. S. (1985). Optimism, coping, and health: Assessment and implications of generalized outcome expectancies. *Health Psychology, 4,* 219–247.

Schroeder, D. H., & Costa, P. T., Jr. (1984). Influence of life event stress on physical illness: Substantive effects or methodological flaws? *Journal of Personality and Social Psychology, 46,* 853–863.

Shekelle, R. B., Raynor, W. J., Jr., Ostfeld, A. M., Garron, D. C., Bieliauskas, L. A., Liu, S. C., Maliza, C., & Paul, O. (1981). Psychological depression and 17-year risk of death from cancer. *Psychosomatic Medicine, 43,* 117–125.

Tellegen, A. (1985). Structures of mood and personality and their relevance to assessing anxiety, with an emphasis on self-report. In A. H. Tuma & J. D. Maser (Eds.), *Anxiety and the anxiety disorders* (pp. 681–706). Hillsdale, NJ: Lawrence Erlbaum Associates.

Tellegen, A. (in press). *Multidimensional Personality Questionnaire.* Minneapolis: University of Minnesota Press.

Tellegen, A., Lykken, D. T., Bouchard, T. J., Jr., Wilcox, K. J., Segal, N. L., & Rich, S. (1988). Personality similarity in twins reared apart and together. *Journal of Personality and Social Psychology, 54,* 1031–1039.

Tessler, R., & Mechanic, D. (1978). Psychological distress and perceived health status. *Journal of Health and Social Behavior, 19,* 254–262.

Tessler, R., Mechanic, D., & Dimond, M. (1976). The effect of psychological distress on physician utilization: A prospective study. *Journal of Health and Social Behavior, 17,* 353–364.

Watson, C. G., & Schuld, D. (1977). Psychosomatic factors in the etiology of neoplasms. *Journal of Consulting and Clinical Psychology, 45,* 455–461.

Watson, D. (1988a). Intraindividual and interindividual analyses of positive and negative affect: Their relation to health complaints, perceived stress, and daily activities. *Journal of Personality and Social Psychology, 54,* 1020–1030.

Watson, D. (1988b). The vicissitudes of mood measurement: Effects of varying descriptors, time frames, and response formats on measures of positive and negative affect. *Journal of Personality and Social Psychology, 55,* 128–141.

Watson, D., & Clark, L. A. (1984). Negative affectivity: The disposition to experience aversive emotional states. *Psychological Bulletin, 96,* 465–490.

Watson, D., & Clark, L. A. (in press). Extraversion and its positive emotional core. In S. Briggs, R. Hogan, & W. Jones (Eds.), *Handbook of personality psychology.* Orlando, FL: Academic Press.

Watson, D., Clark, L. A., & Carey, G. (1988). Positive and negative affectivity and their relation to anxiety and depressive disorders. *Journal of Abnormal Psychology, 97,* 346–353.

Watson, D., Clark, L. A., & Tellegen, A. (1984). Cross-cultural convergence in the structure of mood: A Japanese replication and a comparison with U. S. findings. *Journal of Personality and Social Psychology, 47,* 127–144.

Watson, D., Clark, L. A., & Tellegen, A. (1988). Development and validation of brief measures of positive and negative affect: The PANAS Scales. *Journal of Personality and Social Psychology, 54,* 1063–1070.

Watson, D., & Slack, A. K. (in press). General factors of affective temperament and their relation to job satisfaction over time. *Organizational Behavior and Human Decision Processes.*

Watson, D., & Pennebaker, J. W. (1989). Health complaints, stress, and distress: Exploring the central role of negative affectivity. *Psychological Review, 96,* 234–254.

Watson, D., & Tellegen, A. (1985). Toward a consensual structure of mood. *Psychological Bulletin, 98,* 219–235.

Wegner, D. M., & Giuliano, T. (1980). Arousal-induced attention to self. *Journal of Personality and Social Psychology, 38,* 719–726.

Westermeyer, J. (1985). Psychiatric diagnosis across cultural boundaries. *American Journal of Psychiatry, 142,* 798–805.

Whitehead, W. E., & Drescher, V. M. (1980). Perception of gastric contractions and self-control of gastric motility. *Psychophysiology, 17,* 552–558.

5
Psychological Reactions to Risk Factor Testing

Robert T. Croyle and John B. Jemmott III

How do individuals react when told they have a risk factor for a disease? This is the central question addressed in this chapter. "Risk factor" is defined broadly as any event or characteristic associated with increased probability of disease. Risk factors that have been associated with increased risk of disease include specific health behaviors, genetic factors, radiation exposure, age, and ethnic group. Risk factor testing involves the measurement of one or more physical signs that indicate an individual's heightened risk relative to individuals who do not show the same sign. Two common examples are blood pressure and cholesterol tests. Each year thousands of individuals are tested for these and other risk factors. A major effort is under way within preventive medicine to develop additional screening procedures for risk factors and early signs of disease. But despite the proliferation of risk factor testing, we know surprisingly little about the psychological impact of these tests.

Psychological reactions to risk factor information are important to understand for a number of reasons. From a public health perspective, reactions play a critical role in the effectiveness of modern disease prevention activities. In one sense, population-based screening programs are psychological interventions, for they are intended to reduce disease incidence by informing and influencing at-risk members of the population. Although physician-based and community-based risk factor testing serves to identify persons who need treatment, the utilization of this treatment depends on psychological factors. In addition, the psychological impact of risk factor testing may have effects beyond those relating to health status. In the sections that follow, we first review research on the impact of risk factor testing in public health settings and note its limitations. We then discuss our own work in this area and attempt to illustrate the utility of controlled experimental research for addressing these complex questions. The experiments we describe have examined in some detail the determinants of cognitive appraisals that occur immediately following a risk factor test. We close the chapter by integrating the basic research with the applied and by providing some suggestions for future research.

Previous Research on Risk Factor Testing

Most of the research literature concerning risk factor testing comes from evaluations of high blood pressure screening programs. Although reactions to a variety of other risk factor tests have been studied, the blood pressure literature is the most frequently discussed and debated within the public health research community, for reasons that will be clear shortly. After discussing the blood pressure screening research, we briefly describe other domains of study. AIDS-related testing is addressed at the end of the chapter.

High Blood Pressure Screening

In 1973, the National Heart, Lung, and Blood Institute launched the High Blood Pressure Education Program. This program, which continues to date, is a nationwide effort to promote the detection, treatment, and control of hypertension. The program was initiated because of the wide consensus among the medical community that hypertension is an important, modifiable risk factor for cardiovascular disease. Once studies of the impact of screening programs on participants began to appear, however, a variety of concerns were raised about the possible deleterious effects of testing.

The study that generated the most concern was reported in an article published in the *New England Journal of Medicine* in 1978. Haynes, Sackett, Taylor, Gibson, and Johnson (1978) studied 208 employees of a Canadian steel company who participated in a blood pressure screening program. The investigators found that illness-related absenteeism trebled from the previous year among newly identified hypertensives. This significant increase occurred whether or not the employees had begun a medication regimen (see also Johnson et al., 1984). These results were consistent with findings from the National Health and Nutrition Examination Survey. In that study, individuals with prior knowledge of their hypertensive status provided poorer self-appraisals of their physical and mental health (Monk, 1981). Again, this difference did not depend on the treatment status of the subject. In explaining their data, Haynes et al. borrowed the terminology of medical sociology, suggesting that "the labeling of a person as hypertensive is deleterious, causing many patients to adopt the 'sick role' and treat themselves as more 'fragile' (p. 743).

The impact of the Haynes et al. study was felt at two levels. On the policy level, it led many public health experts to question the merit of community-based screening programs. At the research level, it stimulated a number of investigators to study further the phenomenon of "hypertension labeling." Presentations at a symposium on the topic held at McMaster University in 1979 confirmed the potential for adverse effects (Sackett, 1981). A follow-up study of the steelworkers, for example, found that labeling led to decreased marital adjustment (Mossey, 1981). As other reports entered the literature, however, it soon became clear that the labeling phenomenon was both complex and elusive. Although hypertension labeling was found to produce decreases in subjective well-being (Bloom & Monterossa, 1981; Milne, Logan, & Flanagan, 1985), psychiatric morbidity was not increased (Mann, 1984), and the absenteeism observed in earlier studies seemed limited to younger subjects (Charlson, Alderman, & Melcher, 1982).

Other Studies of Labeling

Evidence concerning the effects of labeling is not limited to hypertension. Some of the earliest insights into the problem come from studies of children with detected heart murmurs. This population is of interest because most heart murmurs in children are classified as insignificant if subjected to a thorough follow-up. Over 20 years ago, Bergman and Stamm (1967) found that many children who had been mislabeled as having a cardiac disorder because of a murmur encountered parental restrictions and hypervigilance. The investigators concluded that "the amount of disability from cardiac nondisease in children is estimated to be greater than that due to actual heart disease" (p. 1083). Cayler, Lynn, and Stein (1973) found that the effects of "cardiac nondisease" impaired the intellectual development of labeled children.

Adverse labeling effects have also been suggested in studies of sickle cell screening participants. In discussing their results from one such study, Hampton, Anderson, Lavizzo, and Bergman (1974) cited a phenomenon that illustrates the critical role of mental representations in psychological reactions to risk factor testing. They noted that "parents of children who have been screened for sickle cell trait tend not to distinguish between a trait and a disease that markedly shortens life. The symptoms attributed to sickle cell trait are those that occur in sickle cell anemia. It was commonly stated, 'there must be something wrong because the doctor told us about it'" (p. 61).

Limitations of Risk Factor Labeling Research

The public health literature on labeling is characterized by a number of methodological limitations. Many of the studies on hypertension labeling, for example, are cross-sectional rather than prospective. As a result, the causal relationship between awareness of hypertensive status and psychological status is difficult to determine. If health-care utilization is used as an index of illness behavior, the direction of the relationship is ambiguous as well. Wagner and Strogatz (1984), reporting the results of one such study, noted that "labeling may undermine one's sense of well-being, or individuals with greater self-perceived morbidity may visit physicians more frequently and, as a result, have a greater opportunity for a blood pressure elevation to be detected" (p. 943).

Some of the studies rely on self-reports of risk factor status (e.g., awareness of hypertension), and it is unclear whether the labeling was induced by a communication from a health professional or the subject's own suspicions. The studies published to date vary substantially in design, subject population, screening context, and dependent measures. These differences make it especially difficult to explain the varied results concerning labeling.

One reason why the data concerning labeling effects are incomplete is that many of the reports concerning labeling effects rely on ancillary data collected during a clinical trial. As a result, most of the data relevant to labeling are observational rather than experimental. Critical baseline measures of psychological adjustment are rarely included. Participants in clinical studies may be highly selected, constraining the distribution of scores on labeling-related variables.

From a cognitive perspective, the timing and content of the dependent measures used in clinical studies are especially limited. Although the measures used to date reveal some aspects of illness behavior and psychiatric symptomatology, there has been little attempt to measure cognitive appraisals immediately after the result of a screening test is communicated. As theories of coping (e.g., Lazarus & Folkman, 1984) would suggest, it is clear that we need to understand this critical first stage of illness behavior if we are to achieve a thorough understanding of the labeling process. Our review of the public health literature on labeling led us to conclude that a systematic analysis of reactions to risk factor labeling would benefit from a converging sequence of carefully controlled experiments that employed samples of subjects from similar populations. Whereas the public health literature has focused on compliance and indirect measures of psychological impact such as absenteeism, we have focused on the immediate cognitive and motivational processes that are initiated by screening test results. For discussions of the role of cognitive variables in compliance, see Leventhal, Zimmerman, and Gutmann (1984) and Ley (1986).

The TAA Enzyme Paradigm

One of the valuable insights gained from the literature on risk factor labeling concerns the independence of labeling effects. Labeling appears to have a significant psychological impact that is independent of actual risk factor or disease status. This conclusion is derived from data gathered in screening evaluation studies that identified a subgroup of participants who were mislabeled. This allows a comparison between healthy individuals who mistakenly believe they possess a risk factor and those who correctly believe they lack it. For example, Bloom and Monterossa (1981) found that normotensives who were labeled as hypertensive reported more depressive symptoms than normotensives not so labeled.

One reason why risk factor testing is especially interesting is its application to individuals who are largely asymptomatic. Risk factor testing departs from the traditional medical model, which limits intervention to ill persons. Prior to the detection of their condition, most individuals with hypertension or hypercholesterolemia feel well. What is missing is the knowledge that a medical test has detected an abnormal physical sign. The critical issue, then, in the study of labeling effects is the impact of risk factor test results. Once the focus is turned toward the psychological variable of perceived risk status, the tools of experimental psychology can be put to use. Perceived risk status can be manipulated experimentally. Because of the asymptomatic nature of many risk conditions, these processes can be studied in healthy populations.

The first stage of our research program involved the development of a procedure for studying the processes of interest within a controlled laboratory setting. In collaboration with Peter Ditto, we developed an experimental paradigm that has now been used in a number of investigations. In order to control for prior knowledge and experience related to the risk factor test, the procedure involves a test for a fictitious enzyme deficiency.

The procedure is convincing. Subjects are told they are being tested for thioamine acetylase (TAA) enzyme deficiency, a risk factor for pancreatic disorders. Participants are also told that a recently developed test can detect the presence or absence of TAA enzyme in the saliva. In some experiments, subjects self-administer the test. In others, the test is conducted by a medical assistant. The test requires subjects to rinse their mouth with mouthwash, wait one minute, and spit some saliva into a small cup. The saliva is then tested with the "TAA enzyme test strip," which is actually a common urinary glucose test strip. Because a small amount of dextrose has been dissolved in the mouthwash, the test strip changes from yellow to green in response to the saliva. Depending on the experimental condition, this color change is explained to be an indication of either a positive or negative test result. Because of our use of the dextrose and the glucose test strip, diabetics and hypoglycemics are excluded from participation. The use of deception also means that subjects are carefully debriefed before they leave the laboratory. To date, all of the subjects in these studies have been college students.

The TAA enzyme paradigm has been used successfully in number of experiments conducted within a psychology laboratory setting. We have found that a typical small room can be easily decorated with sufficient medical posters and paraphernalia to make the setting credible to student subjects. When the paradigm was used in an experiment conducted at a student health clinic, the findings paralleled those obtained in the laboratory (Croyle & Sande, 1988). For an extensive discussion of the paradigm and its limitations, see Croyle and Ditto (1990).

Results of Studies Using the TAA Enzyme Paradigm

In the first experiment that utilized the paradigm, Jemmott, Ditto, and Croyle (1986) examined the effects of test result and perceived prevalence of the risk factor on subjects' cognitive appraisals of TAA enzyme deficiency. The impetus for this experiment came from the results of a survey of college undergraduates concerning illness beliefs (Jemmott, Croyle, & Ditto, 1988). In that study, the investigators found that individuals who had experienced an illness generally rated it as less serious (life-threatening) than did individuals who had never experienced the condition. Similar findings have been reported in survey studies of medical patients (Jamison, Lewis, & Burish, 1986) and their parents (Marteau & Johnston, 1986). Jemmott, Croyle, and Ditto (1988) also reported that perceptions of seriousness were related to beliefs concerning the prevalence of the health disorders. Individuals who believed that a symptom or disease was rare tended to view that condition as more life threatening than did individuals who believed the same condition was common. This finding is consistent with Zola's (1966) observation that ailments are less likely to stimulate individuals to seek treatment in populations where those ailments are relatively widespread.

The observed relationship between illness history and seriousness ratings raises a number of interesting questions. First, are these two factors causally related? Individuals who have experienced pneumonia, for example, may judge it as less serious than others do for reasons of self-enhancement. By minimizing the seriousness of their health history, individuals may maintain a positive image of their health. On the other hand, experience may lead to additional knowledge about a disease, knowledge that the condition can be cured or coped with. The correlation between perceived prevalence and perceived seriousness also leaves the question of causality unanswered. To address these issues, Jemmott et al. (1986) manipulated diagnostic status and perceived prevalence to test their effects on perceived seriousness.

Half of the subjects in the Jemmott et al. (1986) experiment were led to believe they had TAA deficiency (that the color change was a positive test result) and half were led to believe they did not have it (that the color change was a negative test result). Crossed with this independent variable was a manipulation of the perceived prevalence of TAA deficiency. Although subjects participated in groups of two or three with each individual in a separate room, they were led to believe five subjects were participating in the session. Each subject self-administered the enzyme test and reported the results to the experimenter. In the high-prevalence condition, the experimenter then told the subject that four of the five students had the deficiency. In the low-prevalence condition the subject was told that just one of the five students had the deficiency.

The key dependent measure in the study was the perceived seriousness of TAA deficiency. This measure of cognitive appraisal was embedded within a questionnaire asking subjects to rate the seriousness of several health disorders. The list included some disorders that were factual but unfamiliar to the participants, so that TAA disorder was not the only unusual one. Subjects were asked to rate each health problem on a 100-point scale, from not serious (can be ignored) to very serious (life threatening).

We expected that a positive test result would induce denial. Although denial and other forms of defensiveness are manifested in a variety of ways, one common form of denial observed in medical patients is minimizing the seriousness of the health threat (Janis, 1958; Lazarus, 1983; Lipowski, 1970). If minimization results from a motivation to defend the self against threatening information, then individuals who are told they have a health disorder should rate it as *less* serious than individuals who are told they do not have the disorder. This prediction was strongly supported. Subjects who believed they had the deficiency appraised it as less life threatening than did subjects who believed they did not have the deficiency.

Another way to deny diagnostic information is to denigrate the methods that produced the evidence. Bad news may lead to a perception of the physician as incompetent or untrustworthy. Or the patient may be motivated to view the medical tests as flawed or improperly administered. This latter form of denial was also apparent in the experiment. Subjects were asked to rate the accuracy of the TAA test on a nine-point scale. Subjects who were told their test results indicated TAA deficiency rated the test as less accurate than did subjects whose test results indicated that they did not have the deficiency. That this effect is due to denial is further supported by the finding that the tendency to denigrate the accuracy of the test was particularly pronounced when subjects believed that they alone had received a positive test result.

Prevalence information also played a role in subjects' appraisals of the health threat. When subjects believed only one of five students had tested positive for TAA deficiency, they perceived the deficiency as significantly more serious than when they believed four of the five subjects tested positive. This was true even though the medically significant information about the deficiency was exactly the same in both conditions. The use of prevalence information from an available group of peers provides important empirical support for the role of social comparison information in the interpretation of illness signs (Cacioppo, Anderson, Turnquist, & Petty, 1985; Sanders, 1982).

A Scarcity Heuristic in Risk Factor Appraisal

One of the virtues of the TAA enzyme paradigm is that it provides an involving context within which to examine more general processes of cognition and motivation. The use of prevalence information in the study just described, for example, may be but one example of a general heuristic used to evaluate a number of personal characteristics. Ditto and Jemmott (1989) hypothesized that perceived scarcity has an "extremitizing" effect on both positive and negative information. Valued characteristics may increase in their desirability to the extent that they are rare. Similarly, negative characteristics may be especially undesirable when they are unusual.

In two studies, Ditto and Jemmott (1989) told some participants that the enzyme condition was a negative health characteristic while others were told it was a positive health characteristic (that it made one less susceptible to pancreatic disease). Information concerning the prevalence of the characteristic was varied as well. The results confirmed the notion that scarcity information has an extremitizing effect on appraisals. When the enzyme condition was defined as a positive characteristic, it was appraised as more beneficial when it was thought to be rare than when it was thought to be common. When the condition was defined as a negative characteristic, perceived rarity served to increase negative appraisals.

From these and other data, the authors argued that the effect of prevalence information on evaluations of the seriousness of health disorders comes from our reliance on a simple heuristic. This cognitive heuristic links the perceived prevalence of objects and characteristics to their evaluative extremity. Rarity increases the positivity of valued characteristics and the negativity of undesirable characteristics. As is the case with judgmental heuristics in other domains (Tversky & Kahneman, 1974), this heuristic may be useful in many situations but lead to systematic bias and error in others.

One concern regarding basic research on illness cognition is the link between judgments and behavior. The Ditto and Jemmott study included dependent measures of behavior as well as judgments. After receiving their test result, subjects were given the opportunity to sign up to receive any of a number of informational services regarding TAA enzyme. The available services consisted of a free pamphlet, a booklet costing 50 cents, and a free physical exam including a complete pancreas workup. Subjects were asked to indicate their interest in receiving these services by checking the appropriate box and leaving their name, address, and telephone number. The number of services each subject requested was summed to form an index of information-seeking behavior. The results indicated that subjects in the negative health characteristic groups requested more information when the condition was perceived to be rate than when it was perceived to be common.

Is It Really Denial?

The development of the TAA enzyme paradigm has permitted a more thorough experimental investigation of the cognitive and motivational processes induced by risk factor testing than previously achieved. One focus of this line of work has been to test competing explanations for the effect of test results on cognitive appraisal. Are these findings a manifestation of a defensive motivational process like denial, or are they due to a more rational aspect of information processing?

If the minimization observed in the Jemmott et al. experiment was due to motivated denial, it is possible to derive some counterintuitive predictions concerning the effects of treatment information. Research and theory from the stress and coping literature suggest that denial and other forms of defensiveness are most likely to occur when an individual has no means of immediately reducing the threat (Janis, 1984; Lazarus, 1983; Leventhal, 1970). So what should we expect in a diagnostic situation where information concerning treatment was immediately available to the "patient"?

Two lines of reasoning provide two competing predictions. If we adopt the model of a rational actor, it is reasonable to assume that a treatable disease is usually perceived as less threatening than an untreatable one (unless the treatment itself is aversive). But if threat has been significantly minimized by a patient as part of a motivational process, an awareness that the threat can be reduced in the future may allow the patient to acknowledge the seriousness of that threat. Following this reasoning, if motivated denial is operating, information indicating that a given disorder is treatable should lead to an *increase* in how threatening the patient perceives that disorder to be.

Ditto, Jemmott, and Darley (1988) examined this question. Some participants in their experiment were led to believe they had TAA deficiency; others were led to believe they did not. But before the risk factor test was conducted, the investigators gave half the subjects additional information concerning the treatability of TAA deficiency. Subjects in the treatment-informed condition were told, "Fortunately, treatment for TAA deficiency is relatively simple and painless. A short-term medication program has been found to correct the deficiency in most people by stimulating TAA production."

The results supported a denial explanation of biased judgment. Subjects who believed they had the deficiency and were not provided with treatment information made a series of judgments that downplayed the significance of their test result. For example, compared to subjects in the other three conditions, positive-result, treatment-uninformed subjects rated the TAA test as less accurate (giving elevated estimates of the test's false positive rate) and both TAA deficiency and pancreatic disease as less life threatening. In contrast, the highest mean rating of the seriousness of pancreatic disease was observed among subjects who believed they were afflicted with the enzyme deficiency but had been provided with treatment information.

The investigators also considered the possibility that denial might be manifested by perceptual distortion. Subjects in the Ditto et al. experiment were asked the color of their "TAA test strip. Recall that all test strips turned from yellow to green in response to the sugar in the subject's saliva. To assess perceptual bias, subjects were asked to recall the color of their test strip and rate it on a 10-point color scale (from light green to dark green). Consistent with the other measures of denial, subjects in the positive-result, treatment-uninformed group tended to remember their test strip as "less green" than other subjects. This perceptual distortion is similar to anecdotal reports from clinical studies. By claiming that the color reaction of the test paper was minimal, these subjects could have concluded that their result indicated a less severe form of the disorder or, perhaps, that their test result was not positive at all.

Biases in Health Judgments: The Role of Expertise

The demonstration of a motivational basis for many biases and errors in the health domain does not exclude a possible role for other processes. Participants in the TAA enzyme experiments are faced with an ambiguous and unfamiliar threat. They have very little knowledge and experience directly related to the threat. For our purposes, this is an advantage. By studying health judgments under these conditions, we maximize the likelihood that subjects will have to rely on heuristics and generalizations, which then become manifest. A similar strategy has been used to study perception in a variety of domains. Experiential factors are clearly important in everyday judgments, but we have chosen to control these in our experimental research in order to gain clarity and precision.

One way to examine the role of knowledge concerning a health threat is to compare the judgments of experts and nonexperts. Experts may use different decision rules than nonexperts, or they may rely on information not readily available to nonexperts. If the biases manifested by experts and nonexperts are the same, this would suggest that these biases are especially robust and that laypersons' judgments may be resistant to additional information. On the other hand, a differentiation of judgments would suggest that experts have different mental representations of the object or problem being evaluated.

In one comparison study, Jemmott, Croyle, and Ditto (1988) administered questionnaires to both college students and physicians. The respondents provided judgments of the seriousness and prevalence of several health problems. They also indicated whether they had experienced the problem. The findings from the students were mentioned earlier. The disorders they perceived as more common were rated as less serious, as were the disorders they had personally experienced. In contrast, the seriousness ratings of physicians were not related to their personal health history or to their perceived prevalence. Therefore, it appears that the special knowledge that physicians have about medical disorders disengages the typical relationship between personal experience and perceived seriousness.

For one of the biases studied, however, physicians displayed an effect of personal experience comparable to that observed among college students.

When physicians were asked to estimate the prevalence of each of the health disorders, they, like the students, displayed a "false consensus effect" (Ross, Greene, & House, 1977). Physicians who had experienced a health problem provided higher estimates of its prevalence than did physicians who had never experienced the problem. For example, consider the prevalence estimates for herpes simplex of the lips. The average total-population prevalence estimate provided by doctors who had herpes simplex of the lips was 52%. Physicians who had never experienced the same problem estimated its prevalence to be only 15.1%.

These findings have startling implications. Several studies have shown that diagnostic reasoning is biased towards hypothesis confirmation (Elstein, Shulman, & Sprafka, 1978; Snyder, 1984). To the extent that initial hypotheses are shaped by beliefs concerning prevalence (as medical textbooks say they should), medical diagnoses and treatment may be significantly influenced by a physician's personal experience. In the case of risk factor labeling, this suggests that physicians' beliefs concerning their own risk status may have a direct or indirect influence on their identification of important risk factors in their patients. Although the effect of risk factor labeling on physicians' prevalence judgments has not been examined experimentally, recent evidence indicates that test results can produce false consensus effects among laypersons. Croyle and Sande (1988) found that subjects who "tested positive" for TAA deficiency gave significantly higher prevalence estimates of the disorder than did subjects who were assigned negative test results.

The Paradoxical Effects of Labeling

The findings of the public health research described earlier appear to be inconsistent with the results of the laboratory studies using the TAA enzyme paradigm. The larger field studies suggested that labeling increases symptom reporting and sick role behavior. On the other hand, the denial observed in the laboratory studies might lead one to expect the opposite effect, an attenuation of symptom reporting by subjects who test positive.

Leventhal and his colleagues (Leventhal, Meyer, & Nerenz, 1980; Leventhal, Nerenz, & Steele, 1984) have proposed a model of illness cognition and behavior that provides an explanation for this paradox. The model states that a diagnostic label initiates parallel processes of cognition concerning the disease itself and emotional reactions to the threat (see Bishop, this volume, and Schober and Lacroix, this volume, for further descriptions of the model). Mental representations of the illness are especially important in guiding the hypotheses individuals test as they examine symptoms and other signs (see also Pennebaker, 1982). Because individuals tend to apply acute models of disease to chronic asymptomatic problems, labeling can increase symptom reporting. At the same time, individuals must cope with their emotional reaction to the diagnostic label, and denial is one strategy for accomplishing this.

In an experiment conducted by Croyle and Sande (1988), participants were asked to respond to a symptom checklist after receiving their TAA test result. Subjects were told the symptoms were indicative of TAA deficiency. One reason these additional data were collected was to rule out an alternative explanation for the minimization observed in the earlier studies. In all of those studies, the subjects were healthy college students. Participants who were tested for and labeled as having TAA deficiency therefore had special knowledge about it—that people with the disorder do not feel ill. They might have discounted the seriousness of TAA deficiency because they were unable to uncover any symptom experiences associated with the diagnosis.

Contrary to this alternative explanation, Croyle and Sande found that subjects were able to uncover substantial evidence from memory to confirm the presence of TAA deficiency. Subjects in the positive test result group tended to recall more diagnosis-consistent symptoms than other subjects. Furthermore, positive-result subjects also recalled more behaviors that were labeled as increasing the risk of TAA deficiency. Not only to these data provide further support for the motivated denial explanation of our minimization effects, but they also confirm an important prediction derived from Leventhal's self-regulation model of illness behavior, that "given symptoms, an individual will seek a diagnostic label, and given a label, he or she will seek symptoms" (Leventhal et al., 1980).

One question raised by the hypertension labeling studies was whether risk factor labeling can alter memories of health events that occurred before the screening. This possibility has been a concern of some epidemiologists who conduct case control studies (Raphael, 1987). The experimental demonstration of a labeling-induced recall bias raises further concerns about the validity of self-reports in case control studies in epidemiology.

The Croyle and Sande study also replicated the minimization effect observed in the earlier TAA enzyme studies. Subjects diagnosed as having TAA deficiency appraised the disorder as a less serious threat to health than did subjects who were provided with negative test results. Furthermore, the former viewed the test as less accurate than did the latter. Because this experiment was conducted at a student infirmary rather than in a psychology lab room, the findings increase our confidence that the earlier findings are indicative of real-world reactions to risk factor testing.

One other finding from this study provides evidence relevant to the denial issue. Half the subjects in the study were told that the TAA enzyme test was 95% accurate while the other half were told it was 75% accurate. When asked whether they would like to take a definitive follow-up test, subjects who tested positive were more likely to do so when their result was described as 95% accurate. Only 1 of 18 subjects who received an unreliable positive result requested the more definite test. It seems, then, that the ambiguous feedback allowed subjects to employ an avoidant strategy, rather than motivating them to employ an information-seeking strategy.

Extensions to Actual Risk Factors

Blood Pressure Screening

Although the TAA studies consistently demonstrated that minimization is a common initial reaction to risk factor labeling, it was important to determine whether this effect was limited to an unfamiliar disorder. Coping theorists have suggested that denial is most likely to be utilized when an individual is faced with an unfamiliar threat (Lazarus, 1983). Croyle (1990) conducted two experiments to determine whether minimization can be induced by high blood pressure screening. In the first experiment, 40 college students had their blood pressure measured and were told either that it was "high, 140 over 97" or "normal, 110 over 80." Afterward, they completed a questionnaire that included that standard seriousness rating scale. The results replicated the findings of the TAA experiments. Subjects who were told they had high blood pressure readings rated high blood pressure as a less serious threat to health than did subjects who were told they had normal readings. This finding was replicated in a second experiment that employed student participants from another college.

Croyle's second experiment also examined a possible limiting condition for the occurrence of minimization following blood pressure testing. Research by Meyer, Leventhal, and Gutmann (1985) showed that patients' mental representations of hypertension were characterized by one of three types of beliefs concerning the time course of the disorder. Some individuals with hypertension (especially those new to treatment) believed that hypertension was an acute disorder. Others adhered to a cyclical model of the disease, believing that hypertension comes and goes. A third group accepted the medical model of a chronic disease that requires ongoing monitoring and treatment.

After they received their blood pressure test results, subjects in Croyle's second experiment were asked whether they believed hypertension was an acute, cyclical, or chronic disorder. The data revealed that the test feedback influenced mental representations. Subjects who were told their blood pressure was high were less likely to endorse a chronic model of hypertension. Similar results have been obtained by Baumann, Cameron, Zimmerman, and Leventhal (1989). The findings also showed that minimization among those in the high-feedback group was related to subjects' mental representations of the time course of hypertension. Minimization occurred only among subjects who believed that hypertension is an acute or cyclical problem.

The effect of feedback on symptom reporting has also been demonstrated within the context of blood pressure testing. Baumann et al. (1989) recently reported confirmatory symptom reporting in an experiment using randomly assigned feedback on a measure of blood pressure. Subjects who were told their blood pressure was high reported more symptoms laypersons commonly associate with hypertension, especially when they attributed their reading to stress.

Croyle and Williams (in press) provided evidence to suggest that symptom reports induced by blood pressure feedback are influenced by illness stereotypes. They first conducted a small survey and found that individuals who rated high blood pressure as a less serious threat to health also tended to associate the disorder with positive personal characteristics (e.g., professional employment, high intelligence). This relationship was then examined in a laboratory experiment. Participants in the experiment read information about high blood pressure that indicated the disorder was correlated with certain personality characteristics. For some subjects, high blood pressure was associated with undesirable personality traits, such as a tendency to panic under pressure. Others read that the condition was associated with positive characteristics. The experimenter then took the subject's blood pressure and administered a questionnaire that included a checklist of symptoms supposedly associated with high blood pressure. The findings indicated that experimentally induced stereotypes affected symptom reporting. Subjects provided with false feedback that their blood pressure was high were less likely to report symptoms when they had read the negative description. Because other studies have shown that labeling typically increases symptom reporting, these data suggest that lowered symptom reporting occurs only when the diagnostic label carries a stigma.

Cholesterol Screening

One of the premises of risk factor screening is that it provides an effective venue for educating individuals about their health and ways to improve it. Little is known about the impact of screening on this educational process. In 1984, a consensus conference of the National Institutes of Health recommended that all individuals with high cholesterol be identified and offered treatment (Consensus Development Conference, 1985). The National Cholesterol Education Project, launched by the National Heart, Lung, and Blood Institute, has since promoted the widespread use of cholesterol screening as a way to identify and educate individuals with elevated cholesterol. Like the large-scale screening programs of the past, this one has raised concerns about the possible adverse impact of labeling (Lefebvre, Hursey, & Carleton, 1988).

If risk factor test results have an immediate emotional impact on the individual, they might also indirectly influence the individual's ability to remember information concerning the disorder and its treatment. Hopp and Croyle (1989) investigated the immediate impact of cholesterol test results by randomly assigning study participants to one of three experimental groups:

borderline-high, normal, or no-test control. The study focused on the emotional impact of cholesterol test results and whether this impact mediated the ability of subjects to recall information presented on an audiotape. For subjects in the two feedback groups, this tape was played immediately after they received their test results. This was done to simulate the sequence of events that occurs at a community cholesterol screening.

The findings revealed significant differences in self-reported affect after test results were delivered, with the borderline-high group reporting more negative affect. But despite the impact of test results on affect, there was no main effect of test results on memory scores. Emotional responses were not significantly correlated with later ability to remember information on the tape. Because subjects varied greatly in their prior knowledge concerning cholesterol, further research will need to control for effects of prior knowledge. It may be that the emotional impact of test results undermines the learning of completely new material only. If so, only those who know little about high cholesterol and its treatment would be expected to manifest effects of labeling on a later test of knowledge.

Personality and Reactions to Risk Factor Testing

Perhaps the least studied topic relating to psychological aspects of risk factor testing is the role of individual differences. From a public health perspective, this is not surprising. Because screening programs are targeted to large, diverse populations, the opportunity to assess and address individual-level differences is often limited. From a scientific standpoint, however, an understanding of individual differences is a goal of some importance. Risk factor labeling affects different individuals in different ways, and a sound theory of labeling effects must account for this variation. Research on individual differences can also provide indirect benefits. The literature concerning the role of personality in cardiovascular risk, for example, not only has provided important theoretical insights into health behavior, but has also generated new hypotheses concerning the mechanisms of personality–disease relationships (Krantz & Glass, 1984).

One area of study that might inform work on reactions to risk factor testing is psychological research on personality and coping. Studies that have examined personality traits as moderators of the stress–illness relationship have provided mixed results (e.g., Cohen & Edwards, 1989), and some have argued that the conceptualization of coping as a trait is both empirically and theoretically unsound (Lazarus & Folkman, 1984). On the other hand, laboratory studies of more immediate responses to stressors suggest that personality factors can interact with situational factors to influence appraisal and other microlevel aspects of stress reactions (Houston, 1986). One of the major findings related to risk factor labeling, increased symptom reporting, has been related to neuroticism and related constructs (see Watson & Pennebaker, this volume). Research in personality and social psychology suggests that personality may play a role in the processing of threatening information. Self-esteem and positive adjustment have been related to the use of self-enhancing biases and illusory optimism, although the direction of these relationships is unclear (Sackheim, 1983; Taylor & Brown, 1988).

Croyle and Louie (1990) measured the self-esteem and coping styles of subjects 7 to 14 days before they participated in a cholesterol screening experiment. The Rosenberg (1965) scale was used to measure self-esteem, and the Miller Behavior Style Scale (Miller, 1987) was used to measure blunting and monitoring coping styles. Research by Miller and her colleagues indicates that high blunters prefer avoidant coping when faced with threat, whereas high monitors prefer more information and appear to exaggerate the importance of symptoms (e.g., Miller, Brody, & Summerton, 1988).

Subjects were randomly assigned to receive borderline-high or normal cholesterol readings after receiving a fingerprick method screening test. The main effects of cholesterol test feedback replicated the findings from previous studies that used the TAA enzyme paradigm. Relative to normal-feedback subjects, subjects who were told they had borderline-high cholesterol rated high cholesterol as a less serious threat to health and rated the test as less accurate. A false consensus effect was also observed. As was the case when subjects in the Croyle and Sande (1988) study tested positive for TAA deficiency, participants in the Croyle and Louie study who were assigned elevated cholesterol readings provided higher prevalence estimates of high cholesterol.

Within-cell correlations between the personality scores and cholesterol-related judgments yielded mixed results. Although the investigators expected that high scores on the blunting scale might be associated with lower ratings of seriousness (i.e., denial) among high-feedback subjects, this correlation was not significant. Neither blunting nor monitoring scores were correlated with judgments of test accuracy or seriousness within the high-feedback group. Blunting did have the expected relationship with reported emotional response: Higher blunting scores were associated with lower ratings of distress.

Analyses of the relationship between self-esteem and the other measures produced more interesting results. The findings suggest that high self-esteem is associated with self-enhancing biases in judgment and recall. Among subjects assigned a borderline-high test result, high self-esteem was correlated with increases in prevalence estimates from pretest to posttest. When asked to later recall their cholesterol readings, high-self-esteem subjects who received borderline-high readings were more likely to recall a lower test result. Despite this subtle evidence to support a role for personality differences in reactions to cholesterol test results, self-esteem was unrelated to the primary measure of cognitive appraisal: There was no correlation between esteem and seriousness judgments within either of the experimental groups.

Although more work on the topic is in progress, the likelihood of achieving an understanding of the role of personality in reactions to risk factor testing in the near future appears small. One of the difficulties is that personality variables that predict one aspect of labeling effects (e.g., symptom reporting) may not relate to another (e.g., minimization). The relationship between personality traits and mental representations of illness also needs to be studied. To address these questions, it may be necessary to incorporate personality premeasures into large-scale evaluation studies of screening programs. But before public health researchers can be convinced to deal with the inconvenience of these additional measures, it will be necessary for psychologists to provide more compelling experimental evidence of interactions between personality variables and the effects of risk factor testing.

HIV Antibody Testing

Major efforts are now under way to investigate the impact of HIV antibody testing (e.g., August et al., 1989). As with previous screening programs, HIV testing is intended to have an indirect impact on public health via its psychological impact on the individuals tested. As stated in a recent editorial in the *American Journal of Public Health*, "The benefit of testing depends primarily on the individual's knowledge of his or her test results, not on health authorities' creation of registries of infected person" (Cates & Handsfield, 1988, p. 1534) The results published to date have focused on the behavioral effects of test results on gay men. In general, the data suggest that HIV antibody testing and counseling are associated with small reductions in self-reported risky behaviors (Cates & Handsfield, 1988).

One issue that remains unresolved in the labeling area is the impact of negative results on a screening test. In the case of HIV testing, some men have been found to increase sexual activity after a negative test (Martin, 1987). The possibility of this type of disinhibition effect illustrates the importance of comparing high and normal test groups with a control group that receives no test. A similar issue arises in other types of risk factor screening. An individual with poor health habits who is told he or she has normal cholesterol may be less motivated than a control subject to attend to dietary recommendations. We believe this question deserves greater attention.

Although we know that a positive result on an HIV test has a negative emotional impact, we know little about the relationship between these reactions and preventive health behavior (Becker & Joseph, 1988). One of the limitations of observational studies of reactions to HIV testing is that test results are confounded with a wide array of behavioral and psychological variables (e.g., Winkelstein et al. 1987). Although laboratory studies of labeling effects cannot recreate the extensive impact of such an event, they can identify processes that allow public health researchers to generate more systematic hypotheses concerning the psychological impact of HIV testing. It is also possible to examine experimentally the effects of different types of counseling offered to individuals tested. Counseling of one sort or another has been advocated for participants of all screening programs, and it is likely that many of the processes are similar across disease domains.

Although the data concerning the use of denial among HIV-positive individuals is sparse, the discussion of the phenomenon in clinical reports is not. One example comes from an article by two psychiatrists who have treated HIV-infected patients:

> The therapist working with HIV patients may be surprised or shocked by the patients' denial of the illness or its seriousness. . . . It is not unusual for HIV patients to deny the existence for their illness during periods of relative quiescence. At such times, they may have unprotected sex (sexual intercourse without a condom) or sex in which they fail to inform their partner about the illness. (Adler & Beckett, 1989, p. 204)

Clinical reports such as this support the notion that denial is one important reaction to medical test results. They also suggest that laboratory studies of denial, although artificial in some respects, are unlikely to produce effects that have no parallel in the "real world." If fact, the studies reported here most likely underestimate the psychological impact of medical test results.

Remaining Issues

Health Risk Appraisal

Although the research discussed here has focused on reactions to a test for a single biological risk factor, it is important to note that some public health efforts now rely on multiple risk assessment and feedback. Health risk appraisal has a shorter history than simple risk factor testing, but it has become a popular tool for worksite health promotion (Wagner, Beery, Schoenbach, & Graham, 1982). Health risk appraisal has been defined as "a procedure for using epidemiologic and vital statistics to provide individuals with projections of their personalized mortality risk and with recommendations for reducing that risk" (Schoenbach, Wagner, & Beery, 1987). In a recent review of research concerning the effectiveness of health risk appraisal for motivating health behavior change, Schoenbach et al. (1987) argue that the relevant findings are scattered and inconclusive. Few studies have included appropriate control groups or other design required to achieve a reasonable degree of internal validity.

The complexity of the individualized feedback in health risk appraisal and the massive educational and clinical burdens faced by those who use it on a large scale suggest that laboratory experiments may be the most cost-effective means of studying its immediate impact on attitudes, beliefs, and intentions. This is especially true given that field studies have yet to provide compelling evidence that health risk appraisal has any significant impact on cognitive variables assumed to mediate health behavior change.

Are Reactions to Risk Factor Tests Unique?

One of the important theoretical issues in risk factor testing is whether reactions to risk factor labeling are any different from reactions to any type of negative feedback. In their discussion of illness cognition, Leventhal and Nerenz (1985) caution against the mindless application of theories from one domain of behavior to another. Although we agree that differences in the content of mental representations must not be overlooked, we have been struck by the similarities between our subjects' reactions to risk factor testing and the reports of investigators who study reactions to negative feedback on tests of performance.

Apparent similarities in phenomena can be exaggerated by similarities in method. Our methodology is derived from experimental social psychology. Our measures are derived from social psychological theories and theories of stress and coping. This might be limiting us, and we may be missing important phenomena that are specific to this context. We are now trying to get around this problem by including more varied and open-ended measures of cognitive and affective responses to risk factor testing. For example, subjects in the blood pressure and cholesterol studies have been asked to describe in some detail their thoughts and feelings after they were told their test result. Responses are being subjected to content analyses to determine what aspects of subjects' reactions are not assessed by our measures. One factor that is already apparent in these open-ended responses is prior expectation regarding the test result. Many subjects refer to these expectations and note their importance as a determinant of their emotional reaction. This is consistent with the large body of research on the importance of expectancies in stress and emotion. As a result of these analyses, measures of expectations are being incorporated into the studies of cholesterol screening discussed earlier.

The relationship between cognitive and affective reactions to risk factor testing continues to be a most challenging area of study. As with the study of emotion in general, progress in this area will depend on the further development of reliable, nonreactive measures and innovative statistical techniques.

Conclusion

Most of the work on mental representation in health and illness has used one of two strategies, describing patient cognitions or conducting highly controlled, often experimental, examinations of healthy subjects' representations of illnesses. We hope we have illustrated the utility of a third approach, one that examines experimentally the judgments of subjects who have just discovered they have a risk factor for a disease. This program of research has provided a number of insights into the processes underlying risk factor labeling and illness behavior. As our work continues, we hope to move from the laboratory to the field in order to provide a more comprehensive picture of the psychological consequences of screening programs. This fieldwork is an important prerequisite for the development of credible and theoretically sound recommendations to public health officials concerning ways to attenuate the iatrogenic effects of risk factor test results.

Acknowledgment. The authors thank Deborah Bowen for her comments on a draft of this chapter.

References

Adler, G. A., & Beckett, A. (1989). Psychotherapy of the patient with an HIV infection: Some ethical and therapeutic dilemmas. *Psychosomatics, 30,* 203–208.

August, S., Ironson, G., Laperriere, A., Baggett, H. L., Antoni, M., O'Hearn, P., Goldstein, D., Ingram, F., Schneiderman, N., Carver, C. S., and Fletcher, M. A. (1989, March). *Notification of HIV-1 antibody status: Coping and mood state in healthy gay men.* Paper presented at the annual meeting of the Society of Behavioral Medicine, San Francisco.

Baumann, L. J., Cameron, L. D., Zimmerman, R. S., & Leventhal, H. (1989). Illness representations and the symmetry of labels and symptoms. *Health Psychology, 8,* 449–469.

Becker, M. H., & Joseph, J. G. (1988). AIDS and behavioral change to reduce risk: A review. *American Journal of Public Health, 78,* 394–410.

Bergman, A., & Stamm, S. J. (1967). The morbidity of cardiac nondisease in schoolchildren. *New England Journal of Medicine, 276,* 1008–1013.

Bloom, J. R., & Monterossa, S. (1981). Hypertension labeling and sense of well-being. *American Journal of Public Health, 71,* 1228–1232.

Cacioppo, J. T., Anderson, B. L., Turnquist, D. C., & Petty, R. E. (1985). Psychophysiological comparison processes: Interpreting cancer symptoms. In B. L. Anderson (Ed.), *Women with cancer: Psychological perspectives* (pp. 141–171). New York: Springer-Verlag.

Cates, W., & Handsfield, H. H. (1988). HIV counseling and testing: Does it work? *American Journal of Public Health, 78,* 1533–1534.

Cayler, G. G., Lynn, D. B., & Stein, E. M. (1973). Effect of cardiac "nondisease" on intellectual and perceptual motor development. *British Heart Journal, 35,* 543–547.

Charlson, M. E., Alderman, M., & Melcher, L. (1982). Absenteeism and labelling in hypertensive subjects: Prevention of an adverse impact in those at high risk. *American Journal of Medicine, 73,* 165–170.

Cohen, S., & Edwards, J. R. (1989). Personality characteristics as moderators of the relationship between stress and disorder. In R. W. J. Neufeld (Ed.), *Advances in the investigation of psychological stress* (pp. 235–283). New York: Wiley.

Consensus Development Conference. (1985). Lowering blood cholesterol to prevent heart disease. *Journal of the American Medical Association, 254,* 2080–2086.

Croyle, R. T. (1990). Biased appraisal of high blood pressure. *Preventive Medicine, 19,* 40–44.

Croyle, R. T., & Ditto, P. H. (1990). Illness cognition and behavior. An experimental approach. *Journal of Behavioral Medicine, 13,* 31–52.

Croyle, R. T., & Louie, D. (1990). *Coping with borderline-high cholesterol: Defensive processing of an ambiguous health threat.* Manuscript submitted for publication.

Croyle, R. T., & Sande, G. N. (1988). Denial and confirmatory search: Paradoxical consequences of medical diagnosis. *Journal of Applied Social Psychology, 18,* 473–490.

Croyle, R. T., & Williams, K. D. (in press). Reactions to medical diagnosis: The role of illness stereotypes. *Basic and Applied Social Psychology.*

Ditto, P. H., & Jemmott, J. B., III (1989). From rarity to evaluative extremity: Effects of prevalence information on evaluations of positive and negative characteristics. *Journal of Personality and Social Psychology, 57,* 16–26.

Ditto, P. H., Jemmott, J. B., III, & Darley, J. M. (1988). Apraising the threat of illness: A mental representational approach. *Health Psychology, 7,* 183–201.

Elstein, A. S., Shulman, L. S., & Sprafka, S. A. (1978). *Medical problem solving: An analysis of clinical reasoning.* Cambridge, MA: Harvard University Press.

Hampton, M. L., Anderson, J. A., Lavizzo, B. S., & Bergman, A. B. (1974). Sickle cell "nondisease": A potentially serious public health problem. *American Journal of Diseases in Children, 128,* 58–61.

Haynes, R. B., Sackett, D. L., Taylor, W., Gibson, E. S., & Johnson, A. L. (1978). Increased absenteeism from work after detection and labeling of hypertensive patients. *New England Journal of Medicine, 299,* 741–744.

Hopp, H. P., & Croyle, R. T. (1989, May). *Risk factor labeling: The role of affect.* Paper presented at the annual meeting of the Midwestern Psychological Association, Chicago.

Houston, B. K. (1986). Psychological variables and cardiovascular and neuroendocrine reactivity. In K. Matthews, S. M. Weiss, T. Detre, T. M. Dembroski, B. Falkner, S. B. Manuck, & R. B. Williams (Eds.), *Handbook of stress, reactivity, and cardiovascular disease* (pp. 207–229). New York: Wiley.

Jamison, R. N., Lewis, S., & Burish, T. G. (1986). Psychological impact of cancer on adolescents: Self-image, locus of control, perception of illness and knowledge of cancer. *Journal of Chronic Disease, 39,* 609–617.

Janis, I. L. (1958). *Psychological stress.* New York: Wiley.

Janis, I. L. (1984). Improving adherence to medical recommendations: Prescriptive hypotheses derived from recent research in social psychology. In A. Baum, S. E. Taylor, & J. E. Singer (Eds.), *Handbook of psychology and health* (Vol. 4, pp. 113–148). Hillsdale, NJ: Lawrence Erlbaum Associates.

Jemmott, J. B., III, Croyle, R. T., & Ditto, P. H. (1988). Commonsense epidemiology: Self-based judgments from laypersons and physicians. *Health Psychology, 7,* 55–73.

Jemmott, J. B., III, Ditto, P. H., & Croyle, R. T. (1986). Judging health status: Effects of perceived prevalence and personal relevance. *Journal of Personality and Social Psychology, 50,* 899–905.

Johnston, M. E., Gibson, E. S., Terry, C. W., Haynes, R. B., Taylor, D. W., Gafni, A. Sicurella, J. I., & Sackett, D. L. (1984). Effects of labelling on income, work, and social function among hypertensive employees. *Journal of Chronic Disease, 37,* 417–423.

Krantz, D. S., & Glass, D. C. (1984). Personality, behavior patterns, and physical illness: Conceptual and methodological issues. In W. D. Gentry (Ed.), *Handbook of behavioral medicine* (pp. 38–86). New York: Guilford Press.

Lazarus, R. S. (1983). The costs and benefits of denial. In S. Breznitz (Ed.), *The denial of stress* (pp. 1–30). New York: International Universities Press.

Lazarus, R. S., & Folkman, S. (1984). Coping and adaptation. In W. D. Gentry (Ed.), *Handbook of behavioral medicine* (pp. 282–325). New York: Guilford Press.

Lefebvre, R. C., Hursey, K. G., & Carleton, R. A. (1988). Labeling of participants in high blood pressure screening programs: Implications for blood cholesterol screenings. *Archives of Internal Medicine, 148,* 1993–1997.

Leventhal, H. (1970). Findings and theory in the study of fear communications. In L. Berkowitz (Ed.), *Advances in experimental social psychology* (Vol. 5), pp. 120–186. New York: Academic Press.

Leventhal, H., Meyer, D., & Nerenz, D. (1980). The common sense representation of illness danger. In S. Rachman (Ed.), *Medical psychology* (Vol. 2, pp. 7–30). New York: Pergamon Press.

Leventhal, H., & Nerenz, D. R. (1985). The assessment of illness cognition. In P. Karoly (Ed.), *Measurement strategies in health psychology* (pp. 517–554). New York: Wiley.

Leventhal, H., Nerenz, D. R., & Steele, D. J. (1984). Illness representations and coping with health threats. In A. Baum, S. E. Taylor, & J. E. Singer (Eds.), *Handbook of psychology and health* (Vol. 4, pp. 219–252). Hillsdale, NJ: Lawrence Erlbaum Associates.

Leventhal, H., Zimmerman, R., & Gutmann, M. (1984). Compliance: A self-regulation perspective: In D. Gentry (Ed.), *Handbook of behavioral medicine* (pp. 369–436). New York: Guilford Press.

Ley, P. (1986). Cognitive variables and noncompliance. *Journal of Compliance in Health Care, 1,* 171–188.

Lipowski, Z. J. (1970). Physical illness, the individual and the coping process. *International Journal of Psychiatry in Medicine, 1,* 91–102.

Mann, A. (1984). Hypertension: Psychological aspects and diagnostic impact in a clinical trial. *Psychological Medicine,* Monograph Supplement No. 5.

Marteau, T. M., & Johnson, M. (1986). Determinants of beliefs about illness: A study of parents of children with diabetes, asthma, epilepsy, and no chronic illness. *Journal of Psychosomatic Research, 30,* 673–683.

Martin, J. L. (1987, February). *Sexual behavior patterns, behavior change, and occurrence of antibody to HIV among New York City gay men.* Paper presented at the Conference on the Role of HIV Antibody Testing in the Prevention and Control of HIV Infection and AIDS, Atlanta, GA.

Meyer, D., Leventhal, H., & Gutmann, M. (1985). Common-sense models of illness: The example of hypertension. *Health Psychology, 4,* 115–135.

Miller, S. M. (1987). Monitoring and blunting: Validation of a questionnaire to assess styles of information seeking under threat. *Journal of Personality and Social Psychology, 52,* 345–353.

Miller, S. M., Brody, D. S., & Summerton, J. (1988). Styles of coping with threat: Implications for health. *Journal of Personality and Social Psychology, 54,* 142–148.

Milne, B. J., Logan, A. G., & Flanagan, P. T. (1985). Alterations in health perception and life style in treated hypertensives. *Journal of Chronic Disease, 38,* 37–45.

Monk, M. (1981). Blood pressure awareness and psychological well-being in the health and nutrition examination survey. *Clinical and Investigative Medicine, 4,* 183–189.

Mossey, J. M. (1981). Psychosocial consequences of labeling in hypertension. *Clinical and Investigative Medicine, 4,* 201–207.

Pennebaker, J. (1982). *The psychology of physical symptoms.* New York: Springer-Verlag.

Raphael, K. (1987). Recall bias: A proposal for assessment and control. *International Journal of Epidemiology, 16,* 167–170.

Rosenberg, M. (1965). *Society and the adolescent self-image.* Princeton, NJ: Princeton University Press.

Ross, L., Greene, D., & House, P. (1977). The "false consensus effect": An egocentric bias in social perception and attribution processes. *Journal of Experimental Social Psychology, 13,* 276–301.

Sackett, D. L. (1981). The McMaster symposium on patient labelling in hypertension. *Clinical and Investigative Medicine, 4,* 161–226.

Sackheim, H. A. (1983). Self-deception, self-esteem, and depression: The adaptive value of lying to oneself. In J. Masling (Ed.), *Empirical studies of psychoanalytic theories* (Vol. 1, pp. 101–157). Hillsdale, NJ: Lawrence Erlbaum Associates.

Sanders, G. S. (1982). Social comparison and perceptions of health and illness. In G. S. Sanders & J. Suls (Eds.), *Social psychology of health and illness* (pp. 129–157). Hillsdale, NJ: Lawrence Erlbaum Associates.

Schoenbach, V. J., Wagner, E. H., & Beery, W. L. (1987). Health risk appraisal: Review of evidence for effectiveness. *Health Services Research, 22,* 553–580.

Snyder, M. (1984). When belief creates reality. In L. Berkowitz (Ed.), *Advances in experimental social psychology* (Vol. 18, pp. 248–305). New York: Academic Press.

Taylor, S. E., & Brown, J. (1988). Illusory optimism and psychological adjustment. *Psychological Bulletin, 103,* 193–210.

Tversky, A., & Kahneman, D. (1974). Judgment under uncertainty: Heuristics and biases. *Science, 185,* 1124–1131.

Wagner, E. H., Beery, W. L., Schoenbach, V. J., & Graham, R. M. (1982). An assessment of health hazard/health risk appraisal. *American Journal of Public Health, 72,* 347–352.

Wagner, E. H., & Strogatz, D. S. (1984). Hypertension labeling and well-being: Alternative explanations for cross-sectional data. *Journal of Chronic Disease, 37,* 943–947.

Winkelstein, W., Lyman, D. M., Padian, N. Grant, R., Samuel, M., Wiley, J. A., Anderson, R. E., Lang, W., Riggs, J., & Levy, J. A. (1987). Sexual practices and risk of infection by the immunodeficiency virus. The San Francisco Men's Health Study. *Journal of the American Medical Association, 257,* 321–325.

Zola, I. K. (1966). Culture and symptoms: An analysis of patients' presenting complaints. *American Sociological Review, 31,* 615–630.

6
Laypersons' Judgments of Patient Credibility and the Study of Illness Representations

J. A. Skelton

You listen as your spouse complains about a throbbing headache. A professor listens as a student cites a recent bout of flu to justify a request for an extended term paper deadline. A supervisor listens to an employee's description of back pain that has reduced the employee's productivity. In each case, a perceiver is presented with a report of a victim's health problems and is expected to respond in some fashion, based on secondhand information to which only the illness victim can have direct access. The central problem of this chapter is to explain how perceivers accomplish the daunting task of making sense of victims' reports of illness, pain, and physical symptoms and, specifically, which characteristics of these reports make them more or less credible to perceivers.

I have chosen to focus on judgments about the credibility of reported health problems for two reasons. First, individuals are far more likely to report health problems to family members or nonprofessional peers than to seek out professional treatment. Even when people do decide to seek treatment, it is usually after talking over their pain and symptoms with fellow laypersons (Sanders, 1982). Credibility judgments summarize lay perceivers' views of the causes of patients' self-reported health problems. Problems that are attributed to "legitimate" causes (from the standpoint of perceivers' implicit model of diseases and illness) seem likely to elicit different perceptions of the patient and action toward him or her than are problems attributed to illegitimate or suspicious causes. For example, if the supervisor suspects an employee's pain complaints are more strongly related to job dissatisfaction than to tissue damage, this judgment will probably influence which treatments the supervisor advises, the supervisor's willingness to grant time off from work, and so forth. The second reason is that despite their obvious importance in the just described lay consultation system, credibility judgment processes have not, to my knowledge, been experimentally studied in medicine or the behavioral and social sciences.

My primary objective in this chapter is to elucidate the mental model that perceivers in Western biomedically oriented culture use to assess illness victims' self-reports. I begin with a discussion of what the biomedical disease model implies for assessment of health complaints, and how health care professionals apply the model to understand patients' complaints. Then I review research on lay observers' judgments of illness victims and consider what it tells us about how those judgments are made. In general, I take a critical view of the biomedical model, at least in the way observers apply it to certain patient assessment situations.

Patient Credibility in Contemporary Biomedicine

The Organic–Functional Dichotomy

The basic assumption of our culturally dominant biomedical model is that all diseases have organic causes that manifest as physical signs (Engel, 1977). The diagnostician's task is to identify the signs of disease, using the patient's symptom report as a starting point (Wulff, 1976). For biomedicine, symptom reports are legitimate only if they have an organic basis. Symptoms reported in the absence of physical pathology, however, are viewed as having functional value to the patient, either as displaced expressions of emotional distress (Costa & McCrae, 1985; Watson & Pennebaker, this volume) or as attempts to obtain the social gains associated with occupying the sick role (Dollard & Miller, 1950; Parsons, 1951; Smith, Snyder, & Perkins, 1983). The patient who reports pain or symptoms having no known physical cause may be diagnosed a hypochondriac, a conversion hysteric, or a malingerer (Stevens, 1986). Such labels certify the patient as one whose bodily complaints are literally incredible.

A long tradition in both medicine and the social and behavioral sciences supports the organic–functional dichotomy. The concept of conversion hysteria, systematically articulated in the works of Freud (e.g., Breuer & Freud, 1925/1955), has achieved widespread acceptance. Behavioristic psychology gave us the notion of illness behavior as instrumental activity and, by extension, a model of symptom-reporting as a method for obtaining social reinforcement (e.g., Dollard & Miller, 1950). Social psychology and medical sociology provided a group version of conversion hysteria, mass psychogenic illness (Colligan, Pennebaker, & Murphy, 1982; Kerckhoff & Back, 1968). In addition to these theoretical contributions to our collective representation of illness, an impressive array of data can be marshalled in support of dichotomizing illness complaints and symptom reports into "organic" and "functional" types. For a host of reasons—some motivational, some related to inherent limitations of perceptual and cognitive systems—verbal reports of bodily states are often unreliable indicators of physiological states (for reviews, see Leventhal, 1986, and Skelton & Pennebaker, 1990). Correlational studies have repeatedly demonstrated the tendency for negative affect, stress, and symptom-reporting to covary (Tessler & Mechanic, 1978, provide an illustrative example), and recent applications of experimental methodology (e.g., Croyle & Uretsky, 1987) indicate that the causal arrow points from affect to symptoms: When people are unhappy, upset, or distressed, they are more likely report symptoms—independently of variations in objective health status. In addition, subpopulation variation in symptom- and pain-reporting behaviors is frequently unrelated to physical health (Verbrugge, 1985; Zborowski, 1969; Zola, 1966) but does serve expressive and other social functions. Estimates of the percentage of patients who seek treatment for psychological reasons unrelated to organic disease often exceed 50% (e.g., Jennings, 1986). Taken together, such evidence suggests that patients' reports of bodily complaints should not be taken at face value but instead should be validated against an "objective criterion." For contemporary biomedicine that criterion is the presence of signs of physical pathology.

But relying on pathophysiological signs as the final arbiter of symptom legitimacy has certain limitations. First, diagnostic technology is fallible. Without a perfect correlation between signs and symptoms, negative diagnostic evidence may mean only that the search for signs is incomplete. Unfortunately, unless diagnosticians and other medical staff are sensitive to error rates for diagnostic tests, the subtle difference between "negative signs" and "no organic cause" may be ignored. Second, biomedicine's catalog of known organic syndromes is incomplete. In 1970, a patient who presented for treatment of symptoms of Legionnaire's disease or AIDS-related complex would have been an enigma, because neither syndrome had been classified as a recognizable disease entity. Finally, although the distinction between organic and functional symptoms is meant to underscore the primary role accorded to physical causes of disease, it has the potential to deny validation to patients with demonstrable pathology but who also exhibit psychological problems. That is, a patient who simultaneously reports physical symptoms and psychological distress may appear less credible than a patient who merely reports symptoms—even when both are suffering a valid medical problem.

Health-Care Professionals' Doubts About Patient Credibility

For health-care professionals, patients' subjective reports of pain, suffering, and physical symptoms are problematical (Hackett, 1971). One widely documented result of skepticism toward patient reports is extreme conservatism in administering analgesics to patients in pain, even patients who are terminal (Clark, Springer, Hagar, Drew, & Gordon, 1988). Most hospital-ized patients receive lower-than-recommended dosages of narcotic pain-killers (Marks & Sachar, 1973). Health professionals are properly concerned about iatrogenic addiction and drug abuse by patients (Charap, 1978; Cohen, 1980). But they appear to be overly concerned about the motives of patients who request pain medication (Klass, 1989). The possibility that patient self-reports serve functional goals seems rarely to be far from the surface in medical decision making, as illustrated in the following statement by an NIMH research scientist in a recent *Newsweek* article: "When it comes to pain, there's always the question of whether it's real" (Clark et al., 1988). Clearly, patient credibility is very much at issue for medical staff, and functional explanations for patients' pain-related behavior are readily available.

Further evidence regarding problems of the organic–functional dichotomy comes from Wiener (1975), an anthropologist who observed nurse–patient interactions on an orthopedic ward. All patients suffered from chronic low back pain, a syndrome frequently characterized by an elusive etiology. Wiener observed "psychogenic stereotyping" of these patients—a tendency for staff to regard patients' problems as primarily psychological—even though most patients' pain could be traced to specific physical traumas. The mere availability of functional psychological explanations for patients' pain complaints seemed sufficient to engage use of such explanations.

Burgess (1980) also observed that medical staff were often skeptical of patients' descriptions of physical suffering. Unlike Wiener, however, she applied experimental methods to test her observations by presenting to more than 100 hospital nurses a short vignette describing a hypothetical patient who reports suffering from severe pain. Half the nurse-subjects read a vignette in which the patient's attributes were stereotypical of chronic pain patients: an individual who has suffered from pain for a relatively long time, whose diagnostic results are inconclusive, and who exhibits symptoms of psychological depression (Sternbach, 1974). The remaining vignettes de-scribed a typical acute pain patient whose short-duration suffering was the clear result of documented pathology and who exhibited no depression symptoms. Nurses rated the pain experienced by the two types of patients very differently: "The chronic" patient was estimated to be suffering much *less* than the "acute" patient.

A follow-up experiment was performed to identify which of the attributes differentiating chronic from acute pain patients were responsible for Burgess's results (Taylor, Skelton, & Butcher, 1984). Over 230 practicing nurses read paragraph-long case histories that orthogonally manipulated duration of the patient's pain problem, outcome of diagnostic tests, and presence of depression symptoms. Nurses rated the patient's suffering as less intense when diagnostic signs were inconclusive. "Negative diagnosis" descriptions were carefully worded so that test results were negative; the descriptions deliberately avoided stating that the patient had no organic pathology. Yet nurse-subjects interpreted the negative diagnosis descriptions as if they conclusively demonstrated the absence of pathology.

Taylor et al.'s nurses also estimated suffering as less intense if the patient had a long history of pain problems, independently of diagnostic results. The subjects rated the patient on a variety of trait scales, and ratings were less positive when the patient's pain problem was of long duration. Long-term pain is characteristic of chronic pain patients, so the mere presence of this attribute in the vignettes may have triggered nurses' stereotypes of such patients, leading to denigration of the patient's suffering and personality. Taken together, these findings suggested that medical personnel (1) may misinterpret negative diagnostic results and (2) are dubious about the credibility of patients who even minimally fit a "psychogenic" stereotype. The latter conclusion, of course, assumes that suffering estimates and trait attributions reflect professionals' assessments of patient credibility.

Patient Credibility and the Lay Perceiver

Why Study Patient Credibility?

As noted earlier, lay consultation is the first choice for individuals who are seeking to make decisions about their health problems (Sanders, 1982; also Friedson, 1960). This fact implies that laypersons frequently encounter the self-reported health problems of fellow laypersons. The situation shares some similarities with that of the diagnostic interview between patient and health professional, in that the lay perceiver cannot experience the phenomenal reality of the patient's symptoms. Thus if factors that cause medical staff to doubt patients' self-reports also lead nonprofessional observers to question patients' credibility, then it is at least possible that lay perceivers are using a similar (though perhaps an implicit) biomedical model to that of health professionals in assessing patient complaints.

Noncredible complaints lie outside the boundaries of lay perceivers' mental model of the "ideal" disease. Just as cognitive psychologists have studied perceptual illusions and cognitive biases in order to map "normal" perception and cognition, so it is valuable to examine cases in which lay perceivers find it difficult to believe a patient's illness complaint. By determining the points at which patient complaints trangress the boundaries of the "ideal" disease and prompt disbelief from observers, the study of factors affecting patient credibility may indirectly reveal the structure of laypersons' models of disease and illness.

Similarities Between Lay Perceivers and Health Professionals

Formal and lay illness models within a given culture can be expected to be similar, at least in their broad outlines. In fact, it's difficult to imagine a culture where health-care professionals' mental representations of illness differ radically from those of their patients, because laypersons simply would not grant occupancy of the professional healer role to "heretics." Beyond social-structural considerations, which rely on logical analysis, certain observations suggest that lay perceivers are concerned that illness victims' self-reports are credible accounts. Parents teach children the circumstances in which pain, symptom, and illness complaints are acceptable and when they are not acceptable. When a child falls down and begins to cry, parents may try to assuage the hurt by inspecting arms or legs and saying, "See, it's not that bad. You didn't even break the skin!" The message is that pain should be correlated with the extent of tissue damage—although this message has serious flaws (Leventhal & Everhart, 1979)—and that observable physical pathology is the defining attribute of a legitimate pain report. Moreover, "hypochondriacs" and "malingerers" are stereotyped figures in popular culture (e.g., Felix Unger of *The Odd Couple*) and classic literature (Molière's *Imaginary Invalid*); their recurrence across time and cultures suggests a general awareness by laypersons that illness complaints aren't necessarily objective descriptions of pain and symptoms (also see Schober & Lacroix, this volume).

Research evidence also suggests that lay observers dichotomize symptoms and diseases into physical and psychological categories, akin to the organic–functional distinction made by professionals. For example, Bishop's (1987) subjects classified a variety of symptoms in terms of their co-occurrence in illnesses. A major dimension underlying these laypersons' classifications was whether symptoms were viewed as having physical or psychological causes; subjects were less likely to recommend medical care for symptoms perceived as psychologically caused. This leads naturally to the question, Are lay perceivers apt to see "psychological" symptoms as less indicative of a legitimate disease, and the patient who reports such symptoms as less credible? If so, this would suggest another similarity between professional and lay models of illness.

Differences Between Laypersons' and Professionals' Perspectives

Although lay perceivers and health professionals share a general framework for understanding disease, the common ground upon which perceiver and patient stand must also be examined. Both are amateurs at diagnosis and treatment. Indeed, the major difference between patient and lay perceiver is one of immediate perspective: At this particular instant, person A is experiencing symptoms that he or she reports to person B; these roles, however, could easily be reversed at another moment of time—in other words, a perceiver is a potential patient, and patients are potential perceivers. Given the interchangeability of these roles, it is useful to consider how the patient's and the professional's perspectives in health transactions differ.

First, the availability of organic versus functional explanations for patients' reports of pain and symptoms probably varies for patients and professionals. Although the professional's formal knowledge of disease is more extensive than the patient's, so also is the professional's experience with illness complaints that might be termed suspicious. On the other hand, the phenomenal reality of pain and symptoms is indisputable for the patient but not the professional. As a result, an organic interpretation may be far more available for the patient than a functional one, but both interpretations may be equally available to medical practitoners. Certain features of the patient's presentation may be more likely to trigger doubts about credibility for the practitioner.

Seond, patients and health-care staff may have very different outlooks on the meaning of diagnostic test results. The health professional is a daily user of diagnostic technology, and this immersion may contribute to a blind faith in test results—even negative results. Furthermore, because of aforementioned differences in the salience of symptoms, patients may be less disposed to accept negative test outcomes. Sanders (1981) provides some pertinent data. In his experiment, subjects role-played patients who were suffering from physical symptoms. Some were told that a diagnostic test indicated the symptoms required treatment, and others were told the test revealed no need for medical attention. In rating the likelihood that they would go to a doctor, subjects were unaffected by the negative diagnostic result; they were equally likely to seek treatment, regardless of the test outcome, particularly if they had also received advice from fellow laypersons to go to a doctor. These findings suggest that when negative diagnostic evidence conflicts with advice from lay consultants, patients will follow peers' advice. Laypersons in the patient role seem more willing than health-care staff to consider the possibility that negative diagnoses are indeterminate.

Finally, patients and medical personnel have widely different experience in dealing with symptoms and disease on a day-to-day basis. For the patient, health problems are uniquely personal and hedonically relevant. For staff, a given patient is just one of many sharing a similar "profile." This is not to say that staff are not emotionally invested in health transactions to the same degree as are patients; staff members have strong emotional responses to some patients (Maslach, 1982), especially to those whose problems appear intractable (Davitz & Davitz, 1975). But, as noted earlier, staff members stereotype some classes of patients (Wiener, 1975), and attributes of the patient's presentation and behavior may evoke stereotyped responses from staff.

Which Perspective Do Lay Perceivers Adopt?

Are lay perceivers' judgments of patient credibility more similar to those of the professional or the patient? Another way to phrase the question is, Which is the more important determinant of lay perceivers' credibility assessments:

the shared amateur status and interchangeability of patients' and lay perceivers' roles or the difference in immediate perspectives of the patient and perceiver? There are two reasons to suspect the latter is more potent. First, the availability argument cited earlier is equally applicable to lay perceivers and medical staff. For both classes of observers, the patient's suffering is less salient than it is to the patient, and thus alternative explanations for the patient's health complaints are more likely to be available for consideration by observers—regardless of whether the observer is a layperson or a medical practitioner.

A second, related reason can be extrapolated from an attribution theory framework. When causes of an action are to be explained, the causes chosen by observers (who are attempting to explain the action) differ from those chosen by actors (persons whose actions are to be explained). Observers are more likely to invoke properties or attributes of the actor (Jones & Nisbett, 1972). In the present case, both lay perceivers and medical diagnosticians are observers faced with explaining an actor-patient's illness complaint. Whereas the patient is likely to gravitate toward disease explanations (external to himself or herself), observers may be more likely to wonder, What about the patient is causing her (or him) to report this problem? Although lay perceivers and health professionals may differ in the precise details of their illness models, both are aware that illness complaints may serve functional psychosocial needs of the patient. If the patient's description allows the possibility of a functional interpretation, both lay and professional observers may be drawn toward a patient-centered explanation and away from a disease-centered explanation. To use the terms of Kelley's (1973) theory of causal schemata, observers may *discount* organic explanations of patients' self-reported health problems when a plausible functional explanation is equally available. The research program reported in the remainder of this chapter traces the implications of the discounting hypothesis for laypersons' judgments of patient credibility.

Research Evidence on Lay Perceptions of Patient Credibility

Overview

To date, my students and I have conducted six studies of patient credibility involving over 500 college student subjects. Three common features unify the experiments. First, subjects receive a description of a male college student who presents to the Health Center for treatment of a sore throat. Second, data about outcomes of diagnostic tests and personal, nonmedical problems the patient has been experiencing are embedded in the descriptions. Finally, both the perceived severity of the patient's health problem and the credibility of his complaint have been assessed in all studies. Each experiment, however, has differed from the others in important ways. For example, the format of patient descriptions has ranged from short paragraphs (Skelton, 1987) to Health Center records and nurse–patient interview transcripts (Skelton, Conklin, Ralston, & Loughlin, 1989). The patient's personal problems have included a range of everyday difficulties with which college-age subjects can identify—romantic breakups, family health crises, upcoming exams, and insomnia. Such variations have aimed to test the construct validity of independent variables. Most recently, measures of patient credibility have been revised to establish their distinctiveness from measures of psychological versus physical causation and patient blame, thereby testing the construct validity of dependent variables.

Initial Demonstrations

Our beginning efforts were aimed at determining whether lay perceivers doubt the credibility of patients (1) whose diagnostic test results are negative and (2) who experience psychosocial distress, even with positive diagnostic outcomes.

Experiment 1

Our first venture was a modest experiment involving 114 subjects and using an admittedly impoverished methodology. We constructed short scenarios describing a hypothetical patient, a college student suffering from a sore throat. Three factors were systematically varied in the descriptions. First, the patient did or did not have a heavy load of class-related assignments. Second, the patient was described as having recently experienced a romantic breakup or as having a satisfactory lovelife. Besides indicating the presence (or absence) of these nonmedical problems, the description stated that medical examination and testing had or had not revealed signs of a throat infection. We did not state that the patient had *no* infection but, instead, that there was *no evidence* of an infection. The scenario's wording is shown in Table 6-1.

Following the scenario were four rating questions, each scored on 0 to 21-point scales: "How painful do you think JTA's sore throat is?," "How serious is JTA's sore throat?," "How much do you think the problem is 'all in JTA's mind'?," and "How much do you think JTA's problem is just an excuse to avoid coursework?" The mean of the first two items measured the perceived severity of the patient's health problem. The mean of the latter two, when reverse-scored, constituted the credibility measure.

Figure 6-1 illustrates the results for both measures. Only diagnostic test results affected severity scores. Subjects rated the patient's sore throat as significantly more severe when the test revealed positive infection evidence (mean = 11.9) than when the test result was negative (mean = 9.3). The presence of nonmedical problems had little influence on perceived severity of the patient's health problem. Credibility scores, however, were affected both by diagnostic outcome and by information about the patient's nonmedical

Table 6-1. Scenario for First Patient Credibility Experiment

JTA is a student at XYZ College. JTA's workload this semester is *about normal—four courses, with no tests scheduled during the last week or for the next three weeks* (**Alternative**: very heavy—five courses, with midterm exams in four of the five courses during the next three days). JTA has been involved in a romantic relationship since last year which *has been very satisfying* (**Alternative**: broke up just last week).

JTA has had a sore throat for the last three days. JTA goes to the Student Health Center for an examination and tells the nurse that the sore throat is very painful. The nurse runs some tests and finds *evidence of a throat infection* (**Alternative**: no evidence of any throat infection).

Note: Italicized phrases are the independent variable manipulations.
Source: From Skelton, 1987.

problems. Figure 6-1 shows credibility scores decreasing in response to information about the patient's problems. Overall, perceived credibility was lower when diagnostic results were negative (the right panel of Figure 6-1); but it also decreased when the test revealed positive signs of infection and patient problems were mentioned in the scenarios (the left panel). Thus the mere mention of nonmedical problems undermined the patient's credibility, even when the patient was legitimately "sick" by biomedical standards.

Subjects also rated the patient on a series of bipolar trait scales. Two of these, calm–anxious and happy–sad, were averaged to measure how much

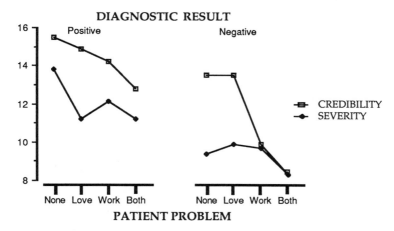

Figure 6-1. Ratings of patient credibility and disease severity in Experiment 1. *Key:* None = no nonmedical problems mentioned in patient description; love = romantic problems mentioned in patient description; work = classwork demands mentioned in patient description; both = romantic and classwork problems mentioned in description.

subjects felt the patient was distressed. The more the patient was perceived as distressed, the lower was his credibility score, $r = -.51$.

Experiment 2

Our first experiment yielded some provocative findings, especially the tendency for patients' nonmedical problems to cause decreases in credibility estimates even with positive diagnostic results. We wondered, however, whether our results were peculiar to romantic and school-related problems, so we followed up with an experiment in which some scenarios mentioned a third source of distress, ill health among members of the patient's family. Specifically, the scenarios were modified to include one of the following statements, in addition to those shown in Table 6-1: "In general, the members of JTA's family have no serious health problems" or "Recently, a member of JTA's family back home was hospitalized due to injuries suffered in a serious accident." All scenarios stated that diagnostic test results were positive; the patient had a documented throat infection. Severity and credibility measures were obtained using the same scales as in Experiment 1. The former were virtually unaffected by the presence of patient problems, so these are ignored. Subjects' ($N = 94$) credibility ratings, however, are shown in Figure 6-2.

As in our first experiment, credibility estimates decreased when patient problems were mentioned. All but two groups' mean credibility scores were

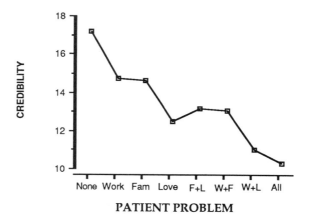

PATIENT PROBLEM

Figure 6-2. Ratings of patient credibility in Experiment 2. *Key:* None = no nonmedical problems mentioned in patient description; work = classwork demands mentioned in patient description; love = romantic problems mentioned in patient description; fam = family illness problem mentioned in patient description; F+L = both family and romantic problems mentioned; W+F = both classwork and family problems mentioned; W+L = both classwork and romantic problems mentioned; all = romantic, classwork, and family problems mentioned in description.

significantly lower ($p < .02$, one-tailed t tests) than that of the group in which no patient problems were mentioned. Credibility scores were marginally lower in the groups where only classwork or family health problems were mentioned. A notable feature of Figure 6-2 is the tendency for credibility scores to decrease as more nonmedical problems were mentioned in the patient scenarios. We combined the one-problem (work, lovelife, and family) groups and the two-problem combination (work + lovelife, work + family, and family + lovelife) groups and then tested for polynomial trends. There was a highly significant ($p < .001$) descreasing linear trend in credibility scores as a function of the number of nonmedical problems (none, one, two, all three) and no quadratic or cubic trend (Fs < 1). This suggests that lay perceivers may factor not only the *kinds* of problems patients experience but also the sheer *quantity* of patient problems into credibility estimates—the "patient doth protest too much" effect.

Clarifying the Processes Underlying Credibility Judgments

The two demonstration experiments suggested that lay perceivers employ a *subtractive* algorithm to judge patient credibility. Negative diagnostic results seemed to cause perceivers to make a "deduction" from baseline estimates of how much to credit the patient's illness complaint. But when perceivers could infer that a patient was also experiencing psychosocial problems, they made further deductions—independently of those prompted by diagnostic evidence. Two additional experiments were conducted to obtain information about how perceivers use diagnostic evidence and to test the generality of our initial findings.

Experiment 3

In this experiment (Skelton et al., 1989), we adopted a more complex method of presenting information about the patient. Subjects ($N = 170$) received multipage file folders containing a symptom checklist and health history form, both allegedly completed by a male patient who visited the College Health Center because of a sore throat, and notes on the patient's visit, purportedly written by a Health Center nurse. Notes in half the folders stated that results of a throat culture were positive; in the remainder, the diagnostic results were described as negative. Other notes orthogonally manipulated information about the patient's nonmedical problems: One stated that the patient mentioned that he had recently broken up with his girlfriend; another stated that the patient mentioned a heavy courseload. Some folders contained neither note, others contained one, and the remainder contained both notes. After examining their folder for three minutes, subjects completed a variety of rating scales.

Two items directly tested perceptions of diagnostic accuracy: "How likely is it that the student has a throat infection?" and "How accurate do you think the throat culture results are?" Each was rated on a 0 to 10-point scale and included a "Can't tell from the information given" option. Only four subjects used the "Can't tell" option for the likelihood-of-infection item. Subjects who received the positive results noted rated the likelihood of infection as very high (mean = 9.6), compared to those who read the negative throat culture note (mean = 1.7). When asked about the accuracy of the throat culture test, 22 subjects chose "Can't tell"; they were equally distributed across the positive and negative results groups. Of those who rated the item, confidence in the test was relatively high (mean = 7.9). But it was significantly higher ($p < .001$) in the positive than the negative groups (means = 8.7 vs. 7.1). Patient problems had no effects on either measure.

Subjects were also asked to rate the likelihood (on 0 to 10-point scales) that they would recommend each of seven actions in response to the patient's sore throat. Two indirect accuracy measures were embedded among the action recommendations: "Refer the patient to a hospital for further testing" and "Perform another throat culture to test for infection." None of the independent variables, including diagnostic results, affected retest likelihoods. Subjects generally saw little need to refer the patient for hospital-based testing, but positive results subjects were more likely to advocate this option than were negative results subjects (means = 2.6 vs. 1.7). A hospital referral would seem logically to be at least as informative in the case of negative signs as positive signs, but negative results subjects apparently did not see things this way. Overall, subjects seemed to take diagnostic test results at face value. Although they were somewhat less likely to see negative diagnostic results as accurate, their action recommendations indicated little motivation to verify the accuracy of negative findings. The perceiver role apparently caused subjects to adopt a perspective similar to that of health professionals, rather than that of the patient.

Measures of patient credibility and disease severity from Experiments 1 and 2 were employed here. The results are shown in Figure 6-3 and are strikingly similar to those of Experiment 1. Only diagnostic results significantly affected perceivers' severity estimates. The patient's credibility, however, was independently influenced by diagnostic results and the presence of nonmedical, psychosocial problems. Regardless of whether the patient had a medically validated infection, subjects viewed him as less credible if romantic or work problems appeared in the nurse's notes.

As in Experiment 1, subjects rated the patient on several bipolar trait scales, and calm–anxious and happy–sad ratings were averaged to produce a "perceived distress" score. The more subjects rated the patient as distressed, the lower they also rated his credibility, $r = -.39$.

Experiment 4

Whereas Experiment 3 showed that lay perceivers are as likely as their professional counterparts to accept diagnostic test results without much

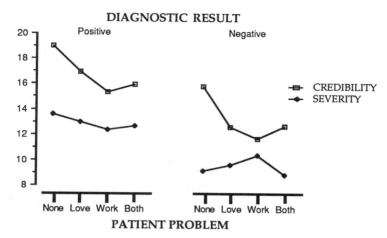

Figure 6-3. Ratings of patient credibility and disease severity in Experiment 3. *Key*: None = no nonmedical problems mentioned in patient description; love = romantic problems mentioned in patient description; work = classwork demands mentioned in patient description; both = romantic and classwork problems mentioned in description.

question, Experiment 4 (Skelton et al., 1989) was primarily intended to clarify the meaning of "credibility." All our previous experiments measured credibility in terms of responses to two questions: "How much do you think the symptom is 'all in the patient's mind'?" and "How much is it just an attempt to avoid coursework?" The first item can be construed as a measure of physical versus psychological causation, and so it begs the question of whether "psychologically"-caused symptoms are less credible. The second item, of course, is a highly leading question for subjects who receive information about the patient's work-related problems. Our previous credibility measure may also have tapped tendencies to blame patients for their health problems. Victims are often blamed for their misfortunes (Coates, Wortman, & Abbey, 1979), especially if they express negative reactions to the misfortune (Westbrook & Nordholm, 1986), and patient derogation varies directly with the degree that health problems are thought to be preventable (Crawford, 1977; Gruman & Sloan, 1983); thus patients who experience both symptoms and nonmedical, psychosocial problems may be viewed as especially blameworthy. Experiment 4 used separate measures of credibility, psychological versus physical causation, and patient blame to establish the discriminant validity of credibility scores.

Experiment 4 also differed from previous studies in that a new nonmedical problem, insomnia, was included in the patient's case history, and patient information was conveyed in the form of a "transcribed interview" between a patient and a Health Center nurse. In some interviews, the patient reported only the symptoms, sore throat and nasal congestion. In others, he also reported a heavy exam schedule, a bout of insomnia, or both. In contrast to all previous experiments, information about the patient's personal problems was elicited through rather aggressive probing by the interviewing nurse, rather than being stated as simple matters of fact (Experiments 1 and 2) or being volunteered spontaneously by the patient (Experiment 3). All interviews indicated that a diagnostic test had revealed a strep infection.

Subjects ($N = 62$) read one of four versions of the nurse–patient interview. Then they responded to a series of rating items. The mean of three items constituted the credibility score: "How believable is the student?," "How much is the student overreacting?" (reverse-scored), and "To what degree does the patient have ulterior motives?" (also reversed). The items "How much is the problem caused primarily by some biological factor?,"

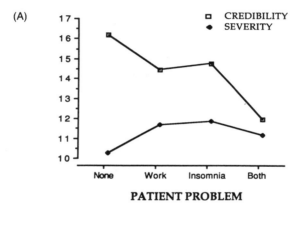

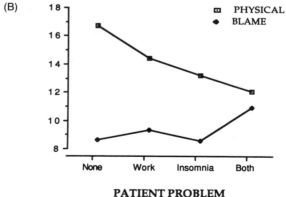

Figure 6-4. (A) Patient credibility and disease severity in Experiment 4. (B) Psychological vs. physical causes and patient blame in Experiment 4.

". . . caused primarily by some psychological factor?," and ". . . all in the student's mind?" were averaged to produce a psychological versus physical cause score, with high scores representing physical causation. Severity was measured by two items, "How serious is the patient's problem?" and "How unpleasant is . . . the problem?" Finally, "How much [is] the problem caused by the student's own behavior?" and "How much is the student to blame for his problem?" comprised the blame score. Subjects also completed bipolar trait ratings similar to those in Experiments 1 and 3. From these ratings were derived scores representing the degree to which the patient was perceived as distressed and as dishonest.

Results for the four major measures are seen in Figure 6-4. Panel A shows that credibility ratings, as usual, decreased when information about the patient's nonmedical problems appeared in the interview. Perceived severity of the patient's health problem was unaffected by the presence of nonmedical sources of patient distress. Panel B shows that the profile of psychological versus physical cause scores was quite similar to that of credibility scores. In fact, the correlation between the two measures was .66. There were no significant group differences, however, in blame scores. In addition, the credibility score was substantially and negatively related to ratings of the patient's dishonesty, $r = -.52$, providing evidence of the credibility measure's concurrent validity. Finally, the correlation between patient distress and credibility was $-.35$, similar in magnitude to the relationships found in Experiments 1 and 3.

Summary

The studies described thus far permit these empirical conclusions:

1. Diagnostic test results are important determinants of credibility assessment outcomes (Experiments 1 and 3).
2. The distinction between negative diagnostic results and "no organic causes" is elusive and blurred for lay perceivers (Experiment 3).
3. The co-occurrence with patient-reported symptoms of nonmedical, psychosocial problems can independently undermine perceived credibility, regardless of the format for presenting such problems (all experiments).
4. Laypersons' credibility judgments can be described reasonably well by a simple, decreasing linear function of the *number* of nonmedical problems the patient experiences (Experiments 2 and 4).
5. The more a patient is perceived as psychologically distressed, the less credible is the patient's health complaint (Experiments 1, 3, and 4).
6. Although credibility and the belief that health complaints have physical causes are related, patient credibility is conceptually distinct from disease severity (all experiments) and from patient derogation (Experiment 4).

I asked earlier, "Whose perspective does the lay perceiver adopt in assessing patients' illness complaints: the patient's or the health professional's?" The findings summarized here indicate the answer: "The profession-al's." Both lay perceiver and professional distinguish patients' symptom reports on the basis of whether the most plausible cause is organic or functional. Both seem relatively insensitive to the indeterminacy of negative diagnostic outcomes. Both tend to question patient complaints when the patient's history provides even minimal evidence consistent with a "psychogenic" or functional interpretation—specifically, any evidence that would lead to the conclusion that the patient is distressed, even when there exists clear evidence of physical pathology. These similarities make a strong case for broad agreement among laypersons with biomedical conceptions of illness.

In addition, our results to date are fully consistent with a discounting interpretation of credibility judgment. Differences between the perspectives of patient and perceiver make symptoms and disease-based explanations less salient for the perceiver, freeing processing capacity for consideration of other factors that might prompt the patient's self-report. The biomedical model makes some of these alternative factors readily available to the perceiver, namely, the expression of negative affect and/or the acquisition of social reinforcers associated with illness. As the sheer number of alternative explanations grows, perceivers' faith in face-value interpretations of patients' symptom reports declines. In Kelley's (1973) language of causal schemata, alternative explanations are *facilitative causes* that undermine perceivers' confidence that patients' symptoms are simply reports of a disease-related pathological process. Thus does the biomedical model lead to a reluctance to validate patients' claims of illness.

Boundary Conditions

The purpose of examining credibility assessment is to reveal lay models of illness and disease. My method until now has been to focus on cases in which the patient's symptom is relatively minor, so that there exists latitude for perceivers to entertain the possibility of alternative explanations for the complaint. But it is perhaps equally revealing to look at cases in which the organic–functional dichotomy should not be expected to be invoked. For example, are there cases where the evidence of organic disease is so overwhelming that perceivers' credibility judgments are unaffected by the presence of patients' nonmedical problems? Does the social context in which symptoms are reported influence perceivers' use of the logic of discounting? Some of my students have performed experiments that address these questions.

Experiment 5

Conklin (1987) used the "health folder" approach of Experiment 3 in an experiment in which subjects ($N = 62$) received information about a male patient. In half the folders, the patient's sole symptom was the usual sore throat; in the remainder, the patient presented to the Health Center with multiple symptoms, including sore throat, high fever, and vomiting. The presence of nonmedical problems (a romantic breakup and schoolwork demands) was manipulated orthogonally. All folders indicated positive diagnostic findings. The two groups in which the patient reported a single minor symptom replicated the outcome of our previous studies: Subjects' credibility estimates decreased when nonmedical problems were cited, relative to estimates by subjects who did not read about the patient's problems. However, when there were several serious symptoms, the presence of nonmedical personal problems did not lead to decreases in perceived credibility. Conklin's findings suggest that there are limits to perceivers' using the logic of discounting on patient complaints. When there is overwhelming evidence of serious disease, the co-occurrence of psychosocial distress may have no effect. One problem with this experiment, however, is that the seriousness of the patient's health problem is confounded with the number of symptoms presented. We are now working on ways to design a manipulation of disease seriousness that is independent of the number and/or types of symptoms reported by patients.

Experiment 6

Although most of our research has dealt with situations in which a patient reports physical symptoms in a medical context, people also suffer from and report *psychological* symptoms to friends or to professional counselors. To the degree that mental representations of "physical" and "mental" illness are different, it's reasonable to expect perceivers' reactions to nonmedical personal problems to be very different when these are reported in a psychological counseling situation. Whereas a patient who reports psychosocial problems in a medical context risks his or her credibility, it seems unlikely that this would occur in a more appropriate social setting. Ralston and Loughlin (1988) adapted the nurse–patient interviews used in Experiment 4 to explore patient credibility in counseling settings.

In this experiment, a student-patient reported an overtly psychological symptom, insomnia, during an interview with a college Counseling Center staff member. In some versions of the interview, it was also revealed that the patient had a number of upcoming exams in his classes. In addition, the patient mentioned in some versions that he had been suffering from a sore throat for several days. In effect, this experiment reversed the roles assigned to sore throat and insomnia in Experiment 4: In the earlier study, the physical symptom was primary and the psychological symptom was mentioned secondarily. In all other respects, the counselor–patient interview was as identical as possible to that used in Experiment 4.

Subjects ($N = 60$) completed ratings measuring the patient's credibility, the severity of his problem, the degree to which the problem was psychologically versus physically caused, and how much the patient was to blame for the problem. The change in the interview context completely altered the outcome, relative to Experiment 4. Subjects did not devalue the patient's credibility at all when schoolwork problems, the secondary physical symptom, or both were mentioned in the interview. The only measure to show any effects of the manipulations was the psychological versus physical score: When the patient mentioned having a sore throat, subjects tended to rate his problem as more "physical" ($p < .07$). Because reporting personal problems is socially appropriate in the context of a counseling session, it is none too surprising that such problems do not detract from perceived credibility. This perhaps sheds further light on why perceivers react so negatively when a medical patient mentions the psychosocial stressors in her or his life. The lay view of the medical treatment setting is so dominated by biomedical assumptions about what constitutes a legitimate medical problem that the patient who violates these assumptions is regarded with suspicion.

Conclusion

Lay Reasoning About Illness

In common with the biomedical reasoning of health-care professionals, lay perceivers rely on the presence of positive organic signs in order to validate patients' complaints. Such reliance is, by itself, neither surprising nor reprehensible. But if we liken the process of diagnosis to that of testing scientific hypotheses, lay perceivers seem to be devoid of the concept of Type II error. They overinterpret the absence of positive physical findings and fail to see the ambiguity of negative diagnostic results.

Lay perceivers also overinterpret patient statements concerning the presence of stress and personal problems, failing to recognize that the *absence* of such statements doesn't mean that patients aren't experiencing these problems. Such misuse of negative information is widespread in human cognition (see the review by Nisbett & Ross, 1980, especially Chapters 3 and 5) and has been called the *feature-positive effect* (e.g., Allison & Messick, 1988).

Both of these are relatively minor problems, however, compared to perceivers' gross misuse of positive information about patients' personal problems. Although there is growing evidence that the sorts of stressors represented by our manipulations of patient problems can precipitate disease by undermining the immune system (Laudenslager & Reite, 1984), lay perceivers continue to view such stressors through the dichotomizing lens of biomedicine's organic and functional categories. Patient distress leads observers to question patients' symptom complaints. In effect, laypersons act as amateur "psychosomatic" theorists, inferring that symptoms are "really" psychologically or gain-motivated defensive reactions to stressful events. What is wrong with this sort of reasoning?

There are three possible meanings of observers' discounting physical causes and patient credibility in the face of positive diagnostic results. First, if observers believe symptoms are imaginary or fabricated (Weiss, 1977), then they are clearly wrong when diagnostic results are positive. Second, if they believe that symptoms are real but the patient's reaction is exaggerated, I find it difficult to understand why seeking treatment for a physical symptom is perceived as exaggerated when patients have personal problems but not when they have no such problems. Finally, even if observers are making the relatively sophisticated observation that psychosocial problems may have rendered the patient more susceptible to disease, it makes little sense to regard the symptom as less physical or the patient as less credible; to paraphrase Weiss (1977), in what way is a stress-facilitated infection less real than any other infection? In short, if observers' reactions to patients who suffer psychosocial distress represent attempts to apply naive psychosomatic theories, then those theories lack logical consistency. This raises questions about whether biopsychosocial models of illness (Engel, 1977) can be accommodated within conventional biomedical thinking, at least as practiced by lay perceivers.

The Study of Illness Representations

The contemporary study of lay illness representations, at least in psychology, has relied primarily on a "patient-as-subject" approach. For example, Leventhal and his associates have studied hypertensive patients' compliance with treatment and hospital patients' delays in seeking treatment as a means of revealing patients' understanding of their disease (Leventhal, Meyer, & Nerenz, 1980; Safer, Jackson, Tharpes, & Leventhal, 1979). Jemmott, Croyle, and their co-workers have studied subjects' perceptions and actions following the diagnosis of a plausible but fictitious disease (Croyle & Sande, 1988; Ditto, Jemmott, & Darley, 1988; Jemmott, Ditto, & Croyle, 1986). Bishop has examined the categorical dimensions of symptoms and diseases, memory for symptoms, and treatment-seeking choices in role-playing situations (Bishop, 1987; Bishop & Converse, 1986). Such worthwhile efforts can reveal much about everyday illness cognition but do not let us determine whether dimensions for representing illness differ in salience when people are in the patient or observer role. In light of these other studies, the research reported here indicates that the perspective one adopts in the patient–observer transaction may make a crucial difference in the explanations of illness that are most available. This implies that a comprehensive view of illness representation processes needs to account for such perspective differences.

Research that does center on lay perceivers' reactions to illness victims focuses either on social comparison and lay referral networks (Sanders, 1982) or on blame-related questions (Gruman & Sloan, 1983; Russel et al., 1985). The former has been useful in identifying the breadth, depth, and outcomes of consultation between nonprofessional peers but has been silent on the crucial issue of what causes the lay perceiver to take a patient's complaints seriously in the first place. The latter tells us some interesting things about the generality of victim blame but little about how perceivers validate patient complaints. The work described in this chapter can be viewed as helping to establish one of the bases for lay consultants' decisions about the advice they offer patients; it remains to be seen how patient credibility affects the advice-giving process.

Future Directions

It has been assumed on logical grounds that credibility is primarily an issue for perceivers, not patients. We need to demonstrate empirically that the assumption is warranted; for example, does observer acquaintance with the patient mitigate the appearance of credibility questions in observers' judgments? We also need to determine whether doubts about credibility emerge naturally from patient–perceiver interaction or instead are an artifact of a rating methodology that directly raises questions about the patient's credibility. In an experiment that is now in progress, subjects are writing open-ended reactions to a nurse–patient interview. These reactions will be analyzed for evidence of spontaneous expressions of doubts about the patient's health problem. If credibility questions do arise spontaneously, we shall have gone a long way toward demonstrating the ecological validity of our research program.

Perhaps the most important unresolved issue concerns the consequences of credibility judgments for patients and their treatment. In seeking to establish the parameters of a believable illness complaint, we have virtually ignored the interpersonal effects of observers' deciding that a patient's complaint is (or is not) to be fully credited. As noted, credibility judgments may mediate lay advice-giving, treatment recommendations, and so forth. In addition, judgments about the patient's character and desirability as a person as well as behavior toward the patient may vary in response to differential perceived credibility. Such issues have potentially grave implications and provide a strong incentive for continued efforts to understand the process and outcomes of laypersons' reasoning about patient credibility.

References

Allison, S. T., & Messick, D. M. (1988). The feature-positive effect, attitude strength, and degree of perceived consensus. *Personality and Social Psychology Bulletin, 14,* 231–241.

Bishop, G. D. (1987). Lay conceptions of physical symptoms. *Journal of Applied Social Psychology, 17,* 127–146.

Bishop, G. D., & Converse, S. A. (1986). Illness representations: A prototype approach. *Health Psychology, 5,* 95–114.

Breuer, J., & Freud, S. (1955). Studies on hysteria. In J. Strachey (Ed. and Trans.), *Standard edition of the complete psychological works of Sigmund Freud* (Vol. 2). London: Hogarth Press. (Original work published in 1925.)

Burgess, M. M. (1980). *Nurses' pain ratings of patients with acute and chronic low back pain.* Unpublished master's thesis, University of Virginia School of Nursing, Charlottesville, VA.

Charap, A. D. (1978). The knowledge, attitudes, and experiences of medical personnel treating pain in the terminally ill. *Mount Sinai Journal of Medicine, 45,* 561–580.

Clark, M., Springer, K., Hagar, M., Drew, L., & Gordon, J. (1988, December 19). Cancer hurts before it kills. *Newsweek,* pp. 58–59.

Coates, D., Wortman, C. B., & Abbey, A. (1979). Reactions to victims. In I. H. Frieze, D. Bar-Tal, & J. S. Carroll (Eds.), *New approaches to social problems* (pp. 21–52). San Francisco: Jossey-Bass.

Cohen, F. L. (1980). Postsurgical pain relief: Patients' status and nurses' medication choices. *Pain, 9,* 265–274.

Colligan, M. J., Pennebaker, J. W., & Murphy, L. R. (1982). *Mass psychogenic illness: A social psychological analysis.* Hillsdale, NJ: Lawrence Erlbaum Associates.

Conklin, H. E. (1987). [Disease seriousness and observer judgments of illness victims]. Unpublished raw data.

Costa, P. T., & McCrae, R. R. (1985). Hypochondriasis, neuroticism, and aging: When are somatic complaints unfounded? *American Psychologist, 40,* 19–28.

Crawford, R. (1977). You are dangerous to your health: The ideology and politics of victim-blaming. *International Journal of Health Services, 7,* 663–680.

Croyle, R. T., & Sande, G. N. (1988). Denial and confirmatory search: Paradoxical consequences of medical diagnoses. *Journal of Applied Social Psychology, 18,* 473–490.

Croyle, R. T., & Uretsky, G. (1987). Effects of mood on the self-appraisal of health status. *Health Psychology, 6,* 239–253.

Davitz, L. J. & Davitz, J. R. (1975). How do nurses feel when patients suffer? *American Journal of Nursing, 75,* 1505–1510.

Ditto, P. H., Jemmott, J. B., III, & Darley, J. M. (1988). Appraising the threat of illness: A mental representational approach. *Health Psychology, 7,* 183–201.

Dollard, J., & Miller, N. E. (1950). *Personality and psychotherapy.* New York: McGraw-Hill.

Engel, G. (1977). The need for a new medical model: A challenge for biomedicine. *Science, 196,* 129–136.

Friedson, E. (1960). Client control and medical behavior. *American Journal of Sociology, 65,* 377.

Gruman, J. C., & Sloan, R. P. (1983). Disease as justice: Perceptions of the victims of physical illness. *Basic and Applied Social Psychology, 4,* 39–46.

Hackett, T. P. (1971, February). Pain and prejudice: Why do we doubt that the patient is in pain? *Medical Times, 99,* 130–141.

Jemmott, J. B., III, Ditto, P. H., & Croyle, R. T. (1986). Judging health status: The effects of perceived prevalence and personal relevance. *Journal of Personality and Social Psychology, 50,* 899–905.

Jennings, D. (1986). The confusion between disease and illness in clinical medicine. *Canadian Medical Association Journal, 135,* 865–870.

Jones, E. E., & Nisbett, R. (1972). The actor and the observer: Divergent perceptions of the causes of behavior. In E. E. Jones, D. E. Kanouse, H. H. Kelley, R. E.

Nisbett, S. Yalins, & B. Weiner (Eds.), *Attribution: Perceiving the causes of behavior* (pp. 79–93). Morristown, NJ: General Learning Press.

Kelley, H. H. (1973). The processes of causal attribution. *American Psychologist, 28,* 107–128.

Kerckhoff, A. C., & Back, K. W. (1968). *The June bug: A study of hysterical contagion.* New York: Appleton-Century-Crofts.

Klass, P. (1989, January). Prosecuting the patient. *Discover,* pp. 12–14.

Laudenslager, M. L., & Reite, M. L. (1984). Losses and separations: Immunological consequences and health implications. In P. Shaver (Ed.), *Review of personality and social psychology* (vol. 5, pp. 285–312). Beverly Hills, CA: Sage Publications.

Leventhal, H. (1986). Symptom reporting: A focus on process. In S. McHugh & T. M. Vallis (Eds.), *Illness behavior: A multidisciplinary model* (pp. 219–237). New York: Plenum Press.

Leventhal, H., & Everhart, D. (1979). Emotion, pain, and physical illness. In C. E. Izard (Ed.), *Emotions in personality and psychopathology* (pp. 263–299). New York: Plenum Press.

Leventhal, H., Meyer, D., & Nerenz, D. (1980). The common sense representation of illness danger. In S. Rachman (Ed.), *Contributions to medical psychology* (Vol. 2, pp. 7–30). New York: Pergamon Press.

Marks, R. M., & Sachar, E. J. (1973). Undertreatment of medical inpatients with narcotic analgesics. *Annals of Internal Medicine, 78,* 173–181.

Maslach, C. (1982). Burnout in the health professions: A social psychological analysis. In G. S. Sanders & J. Suls (Eds.), *Social psychology of health and illness* (pp. 227–251). Hillsdale, NJ: Lawrence Erlbaum Associates.

Nisbett, R. E., & Ross, L. (1980). *Human inference: Strategies and shortcomings of social judgment.* Englewood Cliffs, NJ: Prentice-Hall.

Parsons, T. (1951). *The social system.* New York: Free Press.

Ralston, E. S., & Loughlin, C. A. (1988). [Co-occurring psychological symptoms and patient problems in a counseling interview: Effects on patient credibility]. Unpublished raw data.

Russell, D., Lenel, J. C., Spicer, C., Miller, J., Albrecht, J., & Rose, J. (1985). Evaluating the physically disabled: An attributional analysis. *Personality and Social Psychology Bulletin, 11,* 23–31.

Safer, M. A., Tharpes, Q. J., Jackson, T. C., & Leventhal, H. (1979). Determinants of three stages of delay in seeking care at a medical clinic. *Medical Care, 17,* 11–28.

Sanders, G. S. (1981). The interactive effect of social comparison and objective information on the decision to see a doctor. *Journal of Applied Social Psychology, 11,* 390–400.

Sanders, G. S. (1982). Social comparison and perceptions of health and illness. In G. S. Sanders & J. Suls (Eds.), *Social psychology of health and illness* (pp. 129–161). Hillsdale, NJ: Lawrence Erlbaum Associates.

Skelton, J. A. (1987, May). Legitimating "second-hand" symptoms: Observers' judgments of illness victims: In R. T. Croyle (Chair), *Illness appraisal: Social and cognitive processes.* Symposium conducted at the 59th annual meeting of the Midwestern Psychological Association, Chicago.

Skelton, J. A., Conklin, H. E., Ralston, E. S., & Loughlin, C. A. (1989). *Lay observers' judgments of symptom legitimacy.* Manuscript submitted for publication.

Skelton, J. A., & Pennebaker, J. W. (1990). The verbal system. In J. T. Cacioppo

& L. G. Tassinary (Eds.), *Principles of psychophysiology: Physical, inferential, and social elements* (pp. 631–657). Cambridge: Cambridge University Press.

Smith, T. W., Snyder, C. R., & Perkins, S. C. (1983). The self-serving function of hypochondriacal complaints: Physical symptoms as self-handicapping strategies. *Journal of Personality and Social Psychology, 44,* 787–797.

Sternbach, R. A. (1974). *Pain patients: Traits and treatment.* New York: Academic Press.

Stevens, H. (1986). Is it organic or is it functional? Is it hysteria or malingering? *Psychiatric Clinics of North America, 9,* 241–254.

Taylor, A. G., Skelton, J. A., & Butcher, J. (1984). Duration of pain condition and physical pathology as determinants of nurses' assessments of patients in pain. *Nursing Research, 33,* 4–8.

Tessler, R., & Mechanic, D. (1978). Psychological distress and perceived health status. *Journal of Health and Social Behavior, 19,* 254–262.

Verbrugge, L. (1985). Triggers of symptoms and health care. *Social Science and Medicine, 20,* 855–876.

Weiss, J. M. (1977). The current status of the concept of a psychosomatic disorder. In Z. J. Lipowski, D. R. Lipsitt, & P. C. Whybrow (Eds.), *Psychosomatic medicine: Current trends and clinical applications* (pp. 162–171). New York: Oxford University Press.

Westbrook, M. T., & Nordholm, L. A. (1986). Reactions to patients' self- or chance-blaming attributions for illnesses having varying lifestyle involvement. *Journal of Applied Social Psychology, 16,* 428–446.

Wiener, C. L. (1975). Pain assessment on an orthopedic ward. *Nursing Outlook, 23,* 508–516.

Wulff, H. R. (1976). *Rational diagnosis and treatment.* London: Blackwell Scientific.

Zborowski, M. (1969). *People in pain.* San Francisco: Jossey-Bass.

Zola, I. K. (1966) Culture and symptoms: An analysis of patients' presenting complaints. *American Sociological Review, 31,* 615–630.

7

Illness Representations in Medical Anthropology: A Critical Review and a Case Study of the Representation of AIDS in Haiti

Paul Farmer and Byron J. Good

Anthropologists and psychologists writing about illness representations during the past decade share many concerns: How do individuals conceive illness and symptoms? How do they view their cause, potential consequences, and likely effects on their lives? How do these perceptions influence psychological and behavioral responses? A cursory reading of the literature in health psychology and medical anthropology, however, indicates important differences in the concerns, approaches, and methods of these disciplines. Anthropologists are ethnographers, researchers for whom "the field" is a foreign cultural environment to be experienced, understood, reported on, and analyzed; this is assumed, whether their research site is a remote village in the highlands of New Guinea, a mental health center treating victims of violence in Central America, or an oncology practice in a Boston hospital. Anthropologists from diverse theoretical backgrounds, working in very different settings, thus bring to their research assumptions and problems that mark their writing on illness representations as distinctively anthropological. Two dimensions of this approach are worth noting here.

First, anthropologists view illness representations as dimensions of *culture*. Different as their theories may be about the nature of social reality, symbolic forms, or representational processes, and widely variant as their methods may be for studying these, medical anthropologists view culture as the matrix for illness representation and the presumed independent variable in much of their research. *Cultures* (plural), not merely individuals, vary as to how symptoms are interpreted and addressed, how bodily sensations or illness labels are evaluated and given meaning, how sufferers and their families respond and seek care. "Common sense" is understood not simply as a lay view of the world but as a cultural system, not only a distinctive perspective on the world (to be contrasted with a scientific or clinical perspective, for instance) but a set of assumptions about the world and how to act in it for members of a particular society, the general shape of a culturally distinctive world (Geertz, 1983). When it comes to warding off illness or managing threatening symptoms, common sense for American college sophomores has little in common with that for adolescents in the New Guinea highlands. Thus, for the anthropologist, "basic psychological processes" are not independent of content or context; culture is neither a single variable nor a moderating influence, but the very stuff of social and psychological process, the grounds for human experience and action. This assumption of the *cultural* constitution of illness representations runs throughout the history of medical anthropology as a discipline and forms its primary problematic; much of the psychology literature, from this perspective, often seems culturally naive.

Second, anthropologists share a common concern about how we represent the cultural representations of others. During the past decade, anthropology has come to focus increasingly on the nature of ethnographic representation, on how ethnographers portray "the other," on the place of the author in ethnographic texts and the "authorization" of the portrayals of others. This is no surprise for a discipline in which terms like savage, magical, mystical, protoscientific, folk, common sense, and popular have all served as adjectives for illness beliefs, for a discipline in which leading figures publish sharply contradictory accounts of the cultural representations of the same society, or for a discipline increasingly aware of its historical ties to colonialism. However, given the current lack of agreement in the field about any particular grand theory, longstanding debates about the relationships between anthropological models and those of the natives, about research methods and the reproducibility of data, and about the validity of interpretation are not easily avoided. During recent years, these issues have resurfaced and produced what Marcus and Fischer (1986, p. 8) labeled a "crisis of representation," which in their view has served as "the intellectual stimulus for the contemporary vitality of experimental writing in anthropology." These larger concerns provide a context for recent writings on illness representations in anthropology, including debates over "meaning-centered" and "critical" approaches to interpreting medical discourse. Questions about the place of the observer in the text, the epistemological status of nonscientific knowledge, the social and historical context of medical knowledge, and the politics of representation, which are common to anthropological writing, will appear odd to the psychologist reader interested in anthropology's contributions to this field.

In the following pages, we provide a critical review of anthropological approaches to illness representations, outlining four alternative "paradigms" that have emerged in the past several decades and the resulting debate among applied, cognitive, "meaning-centered," and "critical" approaches to the field. In the second half of the chapter, we describe research on the evolving representation of AIDS in rural Haiti. We use these data as a basis for outlining six issues in current anthropological research on illness representations, posed as a series of questions, which indicate our view of the direction anthropological studies in this field are taking. It is our overall contention that these issues must be addressed if research on illness representation, whether in anthropology or in psychology, is to attain cross-cultural validity and thus rise above the reproduction of our own commonsense view of human nature.

Historical Background

Although it was scarcely more than 20 years ago that the label "medical anthropology" came to describe a subfield, the history of the anthropological study of illness is as old as the discipline itself. It was at the turn of the century, when physician-anthropologist W. H. R. Rivers began his fieldwork, that illness representations first became the object of systematic and sustained investigation. There is some irony in initiating a discussion of the gap between current anthropological and psychological understandings of illness representations with a consideration of Rivers; though remembered most for his work in ethnography, he was also a physician and the founder of the Cambridge School of experimental psychology (Slobodin, 1978). Wellin (1978, p. 25) underlines two propositions central to Rivers's posthumously published work:

> The first was that primitive medical practices follow logically from underlying medical beliefs, that is, that native medical practices "are not a medley of disconnected and meaningless customs . . . [but rather] . . . are inspired by definite ideas concerning the causation of disease" (1924:51). His second proposition was that native medical practices and beliefs, taken together, were parts of culture and constituted a "social institution . . . [to be studied in terms of the same] . . . principles or methods found to be of value in the study of social institutions in general" (1926:61).

The idea of illness and responses to it as part of culturally constituted systems is one that is widely shared even today. Equally enduring was the insistence that behavior is linked to "underlying beliefs," which are in turn linked to a people's "worldview." From the outset, anthropological studies of illness representations have been contextualizing, insisting on the embeddedness in the social world of all that may be observed or elicited.

If Rivers established illness representations as a topic worthy of study, it should be noted that he was especially interested in concepts of *disease causation*. The continuing influence of this concern is reflected in Clements's *Primitive Concepts of Disease*, which appeared in 1932. The study fit neatly into the already discredited paradigm of historical particularism, which attempted to place various "culture traits"—in this case, etiologic concepts—into larger frameworks of geographical diffusion and chronological sequences. Clements's lengthy tabulations did not provoke emulation, and there were few noteworthy studies in the subsequent decade. During World War II, Ackerknecht began to publish his more influential investigations. His work—that of a trained physician heavily indebted to functionalist anthropology—reified the primitive–modern distinction: "Primitive medicine is primarily magico-religious, utilizing a few rational elements, while our medicine is predominantly rational and scientific employing a few magic elements" (Ackerknecht, 1946, p. 467, cited in Wellin, 1978, p. 30). This radical and frequently repeated distinction did not prevent Ackerknecht from deploying Western categories (e.g., surgery, psychotherapy, obstetrics) to describe "primitive" responses to illness and necessarily impoverished his understanding of the illness categories of other cultures.

In the decades following World War II, what has come to be called "medical anthropology" developed in several relatively distinct phases. Many of the debates over the nature of illness representations, prominent in the literature today, are understandable in relation to this history. The 1950s and 1960s saw the rapid growth of medical anthropology as an applied practical discipline in the field of international public health. For example, George Foster, along with a group of his young students and research associates at the Smithsonian Institution, began active collaboration with public health specialists in the Pan American Health Organization (Foster, 1978). As American foreign aid and international agencies supported public health efforts in the developing world, anthropologists began to find positions in schools of public health and a variety of nongovernmental organizations. Several of Benjamin Paul's students at Harvard continued careers in schools of public health or medicine.[1] Medical anthropology as an applied discipline has continued to grow and has become increasingly specialized, focusing on health education, nutrition, infectious diseases, diarrheal disease, infant mortality, and primary health-care systems, as well as more classic public health interventions. "Illness representations" in this context have taken on special meaning, as described later.

Beginning in the late 1960s, medical anthropology began to take new shape as the comparative study of medical systems, particularly focusing on those societies in which the "great traditions" of non-Western professional medicine have flourished alongside diverse popular medical traditions. With the support of the Wenner-Gren Foundation, Charles Leslie organized the first major research conference on Asian medical systems in 1971 (Leslie, 1976). For the first time, anthropologists tackled the ethnographic study of

---

[1] Hazel Weidman's (1978) study of health culture in Miami led to the creation of mental health services targeted to culturally distinct groups; Weidman also founded the Society for Medical Anthropology. Steven Polgar, who did extensive work on natality and its regulation, worked with the World Health Organization and taught at a school of public health (see Polgar, 1972; Weidman, 1982).

the classical traditions—Ayurveda and Yunani medicine in India, Chinese medicine in several Asian societies, Galenic medicine in both Islamic and Hispanic societies—as well as the interrelations among professional, folk, and popular medical traditions. This research took its place alongside more traditional studies of healing systems of small, nonliterate societies and provided a new focus on medical pluralism, on the plurality of illness representations as well as the diversity of healers and medical institutions. Multiple "idioms of distress," care-seeking strategies that organize behavior in relation to alternative resources, and multiple and often highly contested interpretations of illness and medical authority thus emerge as central issues in the study of illness representations. These studies of plural medical systems have also provided many of the basic concepts and methods for anthropological studies of health care in American society.

The mid- and late 1970s saw the development of a new self-consciousness of theorizing in medical anthropology (beginning, notably, with Fabrega, 1974). Long criticized in the academy for being applied and atheoretical, anthropologists with an interest in medical systems, illness experience and healing, and illness representations have developed an increasingly sophisticated theoretical discourse, bringing medical anthropology to the center of the discipline at large.

Beginning in the 1950s, "ethnoscience," or "ethnosemantics," which contributed to the eventual emergence of the cognitive sciences (Gardener, 1985), used medical phenomena as one source for analysis of cognitive representations. Disease nosologies elicited in the field were construed as hierarchically structured taxomonies held to represent the informants' mental representations of disease. It was asserted that inclusion criteria were largely the presence or absence of distinctive attributes or "features." Frake (1961), for example, borrowed from linguistics the technique of componential analysis to analyze the diagnostic terms for skin disorders by members of one small, nonliterate society. Although few of the early cognitive anthropologists would consider themselves medical anthropologists, today cognitive studies have emerged as one important approach to the study of illness representations within medical anthropology.

Another broad paradigm, often identified as the "meaning-centered," or interpretive, approach, which has been influential since the 1980s, is associated with the work of Arthur Kleinman and the journal *Culture, Medicine and Psychiatry*. A number of medical anthropologists have explored illness representations from the perspectives of symbolic and interpretive anthropology, phenomenology, social constructivist theories, and discourse analysis. Finally, some medical anthropologists have recently called for the development of a "critical" medical anthropology, to be focused more explicitly on the representation of power relations and social inequalities within illness discourse. Contributions from each of these traditions are examined next.

Four Anthropological Approaches to the Study of Illness Representations

The positions that have developed in the field during the past several decades are far from exclusive; methods and theoretical approaches from all are found in the work of many medical anthropologists. However, the logic of analysis of illness representations among anthropologists varies considerably among these approaches and provides the basis for the most prominent debates in the field. A brief outline of four conceptual approaches to illness representations should serve to make sense of the debates among the anthropological tribe and provide a map for reading in this field by nonanthropologists.

Illness Representations as Folk Beliefs: The Applied Tradition

Since the 1950s, anthropologists have collaborated with public health professionals in a wide variety of projects designed to bring services to populations in developing societies and in the United States. Much of this work focused on a deceptively complex problem: how to get local populations to alter their behavior in a fashion that would improve their health. Wells can be dug, vaccinations offered, birth control devices or medications provided, oral rehydration therapies made available, but if these services and technologies are not used or not used appropriately, they will be of little value. Public health officials saw resistance to such obviously effective behaviors as irrational, the result of ignorance, superstitions, or traditional views that conflict with modern medical knowledge and require change. Social psychologists of the same era, collaborating with health specialists facing similar problems, were developing the Health Belief Model as a research and intervention tool. Anthropologists addressed the problem by analyzing health beliefs in relation to a local culture. As Benjamin Paul (1955, p.5) wrote in the introduction to the most important early collection of studies in this tradition:

> What appears from the outside as irrational belief and behavior becomes intelligible when viewed from within. Perceiving the connections between items of belief and behavior as the people themselves perceive them enables us to make better sense of the seemingly capricious pattern of acceptance and rejection, of successful and unsuccessful education efforts.

Indigenous "items of belief," Paul argued, must be understood from the "native's point of view." Only then can the seemingly irrational be understood, and only then can programs of education be developed that work within the local frame of reference. Illness representations, from this perspective, are beliefs with a logic to be uncovered by ethnographic research.

Many of the anthropological contributions to public health work begin with this important, if rather straightforward, set of insights. However, this general approach to the study of illness representations has limitations from both practical and theoretical points of view. First, the behaviors identified are often best understood in relation to structural conditions—gross inequalities, poverty, inferior housing and work conditions—or the irrationalities of health bureaucracies and practitioners, rather than as a result of rational albeit mistaken beliefs. Very often neither the "beliefs" nor the behaviors are under the voluntary control of individuals, as this "Enlightenment" model assumes.

Second, facile recourse to the label "belief" has been challenged on methodological grounds. Items termed beliefs are often deduced from illness narratives, which have been found to vary by social context, the audience of the narrative, and the stage in the illness process in which the account is elicited (Good, 1986). Illness stories told to a doctor differ from those told to friends in the home, and both differ from those told to a researcher. Stories vary before and after diagnosis. They vary when the judgment of the narrator is in question, when important social norms are threatened, or when compensation is being sought. Standardized elicitation methods such as those used by many researchers produce a standard story, but it is far from clear that this story represents "belief."

Third, the very concept "belief" as a frame for analyzing illness representations has been challenged on theoretical grounds (Good, 1986). "Beliefs" in 20th-century philosophy, especially recent linguistic philosophy, have been conceived as propositional, normative, and voluntary. Beliefs are often represented as a set of propositions which can be judged as more or less true, depending on the adequacy of their ostensive representation of the objective world. Folk beliefs about illness are, from this perspective, a kind of protoscience (cf. Horton, 1967), with medical science providing the norm against which they may be judged. Indeed, as Smith (1977, 1979) has shown, since the 18th century "belief" has increasingly been used in Western languages for propositions that either are essentially uncertain or are not true. The view that the earth is round is knowledge, not belief. One can believe AIDS is caused by witchcraft, but *we* know it is caused by a retrovirus. Inquiry into folk "beliefs" thus assumes biomedicine as the norm, authorizing the perspective of the researcher over that of the research subject. Furthermore, this generally rationalist perspective assumes that *beliefs drive behavior*, that individuals weigh the costs and benefits of particular acts based on their beliefs about the threats and potential consequences of behavior, and that they seek to maximize benefits in their behavior. Behavior, as well as beliefs, are thus essentially voluntary characteristics of individuals seeking to maximize their personal good, a theoretical position Sahlins (1976) identifies as "subjective utilitarianism."

The theory of illness representations as folk beliefs has been criticized (Good 1977, 1986; Scheper-Hughes & Lock, 1987; A. Young, 1982) on several grounds. It is far from clear that beliefs are propositional in form or indeed that believing, as we conceive this process, is a universal phenomenon (cf. Needham, 1972). Opinions and the speech acts from which they are deduced are seldom protoscientific, and the "objective reality" to which they refer is not simply the biological world but a socially and culturally constituted reality. A concept of belief that authorizes the knowledge of the researcher over the opinions of those who are the object of study is thus open to epistemological criticism. It also poses subtle methodological problems that challenge the validity of the findings. As Favret-Saada (1980) remarks, when a Parisian intellectual asks a French peasant "Do you believe in witchcraft?," the only response possible is "Of course not, do you take me for a fool?" Finally, the "rational man" theory of motivation and behavior is inadequate, even when rationality is treated as a culturally distinctive form of reasoning. Psychologists as well as anthropologists are increasingly aware of the psychological and structural conditions that undermine the relation between rational understanding and human behavior. Indeed, precisely this disjunction serves as the motive for much of the research in medical psychology.

Although serious questions have been raised about the view of illness representations as folk beliefs, this tradition of applied research has continued vitality, contributes in an extremely important way to efforts to solve global health problems, and is likely to play an ongoing role in applied research. However, the recognition of the theoretical and methodological problems outlined here have contributed to the development of alternative approaches in the field.

Illness Representations as Formal Cognitive Structures: The View From Cognitive Anthropology

Researchers working within the cognitive paradigm have focused on the formal structures of cognitive processing—classificatory systems, prototypes, propositions, schemata, or narrative structures. Within the anthropological tradition, these are viewed as representational forms provided by culture, and an elegant tradition of formal methods has developed to investigate how these forms vary from society to society as well as among individuals.

Some early research in this paradigm focused on medical classification: symptoms of illness, diseases, causes of illness, and types of healers. Culture, it was argued, identifies the distinctive features of such phenomena and provides frames for organizing relations among them. Detailed studies were undertaken to investigate the relations between representations of illness and patterns of health-care seeking (Young, 1981). This tradition has been productive and continues to generate research investigating cultural models—akin to schemas—of particular disorders, their cross-cultural variation, and levels of consensus about them among individuals within a culture.

In a paper entitled "A Propositional Analysis of U.S. American Beliefs About Illness," D'Andrade notes that an earlier study of illness categories among North American and Mexican informants, using a multidimensional scaling feature model, "gave us one representation about what people believe, but not a representation of how people go on believing" (1976, p.155). A revised methodology allowed him to elaborate a model with "generative capacity" by incorporating the "transitivity of subset–superset relations." That is, he felt that he was able to account for informants' ability to evaluate a series of propositions that they had surely never entertained prior to the elicitation session. He further improved his own earlier multidimensional scaling work by determining "some of the specific conceptual relations which link properties" (p. 176). His work spoke specifically to the "feature models" of an earlier generation:

> The attributes of disease with which informants are most concerned and which they use in making inferences about diseases are not the defining or distinctive features, but the connotative attributes of "seriousness," "curability," and the like. For example, what people know about cancer is not what defines a cell as cancerous, but rather that having cancer is often fatal and painful. (pp. 177–178)

D'Andrade went on to note that although a cure for all cancers would not change the defining features of cancer, such a discovery *would* alter dramatically "the way cancer is thought of." And that, he added, "is what is culturally and socially, as well as psychologically, important." His conclusion was that feature models, whether based on componential analysis or multidimensional techniques, do not adequately represent belief systems.

Similar concerns have led to increasing focus on the forms illness representations take and on naturally occurring discourse and its relation to formal cognitive structures. Some cognitivists have thus begun to focus on illness narratives, their cultural shaping, and the cultural models that underlie their production (Price, 1987). Such work has begun to shift attention from the formal properties of illness models to their relation to natural discourse, and thus to context and performance characteristics of illness representations. This growing interest they share with sociolinguists, interpretive anthropologists, and others interested in illness narratives.

Cognitive anthropologists have provided elegant methods and analyses of folk illness beliefs. Their work has shared some of the criticisms, however, of the less methodologically developed approach to illness beliefs in the applied tradition, outlined previously. In particular, illness representations have continued to be seen in mentalistic terms, abstracted from "embodied knowledge," affect, and social and historical forces that shape illness meanings. Illness models are viewed in formal, semantic terms, with little attention to pragmatic and performative dimensions. And the formal methods that lie at the heart of their contribution often raise the specter of artifact, the danger that the methods *produce* the neat cognitive models claimed to be those of the informants or produce a form of illness representations that is highly constrained by the mode of their elicitation.

Illness Representations as Culturally Constituted Illness Realities: The "Meaning-Centered" Tradition

Arthur Kleinman's work, beginning in the late 1970s, marked the emergence of medical anthropology as a systematic and theoretically grounded field of inquiry within the larger discipline. Kleinman designated the medical system a "cultural system," and thus a distinctive field of anthropological inquiry. His work combined an interest in complex medical systems following the Leslie tradition, detailed ethnographic analyses of illness and healing in Chinese cultures, theoretical development linked to symbolic, interpretive, and social constructivist writing, and an interest in applied medical anthropology (Kleinman, 1975, 1980). Here we briefly outline some dimensions of the work on illness representations that have grown out of this tradition.

Kleinman argued that illness representations can be understood as "explanatory models," schemata for understanding illness held by individual sufferers and families as well as clinicians and healers, models available in popular, folk, and professional medical cultures. These models shed light on questions concerning etiology, type and onset of symptoms, pathophysiology, course and consequences of illness, and appropriate treatments. In contrast with cognitive researchers, who tended to rely on formal elicitation techniques, researchers investigating explanatory models often conducted their studies in "clinically relevant" contexts, among the sick and those they consulted during illness or therapeutic interventions. Explanatory models were recognized to emerge in situated discourse, to shift with course of illness, to constitute personal accounts of various dimensions of the illness experience:

> In general, patient explanatory models usually are not fully articulated, tend to be less abstract [than clinicians' models], may be inconsistent and even self-contradictory, and may be based on erroneous evaluation of evidence. Nonetheless, they are comparable to clinical models (also often tacit) as attempts to explain clinical phenomena. . . . Such models reflect social class, cultural beliefs, education, occupation, religious affiliation, and past experience with illness and health care. (Kleinman, Eisenberg, & Good, 1978, p. 256)

Thus research in this tradition tended to be concerned less with the way in which people store and process information about sickness and more with ways in which explanatory models come into play as people attempt to interpret disturbing somatic, psychological, or social experience. Explanatory model research has probed the place of such models in discourse about illness and their role in the elaboration of "illness realities" and the shaping of responses to such realities in the context of socially organized power relations.

Second, practitioners of the meaning-centered approach resisted the formal definition of illness categories in relation to distinctive features, exploring instead the notion that illness representations are multivocal symbols that condense a set of associated meanings and are linked to an underlying "semantic network":

> The meaning of a disease category cannot be understood simply as a set of defining symptoms. It is rather a "syndrome" of typical experiences, a set of words, experiences, and feelings which typically "run together" for the members of a society. . . . This conception of medical semantics directs our attention to the use of medical discourse to articulate the experience of distinctive patterns of social stress, to the use of illness language to negotiate relief for the sufferer, and thus to the constitution of the meaning of medical language in its use in a variety of communicative contexts. (Good, 1977, p. 27)

Unlike the research in psychology on semantic networks, where the term has been used to designate patterns of association of ideas or memories in cognitive storage (Johnson-Laird, Herrmann, & Chaffin, 1984), the anthropological account of semantic networks treats them as *cultural*, as symbols associated at a deep level in culture, associations which both underlie explanatory models and social experience and are built up through historical practice and experience. Although no single formal method has been developed to study semantic networks, studies have been conducted of "heart distress" in Iran (Good, 1977; Good & Good, 1982), disease categories in Ngbandi society in Zaire (Bibeau, 1981), hypertension in the United States (Blumhagen, 1980), madness in Sri Lanka (Amarasingham, 1980), and "bad blood" in Haiti (Farmer, 1988).

Third, drawing on phenomenological and social constructionist theories, medical anthropologists have explored the relation between illness representations and illness "realities." That which is real for members of a society—"diseases" treated by physicians, possessing spirits, vague or neatly defined forms of suffering—are constituted through representational and interpretive processes. The nature of those realities, though often highly contested, is determined not only by the natural history of biological and psychological processes, both of which may play a more or less important role, but also by the representation of illness. Research has thus focused on the role of rhetorical processes in the construction and reconstruction of illness realities (Csordas, 1983; Good & Good, 1981), on the relation of representation to embodied experience (Farmer, 1988), on the historical production, continuity, and change of illness representations (Brandt, 1987; Kleinman, 1986), and on the representation of illness realities in narratives (Kleinman, 1988).

The approach to illness representations outlined here has led to debate both among its practitioners and among those outlining alternative approaches. Explanatory model research has been criticized along lines outlined for the folk belief model as assuming a "rational man" (for a debate, see Young, 1982, and commentaries that followed), although from the beginning explanatory models were seldom seen as fixed models motivating behavior. On the other hand, the methods of the approach are essentially ethnographic and lack the experimental rigor of the cognitivists; they have also been criticized from that perspective. More recently, some have charged that the view that illness realities are constituted through interpretive and representational processes treats such realities as consensual and fails to provide a "critical" stance vis-à-vis illness representations. Some have begun to develop this position as an alternative theoretical frame for the analysis of illness representations.

Illness Representations as Authorized Misrepresentation: Views From "Critical" Medical Anthropology

In contrast to the social constructionist line, some have attempted to develop a neo-Marxist approach to illness representations. One touchstone to the position is Antonio Gramsci's analysis of hegemony and the development of his claim that common sense is ultimately hegemonic, a view of reality developed to justify existing social relations. For Gramsci, hegemony asserted itself subtly, leading to

> the permeation throughout civil society . . . of an entire system of values, attitudes, beliefs, morality, etc., that is in one way or another supportive of the established order and the class interests that dominate it . . . to the extent that this prevailing consciousness is internalized by the broad masses, it becomes part of "common sense." . . . For hegemony to assert itself successfully in any society, therefore, it must operate in a dualistic manner: as a "general conception of life" for the masses and as a "scholastic programme." (Greer, cited in Martin, 1987, p. 23)

A critical medical anthropology forcefully poses the question of when illness representations are actually *misrepresentations* that serve the interests of those in power, be they colonial powers, elites within a society, the medical profession, or empowered men. Forms of suffering grounded in social relations can be defined as illness, medicalized, and brought under the authority of the medical profession and the state. Thus symptoms of hunger or diseases that result from poverty, whether among the North American poor or the impoverished cane cutters of Brazil, are medicalized, treated as a condition of individual bodies—"diarrhea," "TB," "nerves," or "stress"—rather than a collective concern. The transformation of a political problem into a medical one is often akin to "neutralizing" critical consciousness and thus serves the interests of the hegemonic class (e.g., Scheper-Hughes & Lock, 1987; Taussig, 1980). Analysis of illness representations therefore requires a critical unmasking of the dominant interests , an exposé of the mechanisms by which they are supported by authorized discourse: What is misrepresented in illness representations must be revealed.

Idioms of distress and illness representations of those who are suffering may, in turn, be viewed as forms of resistance (Comaroff, 1985; Kleinman, 1986; Martin, 1987; Ong, 1987; Scheper-Hughes & Lock, 1987). Here the critical task would seem to be offering an interpretation of an illness that renders explicit the social and political meanings locked inside a sickness:

> The real task of therapy calls for an archaeology of the implicit in such a way that the processes by which social relations are mapped onto disease are brought to light, de-reified, and in so doing liberate the potential for dealing with antagonistic contradictions and breaking the chain of oppression. (Taussig, 1980, p. 7)

In short, critical analysis must examine how illness representations serve to represent and misrepresent power relations within a society. Development of this approach follows in part a shift within anthropology from a dominant focus on symbols and meaning to a focus on practice (Ortner, 1984). These ideas have not yet been fully explored within medical anthropology. However, they are certain to continue to serve as the nexus for debate about the nature of illness representations.

Although our own work has been grounded in the meaning-centered and critical paradigms, it has not been our aim to argue simply for one position over the others. Indeed, the general positions outlined here are not exclusive to individuals; many medical anthropologists have written from the perspective of more than one analytic framework. Our purpose has rather been to outline the dominant analytic perspectives, the logic of the analysis of illness representations within each, and the debates that have emerged within and among these positions; we hoped to clarify for nonanthropologists what may otherwise seem very parochial debates. A review of recent research in medical anthropology will confirm not only that individuals move across these perspectives in their work, but that however different their theoretical approaches and accompanying methodologies, a set of common concerns is emerging. Nearly all writing in the field today reflects a strong sense of the need for much clearer contextualization—both ethnographic and histori-cal—of the sources of our data and the nature of our interpretations.

Case Study: AIDS Comes to a Haitian Village

In this section we begin with a description of the changing representation of AIDS in rural Haiti, a case that demands both cultural analysis and understanding of historical change and power relations as dimensions of illness representations. We then outline a set of questions that any research on illness representations should be able to address, questions that are the source of research at this time, designed to serve as a set of cautionary tales as applicable to the psychologist researchers as to the anthropologist.

Do Kay, a village of fewer than 1000 persons, stretches along an unpaved road that cuts through the central plateau of Haiti.[2] During the rainy season, the trip from Port-au-Prince can take several hours, adding to the impression of insularity. This perception is misleading, as the village owes its existence to a project conceived in the Haitian capital and drafted in Washington, D. C.: Do Kay is composed substantially for the families of peasant farmers displaced some 30 years ago to make room for building Haiti's largest dam. By all the standard measures, inhabitants of the area are now very poor.

Early in 1987, the first case of AIDS was registered in Do Kay. Because we had initiated investigation of local understanding of AIDS years before, we were able to document the subsequent elaboration of a fairly detailed and widely shared cultural model of AIDS. Another important event occurred during the course of this study. The collapse, in 1986, of the country's longstanding family dictatorship led to political changes that were keenly felt in village Haiti. These changes also had a profound effect on the process of illness representation, though in subtle ways that only longitudinal research can reveal. Interviews dating from 1983 to the present reveal not just the role of culture in the structuring of illness narratives, but the ways in which those narratives are elaborated, how they change over time, the embeddedness of representations—also changing—in narratives, and their significance to the experience of illness.

The case study presented here is based on field research in rural Haiti conducted by the first author of this chapter beginning in 1983 and continuing to the present. The data on changing understandings of AIDS are based on a large corpus of interviews, the vast majority of which are not cited here. At least once during each of the six years of research, the same 20 villagers were interviewed about AIDS, tuberculosis, and "bad blood." Of the 20, two died and one left Do Kay. The interviews took place in a variety of settings, most often the informants' houses. The interviews were open-ended but often focused on specific illness stories, always including discussion of the following topics regarding each of the illnesses: key features (including typical presentation, causes, course, and understanding of pathogenesis when relevant), appropriate therapeutic interventions, relation to other sicknesses common in the area, and questions of risk and vulnerability. In addition to these interviews, the research involved lengthy conversations with all villagers afflicted with AIDS and tuberculosis. Members of their families were interviewed, as were other key actors in the events described here. These qualitative data were complemented by information from structured surveys and an annual census.

[2] "Do Kay" is a pseudonym, as are the names of informants cited. Other geographic names are accurate.

In 1983, when we first began working in Do Kay, the word *sida*, an acronym from the French *syndrome d'immunodéficience acquise*, was often heard in Port-au-Prince. This was the year following the initial linking in the North American press of AIDS with Haiti. The small Caribbean nation, it was erroneously suggested, was the source of the virus that causes AIDS. As the nation's tourist industry collapsed, leaving thousands of urban Haitians without jobs, the word sida took on specific connotations. Few citydwellers were unaware of the syndrome, though the majority of them could not have know individuals with AIDS.

The word sida was not yet well established, however, in the rural Haitian lexicon. In interviews conducted in early 1984, only 1 of 17 informants mentioned sida as a possible cause of diarrhea. The term did not occur in natural discourse about tuberculosis, the most common infection among Haitians with AIDS, nor did it figure in talk about diarrhea or other disorders. When questioned, however, 15 of 20 villagers said that they had heard of sida, and a dozen of them associated certain symptoms or stigmata with this label. But many of these attributes were not, in fact, commonly seen in Haitians with AIDS.

Most of the villagers who spoke of sida noted that they had heard of the disorder on the radio or during trips to the capital. There was considerable disagreement as to what the characteristics of sida might be. In our 1983–1984 discussions, 7 out of 20 informants mentioned three aspects of sida: the novelty of the disorder, its relation to diarrhea, and its association with homosexuality. The majority mentioned one or two of these attributes. Only five noted that sida was lethal. Three thought that it was originally a disease of pigs; three were also of the opinion that, despite the contrary claims of the foreign press, sida had been brought to Haiti by North Americans. Two others asserted that "sida is the same things as tuberculosis." One 36-year-old market woman offered in early 1984 the following commentary, which recalls that of several of her covillagers:

> Sida is a sickness they have in Port-au-Prince and in the United States. It gives you a diarrhea that starts very slowly, but never stops until you're completely dry. There's no water left in your body. . . . Sida is a sickness that you see in men who sleep with other men.

She had little else to say about the syndrome. In Do Kay, illnesses were usually the topic of much discussion; sida was not.[3] In the year following May 1983, any talk about the disorder was prompted by questioning; there were no illness stories or "therapeutic narratives" about sida. In 1985, due largely to radio programming, more may have been known about the syndrome, but it still was not a compelling subject of everyday discourse.

---

[3] When one villager was asked if he and his consociates were reluctant to speak about sida, he responded, "Why should that be? There is no one who says he can't talk about sida. But it is nothing that we have seen here. It's a city sickness (*maladi lavil*)."

Before 1984, then, one would have been hard-pressed to delineate a *collective representation* of AIDS in rural Haiti. Despite several individuals' elaborate explanatory models, the lack of natural discourse regarding sida and the low interinformant agreement regarding its core characteristics suggest that, before 1984, no cultural model of AIDS existed in this part of rural Haiti.

If villagers were aware of but uninterested in sida in 1984, interest in the syndrome was almost universal less than three years later. Narratives about sida were easily triggered, and it was clear that a consensus, albeit tenuous, had emerged. Interviews conducted since 1987 revealed that the semantic network in which sida was embedded had changed substantially. The syndrome was then mentioned by over half of those asked to cite possible causes of diarrhea in an adult. A majority also associated sida with tuberculosis. Further, there was clearly a much more widely shared idea of the way in which it became manifest in the afflicted. The extent of these changes is indicated by the observations of a young schoolteacher, himself a native of the village in which we worked. He was interviewed several times between 1983 and the present. In a 1984 interview, he noted,

> Yes, of course I've heard of [sida]. It's caused by living in the city. It gives you diarrhea and can kill you. . . . We've never had any [sida] here. It's a city sickness.

It was clear from a long exchange recorded late in 1987 that the man's understanding of the syndrome had changed substantially. He also held forth at great length about the disorder. A chief factor seems to have been that he was now able to refer to the death from sida of his fellow schoolteacher, Manno Surpris:

> It was sida that killed him: that's what I'm trying to tell you. But they say it was a death sent to him. They sent a sida death to him . . . sida is caused by a tiny microbe. But not just anybody will catch the microbe that can cause sida.

Manno's illness and death made a lasting contribution to the cultural model of sida that took shape in the past few years. This contribution was not substantially lessened by the subsequent deaths from AIDS of two other villagers.

Manno moved to Do Kay in 1982, when he became a teacher at a large new school established by a Haitian priest. He was then 25 years old. An enthusiastic and hardworking man, Manno came to be held in high esteem by the school administrators. He was entrusted with a number of public—and remunerative—tasks, including taking care of the village's new water pump as well as the community pig project, both of which were administered by the priest who ran the school. That an outsider would be granted such favors was resented by some of the villagers, as became clear after Manno fell ill.

Beginning in early 1986, he had been bothered by intermittent diarrhea. His superficial skin infections recrudesced throughout the summer; the patches would clear up with treatment, only to appear again, usually on the scalp, neck, or face. By December, his decline was drastic, and he began to cough. In January 1987, Manno's physician in Port-au-Prince at last referred him to the public clinic that could perform the test necessary to diagnose HIV infection. In the first week of February, while waiting for the results of an HIV antibody test, Manno revealed his own fear about the disorder:

> Most of all, I hope it's not tuberculosis. But I'm afraid that's what it is. I'm coughing, I've lost weight. . . . I'm afraid I have tuberculosis, and that I'll never get better, never be able to work again. . . . People don't want to be near you if you have tuberculosis.

Manno did indeed have tuberculosis, a disease much feared in Haiti, and initially responded well to the appropriate treatment. By March, he no longer looked ill at all. But he also had antibodies to HIV, which suggested to his physicians that immune deficiency caused by the virus was at the root of his health problems. In a sense, these suspicions were shared by Manno's covillagers. They had additional reasons, however, for believing that his tuberculosis was "not simple," as it was often remarked. Manno's illness had "another cause."

A rumor had circulated around Do Kay, and it was not dampened by Manno's clinical improvement: He was the victim, it was whispered, of sorcery. His illness was the intentional result of some angry or jealous rival. Manno's wife was among those interviewed in 1984. She had then offered the opinion that sida was "a form of diarrhea seen in homosexuals." Informed in February 1987, by Manno's physician, that her husband was infected with HIV, she accepted this as true. But she and her husband also knew Manno to be the victim of sorcery: "They did this to him because they were jealous that he had three jobs—teaching, the pigsty, and the water pump."

Because treatment of a "sent sickness" requires that the perpetrators be identified, Manno and his family were increasingly obsessed not with the course of the disease, but with its ultimate origin. They consulted a voodoo priest, who revealed through divination the authors of the crime. One of those accused of killing Manno was his father-in-law's brother's daughter; another, a schoolteacher, was more distantly related to his wife. The third, the "master of the affair," was also a co-worker of Manno's. But divination and the indicated treatment could not save Manno. By the end of August, Manno's breathing had become labored. Painkillers no longer helped and he was unable to sleep. He vomited after most meals and lost a great deal of weight. Manno succumbed in mid-September, and his death was the chief topic of "semiprivate" conversation for months.

Although a few villagers subsequently cast their analysis in terms of the familiar dichotomy of voodoo versus Christianity, most spoke in less

Manichaean terms. A series of oppositions, rather than one, came to guide many of our conversations: An illness might be caused by a "microbe" or by sorcery or by both. An intended victim might be "powerful" or "susceptible." Some spoke of the night, years ago, when Manno had been knocked out of bed by a bolt of lightning. The shock, they said, had left him "susceptible" to a disease caused by a "microbe" and "sent by someone." An illness might be treated by doctors or voodoo priests or herbalists or prayer or any combination of these.

Although many of the ideas and associations were indeed new, it became clear that the term sida, and the syndrome with which it is associated, came to be embedded in a series of properly Haitian ideas about illness. The "adoption" of a new illness category by older interpretive frameworks is well documented. "As new medical terms become known in a society," notes Good (1977, p. 54), "they find their way into existing semantic networks. Thus while new explanatory models may be introduced, it is clear that changes in medical rationality seldom follow quickly." The causal language used in reference to sida is in many respects similar to that employed when speaking of tuberculosis. For example, the new illness became linked to those diseases that can be caused by malign magic. What was at first tentatively suggested came to be seen as an integral part of the new disorder's reality: Just as it is possible to "send a chest death," that is, a death from TB, so too is it possible to "expedite" an AIDS death to someone. The relation of these understandings to voodoo is unclear, as they were shared by villagers regardless of religious affiliation.[4]

There were other associations with existing patterns of discourse about blood. The significance of this framework led Weidman and co-workers to speak of the "blood paradigm" underlying the health-related beliefs of Haitian informants living in Miami (Weidman, 1978; see also Farmer, 1988; Laguerre, 1987). It is this paradigm that encompasses the causal links between the social field and alterations in the quality, consistency, and nature of blood. In the same manner that sida came to be grouped with illnesses that can be caused by sorcery and microbes, so too did the syndrome come to represent an irreversible pollution caused by the volition of significant others. It must be noted, however, that the contributions of this paradigm to the emerging representations seemed to wane with passing years, and the "tuberculosis paradigm" emerged as the more important of preexisting models.

---

[4] Yet it is in the scholarly literature on voodoo that this form of illness causation is well documented. Metraux refers to the sending of the dead as the "most fearful practice in the black arts." His description of expedition is phenomenologically similar to untreated tuberculosis: Whoever has become the prey of one or more dead people sent against him begins to grow thin, spit blood and is soon dead. The laying on of this spell is always attended by fatal results unless it is diagnosed in time and a capable *hungan* succeeds in making the dead let go" (Metraux, 1972, p. 274).

Further, the term became a prominent part of everyday discourse about
misfortune. Sida was the topic of several popular songs, all of which tended
to affirm associations that were important to the Haitian cultural model of
AIDS. This discourse reveals the semantic network in which the term sida is
embedded, a network that has come to include such diverse associations as
divine punishment, the corruption of the ruling class, and the ills of North
American imperialism. These shifts in the "rhetoric of complaint" were
brought into relief during the political turmoil that surrounded the collapse
of the Duvalier dictatorship. For example, when the military government
organized a carefully policed forum on the mechanics of army-run elections,
the gathering was widely termed a "forum sida," a play on the official term
"forum CEDHA," the acronym designating the army's proposed electoral
machinery. The significance of "conspiracy theories," especially those
linking AIDS to the machinations of rascist "America," has yet to decline.
Although such expressions emanated from Port-au-Prince, it is possible that
in some areas they have had a greater effect on the elaboration of rural illness
realities than has the virus itself. Many areas of rural Haiti have to date
registered no local cases of sida; inhabitants of these regions are nonetheless
familiar with many of these expressions.

As an illness caused by witchcraft, sida stands for local, rather than
large-scale, conflicts. Several villagers referred to sida as a "jealousy
sickness"—an illness sent on one poor person by even poorer person. As
such, the disorder has come to connote a perceived inability of poor Haitians
to develop enduring class solidarity. Such observations often served as codas
in the illness stories recounted in Do Kay. Some are ended with a loud sigh
and the observation, "We've been hating each other since Africa." They are
also important in other parts of Haiti: The most recent pre-Lenten carnival
was marred by widespread rumor of a group of people whose plan was to
spread HIV by injecting revelers with HIV-infected serum. Many observed
that these plans were to be implemented by "poor people hurting their own
brothers and sisters."

Tracing the emergence of sida as a collective representation illuminates
our understanding of AIDS in rural Haiti. Recall that, in 1984, the most
frequently mentioned qualifiers of the new term sida were comments about
the novelty of the disorder, its relation to diarrhea, and its association with
homosexuality. Yet there was little consensus regarding these or any other
features of sida. This lack of consensus and the absence of illness stories
regarding the malady call into question the very notion of a cultural model of
sida at that time. As of October 1988, however, there were many stories to
tell. Two other villagers had succumbed to sida. Their illnesses, though quite
different from Manno's, confirmed many of the tentatively held understandings that were elaborated in 1987. A young woman named Anita seemed to
endure an illness strikingly dissimilar from that of Manno; not only was her
illness clinically different from Manno's, but Anita was poor and locally
perceived as the victim of great misfortune. Moreover, she was a native of Do
Kay. Two persons who had explained to me the nature of Manno's illness

queried rhetorically, "Who would send a sida death on this poor, unfortunate child?"

Despite these disparities, Anita's experience did not weaken the slowly emerging cultural model. How did the nascent representation accommodate the new understandings offered by Anita's sickness? Since the sole case of sida registered in the Do Kay area was already thought to be caused by sorcery, it stood to follow, some initially thought, that Anita could not have sida. Few people believed that Anita was the victim of malign magic, and her father's lack of success in the quest for therapy was seen as an indication not of the power of her enemies but of the virulence of her "natural" illness. Gradually, villagers came to agree that she did indeed have sida, but that it could also be caused "naturally." As one of Anita's aunts put it, "We don't know whether or not they sent a sida death to [her lover], but we know that she did not have a death sent to her. She had it in her blood, she caught it from him."

Based on such discourse and also on more structured interviews, the following points summarize the shared understanding of AIDS in a Haitian village at the close of 1988:

1. Sida is a "new disease."
2. Sida is strongly associated with "skin infections," "drying up," "diarrhea," and, especially, "tuberculosis."
3. Sida may occur both "naturally" (maladi bondje, "God's illness") and "unnaturally." Natural sida is caused by sexual contact with someone who "carries the germ." In the unnatural case, the illness is "sent" by someone who willfully inflicts death upon the afflicted. The mechanism of malice is through "expedition" of a "dead [person]," in the same manner that tuberculosis may be sent.
4. Whether "God's illness" or "sent," sida may be held to be caused by a "microbe."
5. Sida may be contracted by contact with contaminated or "dirty" blood, but earlier associations with homosexuality and transfusion are rarely cited.
6. The term sida reverberates with associations, drawn from the larger political-economic context, of North American imperialism, a lack of class solidarity among the poor, and the corruption of the ruling elite.

The extent to which consensus will emerge remains to be seen, but the rapid rate of change in local understanding of sida would seem to be a thing of the past. Although the current meanings will be contested and change, the foregoing points summarize a cultural model, in that high interinformant agreement regarding the nature of the illness has evolved. And although there is "significant variation" in models that may be elicited from individuals, even these discrepant versions seem to be generated by a schema comprising the preceding points (see Garro, 1988).

It is possible to delineate several factors important in the crafting of such an illness representation. Most important, of course, has been the advent of the illness itself. It was sida's introduction in Do Kay that prompted its residents to talk about the syndrome among one another. Manno's illness served as a sort of "prototypical case"; presentations and course of subsequent cases, though much different, did not quickly alter ideas about the etiology, symptomatology, and experience of sida. The flurry of information that followed the arrival in Haiti of AIDS was also important: although billboards, posters, and T-shirts all proclaim AIDS to be a menace, it was the radio that assured a largely nonliterate population a certain exposure to biomedical understanding of the syndrome, shaping at least the contours of a cultural model of AIDS. This medium contributed to or reinforced some of the early associations—homosexuality, blood transfusions, "America"—and although the radio did not immediately stimulate strong interest in the disease in rural Haiti, it seems to have provided a vague grid upon which genuinely interested villagers would later evaluate their covillager's illness. Less important, but clearly contributory, were the efforts of a local clinic to disseminate—in church, in community council meetings, and at conferences for health workers, injectionists, and midwives—information held to "protect health." These efforts seems far less significant, however, than the preexisting meaning structures into which sida so neatly fit.

The Cultural Context of Illness Representations: Six Questions for the Researcher

As the data on AIDS in Haiti indicate, the representation of illness is shaped by broader structures of meaning, historical forces, political and economic relations, and local experiences with illness. The study of a rapidly changing illness representation in a society such as Haiti brings these processes into focus. During the past decade, however, anthropologists from a variety of theoretical perspectives have increasingly concentrated on the *communicative* context in which data on illness representations emerge. Such research takes us far from stereotyped views of cultural representations as beliefs shared consensually by all members of a society. For the psychologist, anthropological contributions to this topic might read more like an anthology of cautionary tales, which we represent here as a series of questions. In addition to the central query—just what is meant by "illness representations"?—we suggest that the following questions might well be asked of any investigation of this topic, whether conducted by psychologist or anthropologist, and indicate some current anthropological research directed to these issues.

Illness Representations by Whom? Intracultural Variation in Illness Representation

Given the epistemological nature of their discipline, anthropologists usually write about the *collective* representations of a particular culture. But this entity is in large part gleaned from work with individual informants, and the degree of sharedness of certain representations is too often an unexamined question. Are collective representations of illness merely composites of individuals' representations? What makes a model a *cultural* model? "Although no sharp distinction between an individual's model and a cultural model can be made, researchers have generally focused on one or the other," notes Garro (1988, p. 98), "and the relationship between the two remains relatively unstudied."

Using a methodology known as "cultural consensus analysis," Garro examined models of high blood pressure among the Ojibway residing on a Canadian reserve. She presented her informants with a series of previously elicited propositions about high blood pressure and asked whether or not these statements were true. The purpose of this propositional analysis was "to determine the level of sharing and the degree to which individual informants approach the shared standard" (1988, p. 100). Insisting that such contextualizing data were necessary to assess validity, her formally elicited responses were complemented with more open-ended investigations of the explanatory models held by her informants. "In spite of a lot of diversity about what causes and accompanies high blood pressure," concludes Garro (p. 15), "there is a cultural model that gives meaning to many of the experiences and actions associated with this illness. Much of the variation expressed by informants is not idiosyncratic but has its origin in the key concepts of the prototypical model."

Garro's study of Ojibway models of high blood pressure affords us an example of someone working in the tradition of cognitive anthropology but more fully alive to the necessary correctives of open-ended interviewing. A number of questions remain unresolved, however, including the emergence over time of such models and their relation to natural discourse about high blood pressure. We turn to these issues later.

Illness Representations How? Canonical Issues in the Elaboration of Illness Narratives

It has been noted that explanatory models often emerge in situated discourse (Good, 1977, 1986). One common form of such discourse has been termed illness narratives or stories. In rural Haiti, we found that the elaboration of a properly cultural model of sida depended to no small extent on the local salience of illness narratives replete with characteristics and settings and lessons—in other words, stories to tell. Illness stories seem to be a form of natural discourse. Culture shapes both the narrative form and the knowledge encoded in the stories: "Set apart from the conversational flow by certain structural features, [they] encode cultural models of causation, extensive situation knowledge about appropriate behavior when someone is sick, and a vast amount of cultural knowledge about types of treatments and health specialists" (Price, 1987, p. 313; see also Holland, 1985).

To elicit such stories, Early (1982) sat with women in a poor neighborhood of Cairo and recorded naturally occurring discussions of present and past illnesses and encounters with professional or folk specialists. She began to find that these accounts had a particular narrative structure. "Therapeutic narratives," as she called them, were organized to provide biographical context and experiential reference for the perception and diagnosis of illness. These narratives made sense of symptoms or illnesses by relating them to the life histories of the women, connecting troubling life circumstances with shared cultural knowledge about illness. Some narratives, she found, were used to make sense of a current ambiguous situation and negotiate an approach to therapy; others, she found, "form a codified, elaborated version [of past events] affirming cultural truths" about such central concerns as envy and sibling rivalry. Early's research focused on both the structure of these stories and the principles that generated the narrative.

In her study of the narratization of illness episodes among urban, largely poor Ecuadorians, Price (1987) also found that illness stories affirmed cultural truths, particularly those concerning appropriate social roles. She found that structural features of illness narratives include the anchoring of the account in a time and a place; the story's chronological advancement; the presence of "counterexamples," which serve to highlight the distinction between appropriate and inappropriate responses to sickness; and the account's termination in a "coda," or end phrase. Certain topics also seem to be "built in" to the narrative, for example, consideration of questions of etiology and the role of the narrator in the quest for therapy.

Price asks a question relevant to psychologists, cognitive anthropologists, and others employing formal elicitation methods: "How would the system of beliefs about illness that can be distilled from analysis of illness stories compare with the sets of interrelated propositions about illness resulting from a more formal elicitation approach in the same population?" Acknowledging her inability, given the nature of her research, to answer the question, Price (1987, p. 329) nonetheless asserts that there are key elements of cultural models of illness, including moral causation, that are more likely to be uncovered in natural discourse: "Formal elicitation procedures . . . may access beliefs only on a general and rather abstract level: Respondents focus on the unmarked case that is largely detached from knowledge of specific people and is irrelevant to the normal social purposes of the respondent in talking about illness." Her point is amply supported by the material from Haiti, which suggests the extent to which understandings of an illness are linked to meaningful experience; such dimensions of illness representations as the relation of "sent" sida to Manno's status in the village would not easily be revealed through questionnaires.

Illness Representations Why? Rhetorical Ploys as Ends Unto Themselves

Some dictionaries define "rhetoric" as "the art of speaking effectively." For decades, anthropological studies of illness did not attend closely to the manner in which speech about illness comes to have effects. This was due, in part, to the utilitarianism that has long collapsed several important questions into investigations of the "secondary gains" of sickness. It is also due, one suspects, to our culturally reified opposition of "talking" and "doing." But when Quinn and Holland (1987, p. 9) write of "talk as action," they remind us that "talk is one of the most important ways in which people negotiate understanding and accomplish social ends." For example, talk often seemed to be the only action taken by the ill Iberian women we interviewed in urban, working-class France (Gaines & Farmer, 1986). "Speaking effectively" then became the primary goal of a sick person (or the wife or mother of one), seeking to elaborate a public and legitimized recounting of suffering. Pointed questions about specific illness terms, episodes, or events often elicited long, nonspecific narratives that seemed to address far larger, more "existential" questions of suffering. These narratives were most often couched in what was termed a "rhetoric of complaint," highly context-dependent and markedly performative.

In village Haiti, illness narratives become most compelling and effective when the actions of the speaker are defended, or when those of a rival are decried—that is, when moral matters are at stake. One learns a great deal about sida when listening to Manno's wife explain why she consulted one healer rather than another. And it is an airing of these grave matters in illness narratives that is the prime purpose of many of the stories in which illness representations are embedded.

Another example of how speech comes to have its effects is found in Brown's recent analysis of shamanic healing in Amazonian Peru. Noting the romanticism inherent in anthropological images of "the heroic shaman," Brown shows that careful contextualization of shamanism in its "social and political space" reveals the darker side of recourse to such healers: the fear of sorcery, also the province of shamans. Through "textual analysis of rhetoric and counter-rhetoric in an Aguaruna Indian healing session," Brown's study "assesses shamanism's second face" (1988, p. 103). With the help of powerful hallucinogens, the shaman is able to share with the afflicted and their family members his own mental representations of their illnesses. But much of the power of these representations is derived from their embedded-ness in rhetorical speech acts, his and those of others present, which reveal the ambivalence with which any shaman-sorceror is regarded. The result is a setting which Brown's informants experience as both dangerous and therapeutic.

Careful *textual* analysis of illness discourse reveals the contours of rhetorics of complaint and healing; it also suggests the relationships between illness categories and the discourse in which they are situated. Careful *ethnographic* analysis of illness realities and responses to them reveals that talk is indeed action. To again cite Price's work in urban Ecuador:

First, conversation about illness has problem-solving value because it transmits useful technical information about such things as home remedies, disease symptoms, health care specialists. . . . Second, through exposure to the many causal propositions in illness narratives, listeners expand and refine their own theories of disease. Third, many illness stories focus attention on the caretaker role of the narrator. The narrator frequently asserts in an implicit way: "I did the right thing." This public declaration constitutes a way of negotiating the meaning of the illness events and may be an important source of social validation for the narrator. Finally, it may be hypothesized that sharing illness stories reinforces bonds of mutual support among individuals and intensifies friendships. (Price 1987, pp. 314–315; paragraphing altered)

Further, narratized rhetoric often serves as a primary means of encoding affective propositions that are regarded as inappropriate to more direct confrontation. By affording a meaningful framework in which to air gripes, disappointment, disapprobation, and even warning, illness stories often permit the oblique elaboration of affects that might otherwise be too painful or too disruptive of socially sanctioned norms of interaction.

Illness Representations Where? Performative Factors and Representation

Shamanic healing ceremonies underline the fact that the meanings of illness categories are often elaborated in distinctive settings—in the preceding case, one of darkness pervaded by the audible presence of the ill and their family members, and the loud retching the arcane singing of the shaman. Similarly, the meanings of sida were only gradually elaborated in a variety of settings, each with its own performative exigencies. Any assessment of what was idiosyncratic and what was part of the emerging collective representation required that the ethnographer work in a variety of settings: homes, clinics, a church, voodoo temples, and "in the streets."

Insisting upon the importance of setting to ritual is something of a disciplinary forte, and performative factors have been appreciated for as long as anthropologists have elicited the same informants' explanatory models as they sought care in different settings (in "folk" versus professional spheres, for example). As Good (1986, pp. 165–166) notes, "Different contexts within culture may be as important as differences between cultures in determining the nature of symptom presentation of idioms of complaint." It is for this reason that Bibeau (1981, p. 296), although focusing his attention on lexical structuring of illness categories, promises that "the words and terms will be couched within behavioral settings, involving linguistic actors and definite speech situations."

Investigating the issue of somatization in Chinese culture, Cheung, Lau, and Wong (1984) showed that illness narratives in physicians' offices are quite different from those in other settings. It is not that individuals in Hong Kong fail to experience psychological symptoms, they argue, but that social norms and linguistic conventions play a critical role in determining the idiom that will be used in particular communicative contexts. Whereas Cheung et al. focused more on narratives and less on the illness representations deployed in them, Tambiah's study of a Thai healing cult suggests that the representations themselves, which are largely cosmologically given, take much of their power and meaning from the milieu: "As to the performative features of the cult, it cannot be emphasized enough that the cosmological scheme is not simply an abstract mapping in the mind; the meaningfulness of the healing situation stems from the enactments of the ritual and healing process that translate and *create* the cosmology as an experiential reality for the participants" (Tambiah, 1985, pp. 88–89). There is no reason to believe that these assertions do not hold in less clearly ritualized settings. Indeed, they are likely to be true in the professional, the popular, and the folk sectors of health care.

Illness Representations for Whom? The Politics of Image-Making

Painstaking historical studies of sickness have repeatedly underlined the contribution to nascent representations of the witting and unwitting manipulation of meaning (e.g., Brandt, 1987; Kleinman, 1986). One of the most spectacularly manipulated of illnesses has been AIDS. Relevant maneuvers have included the conscious crafting of the way the illness is represented in the major media: One thinks immediately of the attempts of the "Moral Majority" to portray the disorder as a not altogether deplorable "gay plague." The effects of such efforts are difficult to gauge, but it is instructive to follow shifts in the "official" interpretations of AIDS in the United States. For the U.S. Health and Human Services secretary, AIDS was construed, in 1985, as a disorder that must be conquered "before it affects the heterosexual population and threatens the health of our general population" (cited in Panem, 1988, p. 120). The comment generated a furor in the gay community, which had explicitly decried the government's attempt to represent AIDS as a "gay disease." But, as Sontag (1988, p. 82) noted, *general population* "may be as much a code phrase for whites as it is for heterosexuals." The truth is that AIDS has been held to be everything from the "terminal result of a chronic retrovirus infection" to a "punishment from God," from "gay plague" to "African curse," to cite only a few of the more commonly heard attributes.

It is also possible to see how, through counterrhetoric and the generation of their own images and associations, the disempowered (or less empowered) have struck back. In the autumn of 1982, for example, a radical Haitian political faction in exile circulated a flyer denouncing AIDS, a term then freshly coined, as "an imperialist plot to destroy the Third World." The flyer was readily dismissed as paranoid propaganda from a fringe group, but it soon became clear that such thinking was much more common among Haitians than were the politics espoused by the group. We have often heard Haitians suggest that human agency played a role in the creation of HIV, and that it is no accident that it strikes disproportionately the disempowered.

Such understandings are by no means restricted to Haitians. "If the Africans often see in Western discussion of an African origin of AIDS a wish to blame the epidemic on Africa," observes Sabatier (1988, p. 63), "so many Third Worlders have found attractive a counter-blame theory: that AIDS was unleashed on the world by germ warfare experimentation in the U.S. Defence Department laboratory at Fort Detrick, Maryland." These so-called conspiracy theories of AIDS would be incomprehensible without an understanding of the forces that make them attractive to those without access to the dominant media but capable, nonetheless, of contributing to the shaping of representations. Studies of this process must make sense of conspiracy theories in the context of the socially structured power relations in which they are inevitably embedded. These relations all preceded AIDS by decades or longer:

> More often than not the historical development of a given model or set of models reveals hidden preconceptions that have been masked or mutilated through the passage of time. They reveal how the discourse of power uses (or generates) images of illness, for many ends, drawing on this wide repertory of images to isolate, stigmatize, and control. (Gilman, 1988, p. 9)

Gilman's historical approach to images of illness brings us to the last, and perhaps most important, or our cautionary tales—that regarding the changing nature of illness representations.

Illness Representations When? Processual Considerations in Medical Ethnography

To each of the questions thus far posed, we might add a corollary: Illness representations when? In other words, each of these considerations— sharedness of representations, the relation of such representations to situational discourse and performative factors, the politics of representation—may be expected to change over time and across social contexts. Illness representations are grounded in historicity. Therefore, the anthropological study of illness representations is invariably the investigation of a moving target. The need for a more processual approach to the study of illness representations is perhaps most dramatically illustrated when one is witness to the advent of a disorder that is new or previously unknown among one's host community. The case study from rural Haiti demonstrates that, at the beginning of such a process, there is no collective representation of the disorder. But with time and experience, low interinformant agreement gives way to a cultural model. We previously asked, how shared is the model? We now reformulate the question: How does cultural consensus emerge? How do illness representations, and the realities they organize and constitute, emerge? And how are new representations related to preexisting models?

Indeed, the need for a more processual approach to the study of illness representations is evident in each of the studies examined in this section.

Among the Ojibway, for example, we saw that high blood pressure is regarded as a "new disease," one that came with the white man's domination (Garro, 1988). It thus follows that Ojibway representations of the illness have their own history, and it is equally probable that they continue to change. Investigations of illness meanings during a single episode must be alive to what is at stake at a given moment of illness threat and treatment, to performative factors, and to processual considerations. Narratives, the source of much of our information about "representations," are structured for audiences, which shift and change in the illness process. Illness representations emerge in given contexts; contexts change over time. If we are to be accountable to history and political economy, "time" must mean more than the duration of an illness.

Conclusions

The past few decades of psychological and anthropological research have led to increasingly sophisticated understanding of basic cognitive processes related to health and illness. It is clear that a full understanding of illness representations will require the resources of each of those disciplines. Yet an appreciation of the cognitive dimensions of such representations is of limited value, for their relation to volition and action remains poorly understood. We must strive to understand not only what is said, but what is done "on the ground," during illness episodes. Medical anthropology has not turned away from the distinctive accomplishment of its parent field: Anthropology is a radically contextualizing discipline, even when the most basic cognitive processes are the subject of scrutiny.

Regardless of whether they attend most closely to what their informants say or what their informants do, or both, all those who write of "mental representations" are of course inferring the existence and contours of structures that cannot be observed. As Angel and Thoits (1987, p. 468) note, "Assuming phenomenological equivalence based on behavior or reports of symptoms, therefore, requires rather large inferential leaps, since culture in its manifold forms, but especially as language, intervenes between the investigator and whatever objective reality he or she attempts to assess." The "objective reality" in this case demands attention to several key issues: the sharedness of illness representations, the relation of such representations to situated discourse and thus to performative factors, and the politics of representation. Even more humbling is the fact that each of these considerations may be expected to change over time and across social contexts. By sticking to anthropology's concern with context, and appreciating the changing nature of such contexts, we may hope to make a contribution to an understanding of the significance of illness representations in the social construction of illness experience.

Acknowledgment. Thanks to Linda Garro for substantive and editorial comments on this chapter.

References

Ackerknecht, E. H. (1946). Natural diseases and rational treatments in primitive medicine. *Bulletin of the History of Medicine, 19,* 467–497.

Amarasingham, L. (1980). Movement among healers in Sri Lanka: A case study of a Sinhalese patient. *Culture, Medicine and Psychiatry, 4,* 71–92.

Angel, R., & Thoits, P. (1987). The impact of culture on the cognitive structure of illness. *Culture, Medicine and Psychiatry, 11,* 465–494.

Bibeau, G. (1981). The circular semantic network in Ngbandi disease nosology. *Social Science and Medicine, 15B,* 295–307.

Blumhagen, D. (1980). Hyper-tension: A folk illness with a medical name. *Culture, Medicine and Psychiatry, 4,* 197–227.

Brandt, A. (1987). *No magic bullet: A social history of venereal disease in the United States since 1880* (expanded edition). New York: Oxford University Press.

Brown, M. (1988). Shamanism and its discontents. *Medical Anthropology Quarterly, 2,* 102–120.

Cheung, F. M., Lau, B. K. W., & Wong, S. (1984). Paths to psychiatric care in Hong Kong. *Culture, Medicine and Psychiatry, 8,* 207–228.

Clements, F. (1932). Primitive concepts of disease. *University of California Publications in Archeology and Ethnology, 32,* 185–252.

Comaroff, J. (1985). *Body of power, spirit of resistance.* Chicago: University of Chicago Press.

Csordas, T. (1983). The rhetoric of transformation in ritual healing. *Culture, Medicine and Psychiatry, 7,* 333–375.

D'Andrade, R. (1976). A propositional analysis of U.S. American beliefs about illness. In K. A. Basso & H. A. Selby (Eds.), *Meanings in anthropology* (pp. 155–180). Albuquerque: University of New Mexico Press.

Early, E. (1982). The logic of well-being: Therapeutic narratives in Cairo, Egypt. *Social Science and Medicine, 16,* 1491–1497.

Fabrega, H. (1974). *Disease and social behavior.* Cambridge, MA: MIT Press.

Farmer, P. (1988). Bad blood, spoiled milk: Bodily fluids as moral barometers in rural Haiti. *American Ethnologist, 15,* 61–83.

Farmer, P. (1990). AIDS and accusation: Haiti, Haitians, and the geography of blame. In D. Felman (Ed.), *AIDS and culture: The human factor.* New York: Praeger.

Favret-Saada, J. (1980). *Deadly words: Witchcraft in the Bocage.* Cambridge: Cambridge University Press.

Foster, G. (1978). Medical anthropology and international health planning. In M. Logan & E. Hunt (Eds.), *Health and the human condition* (pp. 301–313). North Scituate, MA: Duxbury Press.

Frake, C. (1961). The diagnosis of disease among the Subanun of Mindanao. *American Anthropologist, 63,* 113–132.

Gaines, A., & Farmer, P. (1986). Visible saints: Social cynosures and dysphoria in the Mediterranean tradition. *Culture, Medicine and Psychiatry, 11,* 295–330.

Gardener, H. (1985). *The mind's new science.* New York: Basic Books.

Garro, L. (1988). Explaining high blood pressure: Variation in knowledge about knowledge. *American Ethnologist*, *15*, 98–119.

Geertz, C. (1983). Common sense as a cultural system. In C. Geertz, *Local knowledge* (pp. 73–93). New York: Basic Books.

Gilman, S. (1988). *Disease and representation: Images of illness from madness to AIDS*. Ithaca, NY: Cornell University Press.

Good, B. (1977). The heart of what's the matter: The semantics of illness in Iran. *Culture, Medicine and Psychiatry*, *1*, 25–58.

Good, B. (1986). Explanatory models and care seeking: A critical account. In S. McHugh & T. M. Vallis (Eds.), *Illness behavior: A multidisciplinary model* (pp. 161–172). New York: Plenum.

Good, B., & Good, M. (1982). Toward a meaning centered analysis of popular illness categories: "Fright Illness" and "Heart Distress" in Iran. In A. J. Marsella & G. M. White (Eds.), *Cultural concepts of mental health and therapy* (pp. 141–166). Boston: Reidel.

Holland, D. (1985). From situation to impressions: How Americans use cultural knowledge to get to know themselves and one another. In J. Dougherty (Ed.), *Directions in cognitive anthropology* (pp. 389–411). Urbana: University of Illinois Press.

Horton, R. (1967). African traditional thought and Western science. *Africa*, *37*, 50–71, 155–187.

Johnson-Laird, P. N., Herrmann, D. J., & Chaffin, R. (1984). Only connections: A critique of semantic networks. *Psychological Bulletin*, *96*, 292–315.

Kleinman, A. (1975). Explanatory models in health care relationships. In *Health of the family* (pp. 159–172). Washington, DC: NCIH.

Kleinman, A. (1980). *Patients and healers in the context of culture*. Berkeley: University of California Press.

Kleinman, A. (1986). *Social origins of distress and disease: Depression, neurasthenia, and pain in modern China*. New Haven, CT: Yale University Press.

Kleinman, A. (1988). *The illness narratives: Suffering, healing and the human condition*. New York: Basic Books.

Kleinman, A., Eisenberg, E., & Good, B. (1978). Culture, illness and care: Clinical lessons from anthropologic and cross-cultural research. *Annals of Internal Medicine*, *88*, 251–258.

Laguerre, M. (1987). *Afro-Caribbean folk medicine*. South Hadley, MA: Bergin and Garvey.

Leslie, C. (1976). *Asian medical systems*. Berkeley: University of California Press.

Marcus, G., & Fischer, M. (1986). *Anthropology as cultural critique: An experimental moment in the human sciences*. Chicago: University of Chicago Press.

Martin, E. (1987). *The woman in the body: A cultural analysis of reproduction*. Boston: Beacon Press.

Metraux, A. (1972). *Haitian voodoo* (H. Charteris, Trans.). New York: Schocken.

Needham, R. (1972). *Belief, language and experience*. Chicago: University of Chicago Press.

Ong, A. (1987). *Spirits of resistance and capitalist discipline: Factory women in Malaysia*. Albany: SUNY Press.

Ortner, S. (1984). Theory in anthropology since the sixties. *Comparative Studies in Society and History*, *26*, 126–166.

162   Paul Farmer and Byron J. Good

Panem, S. (1988). *The AIDS bureaucracy*. Cambridge, MA: Harvard University Press.

Paul, B. (1955). *Health, culture, and community*. New York: Russell Sage Foundation.

Polgar, S. (1972). Population history and population policies from an anthropological perspective. *Current Anthropology, 13*, 203–211.

Price, L. (1987). Ecuadorian illness stories: Cultural knowledge in national discourse. In D. Holland & N. Quinn (Eds.), *Cultural models in language and thought* (pp. 313–342). Cambridge: Cambridge University Press.

Quinn, N., & Holland, D. (1987). Culture and cognition. In D. Holland & N. Quinn (Eds.), *Culture models in language and thought* (pp. 3–40). Cambridge: Cambridge University Press.

Rivers, W. H. R. (1924). *Medicine, magic, and religion*. New York: Harcourt Brace.

Rivers, W. H. R. (1926). *Psychology and ethnology*. London: Routledge.

Sabatier, R. (1988). *Blaming others: Prejudice, race, and worldwide AIDS*. Philadelphia: New Society Publishers.

Sahlins, M. (1976). *Culture and practical reason*. Chicago: University of Chicago Press.

Scheper-Hughes, N., & Lock, M. M. (1987). The mindful body: A prolegomenon to future work in medical anthropology. *Medical Anthropology Quarterly, 1*, 6–41.

Slobodin, R. (1978). *W. H. R. Rivers*. New York: Columbia University Press.

Smith, W. C. (1977). *Belief and history*. Charlottesville: University Press of Virginia.

Smith, W. C. (1979). *Faith and belief*. Princeton: Princeton University Press.

Sontag, S. (1988). *AIDS and its metaphors*. New York: Farrar, Strauss & Giroux.

Tambiah, S. (1985). A Thai cult of healing through meditation. In S. Tambiah (Ed.), *Culture, thought, and social action: An anthropological perspective* (pp. 87–122). Cambridge, MA: Harvard University Press.

Taussig, M. (1980). Reification and the consciousness of the patient. *Social Science and Medicine, 14*, 3–13.

Weidman, H. (1978). *Miami health ecology project report: A statement on ethnicity and health*. Miami, FL: University of Miami, Department of Psychiatry.

Weidman, H. (1982). Research strategies, structural alterations and clinically relevant anthropology. In N. Chrisman & T. Maretski (Eds.), *Clinically applied anthropology* (pp. 201–241). Boston: Reidel.

Wellin, E. (1978). Theoretical orientations in medical anthropology: Change and continuity over the past half-century. In M. Logan & E. Hunt (Eds.), *Health and the human condition* (pp. 23–39). North Scituate, MA: Duxbury Press.

Young, A. (1982). Rational men and the explanatory model approach. *Culture, Medicine and Psychiatry, 6*, 57–71.

Young, J. C. (1981). *Medical choice in a Mexican village*. New Brunswick, NJ: Rutgers University Press.

8
A Mental Representation Approach to Health Policy Analysis

K. Mark Leek

Community interventions have become a popular strategy for modifying health behavior and attitudes (Farquhar, 1978; Gesten & Jason, 1987; Green & McAlister, 1984; Kelly, Snowden, & Ricardo, 1977). Nevertheless, the methodological foundations of community intervention have yet to be fully developed. One of the shortcomings of interventions to date has been a tendency to impose a medical model on the members of the targeted community (Leventhal, Cleary, Safer, & Gutmann, 1980). From the perspective of community agenda-building, a successful intervention must be based on a thorough understanding of the values and policy orientations of those whose participation is sought. Only then can mobilization that leads to structural change occur.

In this chapter a mental representation approach to policy analysis is used to examine two relationships that are fundamental to the policy-making process. The first deals with the relationship among policymakers. In many policy-making situations policymakers find it difficult to engage each other for the purpose of working together to address a problem. There is a shared concern but problems are not addressed because they cannot be approached in ways that permit leaders to invest themselves in the search for solutions.

The second relationship that is fundamental to policy-making is the relationship between policymakers and constituents. Policymakers often face a difficult challenge in attempting to fashion programs that are compatible with the needs and values of those whom programs are intended to serve. This is especially apparent in medical situations where approaches to wellness so often depend on the ability of health-care providers to define problems in nonmedical or human terms.

The study of mental representation offers a systematic means to define problems in ways that are compatible with the values and policy orientations of those whose participation is key to effective policy-making. The mental representation approach is defined here as the study of the mental images and orientations of individuals toward a particular subject domain. This includes both the structure and content of mental orientations. This approach offers policymakers what they most lack, that is, an understanding of the conceptual "referents" that they and/or their constituents rely on to define a problem. Edelman defines referential symbols as "economical ways of referring to the objective elements in objects or situations: the elements identified in the same way by different people. Such symbols are useful because they help in logical thinking about the situation and in manipulating it" (1972, p. 6). By bringing to the surface and giving shape to what is often latent, the study of mental representation can assist policymakers in the difficult task of framing problems in ways that can lead to leadership and/or constituent participation in the policy-making process.

This chapter examines these two relationships separately. In the first part a mental representation approach is used to examine the process of agenda-building on behalf of alcohol use and abuse among community leaders. Policymakers find this to be an issue that is difficult to engage because sources of support for program development are often latent and thus difficult to define.

In the second part the study of mental representation is used to examine the doctor–patient relationship among people with multiple sclerosis (MS). Multiple sclerosis lends itself to a mental representation approach because of the important role that human factors associated with disability play in coping. This study looks at the role of the physician as a facilitator in the coping process.

A Mental Representation Approach to Problem-Structuring

Problem-structuring is a term used to describe the process by which problems are defined and is a key component of policy formulation. Problem-structuring is especially important, and often problematic, with respect to what Dunn describes as "ill-structured problems" (1981; also see Rein, 1976). Many health-related problems are of this type. There is conflict among competing goals, and often policy alternatives and outcomes are unknown. Cigarette smoking is an example of this kind of issue. A battle is currently being waged over whether to define cigarette smoking as a health issue or a matter of individual rights. The definition of the problem itself must be viewed as an analytic construct.

A mental representation approach to problem-structuring anchors the definition of a problem in the structure of shared mental images of policymakers or constituents. It is the existence of a shared mental structure that gives the study of mental representation its credibility as an analytic tool. As Moskowitz explains, to serve as a guide to behavior, certain core dimensions "must be held almost universally by the policy makers." In the absence of certain core dimensions, a mental representation approach would amount to no more than "the aggregation of individual attitudes rather than being a systemic trait" (1978, p. 67).

The approach to mental representation used in this chapter is empirical. Subject responses to balanced subsets of statements about a problem were statistically reduced into a few core dimensions. The dimensions depict the shared mental structure of key participants, which represents the conceptual referents that policymakers or constituents rely on to bring order and coherence to a complex policy area (Brown, 1980; Stephenson, 1957). The discovery of a shared mental structure offers policymakers a framework for use in problem-structuring (Gore & Leek, 1987; Kessel, 1983; Leek, 1982; Sabatier, 1989; Williams, Gore, Broches, & Lostoski, 1987).

A Mental Representation Approach to Policy Analysis in the Area of Alcohol Abuse

In this analysis the study of mental representation is used to examine the process of agenda-building in the area of alochol abuse. Agenda-building refers to the process by which problems come to be accepted as legitimate objects of collective action. The analysis begins with a discussion of the type of problem that is best suited to a mental representation approach. It is especially useful with regard to problems that require a broad base of involvement for their solution, as opposed to those that require a rational or overtly political solution.

Mental Representation: A Value-Based Approach to Agenda-Building

Agenda-building is the process by which issues emerge as legitimate objects of collective action. There are two kinds of agendas, one systemic and the other institutional. The systemic, or informal, agenda is the "general set of political controversies that will be viewed as falling within the range of legitimate concerns meriting the attention of the polity." The institutional, or formal, agenda is the "set of concrete items scheduled for active and serious consideration by a particular institutional decision-making body" (Cobb & Elder, 1971, p. 906; see also Cobb & Elder, 1983). The formal agenda will always consist of a subset of those items on the systemic agenda. How problem-structuring affects the movement of issues from the systemic to the institutional agenda is the subject of this chapter.

Three types of agenda-building strategies are available to policymakers. The choice of strategies depends on the type of issue involved and whom the policymaker perceives as his or her primary source of support for collective action. A policymaker can target organized groups, the attentive public, or policy experts and program elites (Figure 8-1). The three can be targeted

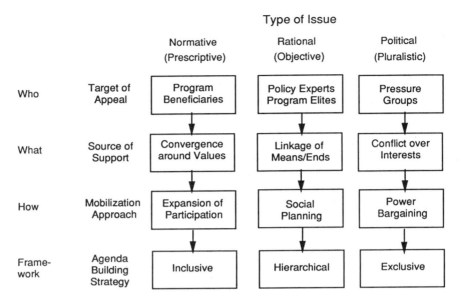

Figure 8-1. Type of agenda-building strategy by issue and source of support for collective action. (This chapter deals exclusively with agenda-building among normative issues.)

individually or in combination with each other, though usually a single strategy is used for each targeted group.

Political issues are defined in terms of the organized groups that identify with them. Support for collective action is obtained through the mobilization of "interests" as different groups and their representatives in government compete with each other for political dominance. Problems are defined as objects of collective action by a single group or coalition if it controls a policy domain, or through bargaining if several groups share or have access to power more or less equally (Allison, 1969; Elmore, 1978; Lindblom, 1965; Majone, 1976). Because agenda-building depends on the ability of policy-makers to manage social conflict in the pursuit of their own ends, policymakers strive to limit participation in the decision process.

Rational issues involve technical problem solving where there is a high degree of consensus over basic policy goals. Decisions involve choices among the "most rational (goalmaximizing) course of action to take" to achieve clearly defined objectives (Rothman, 1972, p. 24). Support for collective action is obtained through the mobilization of expertise as policy experts and program elites compete with each other for policy control. Problems are defined through a process of social planning within a hierarchical framework of decision making (May, 1989). Municipal response to the threat of a hazardous materials accident is an example of this type of decision framework. The public is generally uninvolved in municipal decisions to prevent and respond to a hazardous materials accident and is likely to remain so until city officials demonstrate that they have failed to adequately prepare for an emergency.

Normative issues are framed in terms of values and usually involve quality of life concerns (Inglehart, 1977). As Richardson et al. note, conflict within "policy communities" is increasingly "not (only) about the distribution of material benefits to different sections of society, but is also concerned with what Inglehart has identified as nonmaterialistic values" (Richardson, Gustafsson, & Jordan, 1982, p. 3). Support for collective action is obtained through the mobilization of values as members of the attentive public cooperate with each other "in determining and solving their own problems" (Rothman, 1972, p. 24; also Walker, 1983) Because agenda-building depends on the combined efforts of a broad cross section of people, policymakers strive to expand the scope of participation.

Normative issues present policymakers with agenda-building problems not encountered in other types of issues. In contrast to political and rational issues, policymakers do not possess the means to systematically assess the potential for collective action. With political issues, the "group" provides a conceptual frame of reference for defining potential sources of support. Policymakers assess the potential for collective action by evaluating the strength of the groups associated with competing interests. Rational issues are defined in terms of policy. Policymakers assess the potential for collective action by evaluating how well policy proposals satisfy predetermined decision criteria (Elster, 1985).

Among normative issues, where agenda-building depends on the ability of policymakers to expand the scope of participation, the only apparent characteristic that individuals often share is a concern for the problem. Networks of individuals from diverse organizations and groups cooperate with one another to form what Hjern and Porter describe as "implementation structures" (1981). These structures are problematic from a mobilization standpoint because the conceptual referents that individuals rely on to define a problem do not correspond to existing groups or policy frameworks. As Thrasher notes, this makes it "extremely difficult to design policies anticipating possible implementation structures which might subsequently develop" (1983, p. 376).

A mental representation approach is especially suited to agenda-building among normative issues because of its ability to offer policymakers a conceptual frame of reference in a policy environment that does not otherwise offer stable cues for problem definition. The problem policymakers face is an inability to systematically differentiate among diverse value orientations. They are often aware of widespread concern about a problem but have little means to sort out and bring coherence to conflicting messages and diverse points of view. The discovery of a structure of shared mental images provides policymakers with a conceptual framework for identifying diverse value orientations. It offers a means to structure a problem in a way that responds to, and thus reflects, the values that underlie diverse and often latent network structures. The capacity to identify and target potential implementation structures is crucial to the ability of policymakers to assess the potential for collective action.

The Identification of Diverse Leadership Orientations Toward the Problem of Alcohol Abuse

In this section factor analysis and object typing are used to identify diverse leadership orientations toward the problem of alcohol abuse. Subject selection, instrument design, and data-taking procedures are described in Gore and Leek (1987). Data were obtained from 86 people, 92% of those identified as influential in a small rural community. The community is an unincorporated part of a large Pacific Northwest county. It has a community council that deals mostly with zoning issues. Leadership has a history of taking the initiative. Prior to the study local leaders initiated a series of actions which culminated in the creation of the community's first and only outpatient health clinic.

Data were obtained from subjects' Q sorts of 58 cards that contained balanced subsets of statements concerning the antecedents of alcohol abuse, its social consequences, locus of responsibility, and response. Subject responses were factor analyzed to determine the set of mental images or conceptual referents that leaders rely on to orient themselves to the problem (Table 8-1). (The size of the leadership population limited the number of subjects available for factor analysis.) The BC-Try computer program was used to produce three leadership profiles based on common orientations toward each of the seven factors (Figure 8-2).

Table 8-2 combines the information from Table 8-1 and Figure 8-2 to show how shared mental images (factors) combine to form core dimensions, and how core dimensions combine to form a structure of belief. The factors depict the orientation (plus or minus) of the profiles toward each of the core dimensions.

The "deep (normative) core" of a belief system consists of the "fundamental normative and ontological axioms which define a person's underlying personal philosophy" (Sabatier, 1987, p. 666). It consists of basic conceptions about the nature of man. Fundamental differences in orientations toward alcohol abuse are found at this level. From the moral perspective, alcohol abuse is viewed as a weakness of character; for medicals it is viewed as an illness. Compared to the other profiles, the ambivalents do not have a strong view about the origin of abuse, since they are close to the population mean on both factors.

The "near (policy) core" consists of "fundamental policy positions concerning the basic strategies for achieving normative axioms of (the) deep core" (Sabatier, 1987, p. 667). It consists of beliefs about fundamental relationships such as the "proper scope of government vs. market activity."

Table 8-1. Factor Analysis of Items Defining the Shared Mental Images of Community Leaders Toward the Problem of Alcohol Abuse

Loading	Item
	Factor 1: Alcohol abuse as a public problem
−.76	Drinking is a private matter.
−.72	Too much is made of alcohol abuse in this community.
.67	Negligence, even in one's home, is a matter of public concern.
.63	There is no such thing as a victimless social problem.
	Factor 2: Moralistic perspective
.69	Alcoholism has a chemical/psychological element, but at base it is a matter of character.
.56	I have little sympathy for problem drinkers.
−.46	Alcoholism is a disease.
	Factor 3: Treatment
.63	Local residents should provide treatment for alcoholics.
−.62	Local residents cannot provide all of the services people want.
.58	A small community is an ideal place in which to help people.
.49	Alcoholics need help and understanding.
	Factor 4: Medical perspective
−.70	People have been drinking for centuries and this will continue.
.67	Alcoholism is a disease.
.52	Alcohol education is essential.
−.47	I have no sympathy for those with drinking problems.
	Factor 5: Role of formal authority
.69	The school board should do more to constrain alcohol abuse.
.65	Alcohol abuse is a factor in sending children off-island to school.
.43	Societal permissiveness contributes to alcohol abuse.
.42	Need to stop those who provide alcohol to minors.
	Factor 6: Social constraints on help-seeking
.72	Problem drinkers are anxious about social rejection.
.53	Treatment needs to be calibrated to the whole person.
.49	Community is a social fishbowl.
.48	People are driven to drinking because of intractable difficulties.
	Factor 7: Deterrence
.68	The local court is too easy on those who abuse alcohol.
.53	Treatment is best left to those with professional competence.
.50	People who injure others while intoxicated should make restitution.

170 K. Mark Leek

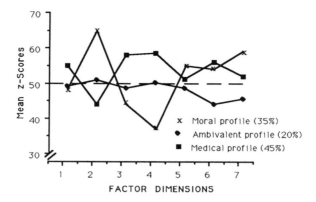

Figure 8-2. Leadership profiles toward alcohol abuse. Factor dimensions: 1, social problem; 2, moralistic; 3, treatment; 4, medical; 5, formal authority; 6, social restraints on help-seeking; 7, deterrence.

Medical and moral profiles take a different view of the obligation of society toward the individual. Medicals view alcohol abuse as a social issue that must be addressed as a public problem. Morals view alcohol abuse as a private matter that should be addressed by the individual. The ambivalents share the moral profile's reluctance to define alcohol abuse as a public problem, but they do so for a different reason. For ambivalents the relationship of society to the individual is mediated by the problem of addiction. Until the individual is ready to seek help the appropriate relation of society to the individual is a moot point.[1]

A second "near (policy) core" component consists of "basic choices concerning policy instruments, e.g., coercion vs. inducement vs. persuasion" (Sabatier, 1987, p. 667). Basic differences are found in orientations toward intervention. Medicals favor treatment, whereas morals emphasize deterrence as the appropriate form of intervention. Ambivalents do not have an action component to their orientation. Apparently their ambivalence about the cause of abuse leads to passivity when it comes to taking a position on how to deal with it.

A third "near (policy) core" component addresses the "proper distribution of authority among various units (e.g., levels) of government" (Sabatier, 1987, p. 667). Fundamental differences are found in orientations toward the role of formal authority as an instrument of public policy. Morals see alcohol abuse among youth as a challenge to the capacity of the school board to address a social problem. For medicals it will not do to isolate the

[1] This interpretation is based on some 20 hours of intensive interviews by the author with a person from the ambivalent profile.

Table 8-2. Structure of Leadership Belief Toward the Problem of Alcohol Abuse

Core Dimensions of Belief	Leadership Perspectives (Profiles) Toward Alcohol Abuse[a]		
	Medical (45%)	Moral (35%)	Ambivalent (20%)
	Deep (normative) core[b]		
Origin of abuse	Disease (+ factor 4)	Character (+ factor 2)	Disease/ character
	Near (policy) core		
Locus of responsibility	Public problem (+ factor 1)	Private problem (− factor 1)	Private problem (− factor 1)
Individual-level intervention	Treatment (+ factor 3)	Deterrence (+ factor 7)	N/A
Group-level intervention	Community based (+ factor 5)	Formal authority (+ factor 5)	N/A
	Secondary aspects		
Constraints on help-seeking	Social (+ factor 6)	Social (+ factor 6)	Individual (− factor 6)

[a] Valence signs indicate the orientation of each perspective (plus or minus) toward each of the factors.
[b] From Sabatier (1987).

problem from the social context in which it occurs. They view the school board as one component of a multifaceted approach.

A third level of belief consists of a set of "secondary aspects" comprising "a multitude of instrumental decisions and information searches necessary to implement the policy core in the specific policy area." It is "the topic of most administrative and even legislative policy making" (Sabatier, 1987, p. 666). In relation to alcohol abuse instrumental decisions address views toward the personal and social constraints that prevent implementation of core beliefs. Morals and medicals both focus on the social constraints that prevent individuals from seeking help (Factor 6). Both focus on the individual's fear of social rejection. For morals, fear of social rejection prevents the individual from taking initiatives on his or her own behalf; for medicals, fear of social rejection creates a wall of isolation that distances the individual from available sources of support. For ambivalents social rejection isn't an issue. The major impediment to seeking help is denial of the problem.

This analysis points to the likely outcome of basing an agenda-building strategy on a definition of alcohol abuse that captures only a single orientation to the problem. How a problem is defined is exceedingly important for the potential for interpersonal cooperation. Mobilization of support for collective action depends on the willingness of individuals to respond to the cues they receive concerning the need to address the problem. If the message they receive is ambiguous about the need for action or contradicts basic assumptions about the nature of the problem and how to deal with it, the potential for personal investment in collective action is diminished. An agenda-building strategy that defines alcohol abuse in either moral or medical terms would fail to address the core values and concerns of a large segment of the leadership population. A large segment of leaders would be unlikely to become involved in agenda-building activities.

Defining alcohol abuse so as to emphasize the area where the medical and moral perspectives converge is also unlikely to elicit much active support. Improving opportunities for confidential help-seeking is peripheral to leaders' core concerns. As a vehicle for change it is important only in the context of some larger conception of the problem and what to do about it. Leaders may condone the efforts of others to address social constraints on help-seeking, but they are unlikely to find it a compelling reason to take initiatives themselves.

The Role of Diverse Leadership Attributes in the Agenda-Building Process

The premise of the argument so far is that the manner in which a problem is defined is crucial to determining the outcome of efforts to move an item from the systemic onto the formal agenda. To mobilize support for collective action, problems must be defined in ways that conform to the values and concerns of key participants. What isn't clear is why agenda-building depends on the involvement of individuals with a diverse range of values and policy orientations. On its face it would seem that the number of people involved is more important than the distribution of views that are represented in the agenda-building process. If enough individuals become involved, it shouldn't particularly matter how the different perspectives are represented in the agenda-building process. The key is to generate enough involvement to move an item onto the formal agenda, where by definition it will become an object of collective action.

This section develops the argument that participation from more than a single perspective is necessary because each perspective contributes to the agenda-building process in a unique way. As a group, leaders possess a pool of leadership attributes. If leadership participation is circumscribed in some manner, for instance, through the systematic exclusion of a segment of the leadership population due to the way that a problem is defined, individuals with leadership attributes that are essential to the agenda-building process will fail to participate.[2]

Differences in the leadership attributes of leaders were investigated empirically. Subjects from each alcohol perspective were asked to examine lists of names corresponding to individuals from each of the medical, moral, and ambivalent profiles taken from the top third of the influence matrix. The lists were unlabeled and each subject's own name was removed prior to the interview. Subjects were asked to describe the leadership attributes of the individuals from each list, both individually and as a group.

Based on subject responses three patterns of leadership attributes emerged. Each pattern describes a unique contribution to the agenda-building process (Figure 8-3). Medicals are agenda initiators. They are described as people who "implant ideas in others." (Quotations are drawn from subject interviews.) Although they are good at "putting things into action," they prefer to "remain in the background" where they are "often involved in some program." Morals are agenda activators. Generally they are "not self-starters" but need to be convinced of the need for action. Once involved they are highly committed. Often they are unwilling "to simply petition titular powers" but will try to "change government in some way if necessary." They actively try to be "change agents." Ambivalents are agenda ratifiers. They are "quiet people who listen as much, if not more, than they talk." "All have ideas and are willing to work through other people" to effect change. While not entirely comfortable with conflict, they can be highly persuasive in presenting their views to others.

The three patterns of leadership attributes interact to form a mutually reinforcing system of initiative-taking. Initiators bring an issue to the attention of activators, who are especially adept at dealing with the large bureaucratic forces that need to be handled in order to pave the way for collective action. Their assertions serve to sanction the problem as a legitimate object of public concern in the eyes of the community. By engaging the problem on a community level, activators sustain the efforts of initiators to engage the problem on a program level. Ratifiers facilitate this process by legitimizing the efforts of other leaders. By engaging the agenda-building process they cue other leaders of the emergence of consensus as a basis for initiative-taking.

---

[2] This is an empirically based claim and is not intended as a normative statement about the conditions associated with agenda-building in all instances. It is not assumed that some optimum balance of leadership attributes must be present for agenda-setting to culminate in the transfer of an item from the systemic to the formal agenda. Rather, if specific leadership attributes are found to exist among leaders, and it can be shown that some of these are absent in situations where agenda-building is problematic, it may be argued that there has been a breakdown in the agenda-setting functions associated with these attributes. See Collins (1973) for a discussion of the shortcomings of a structural–functional approach.

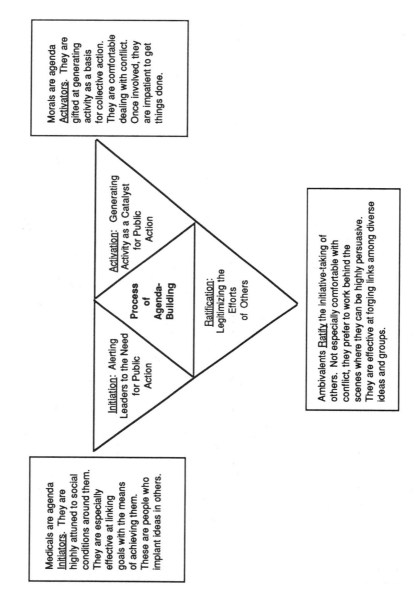

Morals are agenda Activators. They are gifted at generating activity as a basis for collective action. They are comfortable dealing with conflict. Once involved, they are impatient to get things done.

Activation: Generating Activity as a Catalyst for Public Action

Process of Agenda-Building

Initiation: Alerting Leaders to the Need for Public Action

Ratification: Legitimizing the Efforts of Others

Ambivalents Ratify the initiative-taking of others. Not especially comfortable with conflict, they prefer to work behind the scenes where they can be highly persuasive. They are effective at forging links among diverse ideas and groups.

Medicals are agenda Initiators. They are highly attuned to social conditions around them. They are especially effective at linking goals with the means of achieving them. These are people who implant ideas in others.

Figure 8-3. Role of three alcohol perspectives in the agenda-building process.

All three leadership attributes must be present for the agenda-building process to culminate in the movement of an item from the systemic to the formal agenda. For an issue to achieve formal agenda status leaders must be willing to cooperate with one another in a collective effort to translate a mutual concern into a program of action for addressing a problem. Each attribute plays a vital role in sustaining the collective search for solutions. If leaders with unique leadership attributes choose not to participate in the agenda-building process, then initiative-taking as a basis for program development will not occur.[3]

The Implications for Program Development of a Breakdown in the Agenda-Building Process

What does it mean to say that the absence of a diverse range of leadership attributes leads to a breakdown in the agenda-building process and how can such a breakdown occur? This section uses the same case study to explore the implications for program development of a situation in which initiators bring a problem to the attention of community leaders but, because of the way the problem is defined, activators fail to engage the agenda-building process.

Efforts to engage the problem of alcohol abuse in this community centered around the local public school district and the local Community Alcohol Center (CAC), with secondary involvement from a local volunteer coordinating agency. With the focus of the school district on the problem of alcohol use among students, attempts to transform the problem into a community issue depended heavily on the local CAC as a focal point for community involvement. The CAC never lived up to community expectations in this regard. According to one person, the problem was that "the community never said that we need an alcohol treatment center; there was never a groundswell of support." In the absence of commuity support "nothing ever took fire, it was always a lot of hard slogging and footwork."

The source of much of the community's ambivalence toward the CAC lay with the CAC itself. While the CAC staff, in the words of one person, performed a "yeoman's job in keeping the Center alive," it was often at odds with its own board. The CAC board was never able to effectively challenge its own staff for organizational or policy control. Free to do much as it wanted, the staff often acted in ways that undermined its relations with other community groups and organizations. According to one leader the community was receptive to the CAC but the people who ran the Center "didn't know how to use the help they could get." Often they would "get people interested in a project but then not support it."

The failure of the community to support the CAC and the inability of the CAC board to assert managerial control over its own staff are symptomatic of

---

[3] Program development is defined as the mobilization of goal-directed activity for the purpose of addressing a public problem.

a breakdown in the agenda-building process. Alcohol abuse ws presented to the community almost exclusively as a medical problem. The CAC viewed the promotion of the medical model as its primary mission while the legal community offered little counterweight to this dominant view. The local judge was perceived by many as too lenient in his approach to sentencing. Virtually all sentences for DWI were suspended if a person sought treatment at the local CAC.

Because alcohol abuse was defined predominantly in medical terms, support for collective action came primarily from individuals predisposed to initiative-taking in the context of a specific program. Individuals capable of asserting themselves on a community level by forging links among groups and organizations did not feel compelled to take initiatives on behalf of the problem. As a result of their unwillingness to engage the agenda-building process and thereby sanction the problem as a legitimate object of collective action in the eyes of the community, the CAC board was denied the leverage it needed to assert itself in relation to its own staff. The kinds of assertions needed to forge links with diverse groups as a basis for eliciting the support of those with a moralistic orientation to the problem did not occur.

There is evidence that an approach to problem-structuring that incorporated both medical and moral orientations toward the problem might have led to greater community involvement. A community leader with a moralistic orientation recently told the author that for a while community interest in alcohol abuse intensified when local police "became very much more pushy about enforcing the rules," particularly in relation to alcohol use among youths. He noted, however, that recently police had been "slipping" in their enforcement of the rules and enthusiasm for addressing the problem had abated. In his own mind he drew a direct connection between community interest in the problem and a hard-line approach to enforcement. A similar pattern may be seen at the national policy level where a dramatic increase in public awareness and interest in the problem of alcohol abuse has occurred since Mothers Against Drunk Driving (MADD) began its crusade to obtain more severe mandatory sentencing for drinking and driving.

Conclusion

This analysis has sought to show the link between problem-structuring and the potential for collective action. The mobilization of support for collective action depends on the ability of policymakers to effectively challenge program experts and policy elites for policy control. If leadership is unable to assert itself on behalf of collective action, policy control will remain with those who have an organizational interest in limiting the scope of participation. A prerequisite to sustained community involvement is the activation of leaders with diverse points of view. The full range of leadership attributes necessary to sustain the collective search for solutions becomes available to leaders only when diverse value orientations are represented in the agenda-building process. A mental representation approach to problem-structuring offers policymakers a means to overcome organizational inertia through the identification and activation of individuals with diverse value orientations.

The second half of this chapter uses a mental representation approach to problem-structuring to address a different type of value-oriented problem, though one that also involves the indentification of diverse value orientations as a prerequisite to program development. Problem-structuring in the area of health-care delivery is subject to many of the same challenges that confront policymakers in general. Health-care professionals responsible for the development of treatment programs often have little means to systematically evaluate the human dimensions associated with coping. Yet successful adaptation to illness often depends on the ability of patients to invest themselves in their own treatment process. A mental representation approach addresses these concerns by offering providers a means to define health problems and coping strategies in ways that are consistent with patient needs and orientations toward coping.

A Mental Representation Approach to Policy Analysis in the Area of Multiple Sclerosis

This study is highly exploratory. It originated when a few members of a multiple sclerosis support group invited the author and a colleague to join them in applying a mental representation approach to problem-structuring to the study of the relationship between doctors and patients with MS. A general feeling existed that this relationship is not well understood. While individual experiences with health-care providers varied from person to person, almost everyone could recall at least one instance when the health-care system had let them down. Often this memory centered on the anger and frustration they felt in the early stages of the disease process when they knew that something was very wrong but could not obtain a diagnosis. For others the health-care community is a constant source of anger and frustration.

This study was conceived as half of a two-part study. A complementary study would deal with the orientations of health-care providers toward people with MS. Together the two studies would provide an understanding of the patterns of variation in the way doctors and patients relate to coping and to each other. Eventually this might lead to the construction of an instrument for matching patients and physicians with compatible coping orientations. The study is included in this chapter as another example of a mental representation approach to health policy analysis. It is not intended as a definitive statement about the structure of patient orientations toward coping or health-care providers.[4]

Traditional Approaches to the Study of Doctor–Patient Interaction

The need to focus on patient orientations toward coping and wellness is a basic presupposition of those who study doctor–patient interaction. There is a general feeling that more attention needs to be given to the nontechnical or human dimensions of this exchange. For example, Wasserman et al. state that pediatric office visits "have two strikingly different agenda," one technical and other nontechnical. They state that whereas "much is known about the performance and effectiveness of the technical elements of preventive child health visits . . . very little [is known] about the other, nontechnical component" (Wasserman, Inui, Barriatua, Carter, & Lippincott, 1983, p. 171).

For the most part studies of doctor–patient interaction focus on face-to-face encounters. They rely on a variety of observational strategies— direct, videotape, audiotape, or transcript formats—to evaluate verbal and nonverbal interaction processes (Advani, 1973; DiMatteo & Rodin, 1980; Snyder, Lynch, & Gruss, 1976) Typically, encounter processes are correlated with treatment outcomes such as patient knowledge, satisfaction, compliance, and reassurance.

These studies show that the doctor–patient relationship is an ordered process amenable to purposive change. Doctors and patients each contribute to the character of the relationship in systematic and identifiable ways. Wasserman et al. (1983) found evidence to suggest that pediatric clinicians are responsive to variation in level of previsit maternal concerns. Providers showed more empathy and offered more reassurance to mothers who sought information and initiated conversation. Among providers, nurse practitioners more than physicians, and females more than males, were found to offer more empathy and reassurance to mothers. These processes were found to directly affect clinical outcomes. "Mothers exposed to high levels of empathy had higher satisfaction and greater reduction in concerns" (Wasserman, Inui, Barriatua, Carter, & Lippincott, 1984, p. 1047).

If there is a drawback to this approach to the study of doctor–patient interaction it is a tendency to focus almost exclusively on the observable and contextually specific behaviors of doctors and patients. As Wasserman and Inui state, "The most commonly applied analytic strategy has been to develop communicator profiles based on frequency distributions of communication behaviors" (1983, p. 291). This emphasis ignores the role contextual factors may play in determining the character and outcome of

---

[4] Most subjects, perhaps as many as 75% of the total of 113 people interviewed, were recruited from local MS support groups. Respondents are not a representative sample of people with MS or of those who belong to an MS support group.

doctor–patient interaction (Inui & Carter, 1985; Wasserman & Inui, 1983).

This study examines how patient orientations toward coping and wellness may influence patient perceptions of the doctor–patient relationship. The study assumes that there are two broad categories of patient orientations toward coping that may contribute to patient orientations toward health-care providers, one personal and the other environmental. Personal factors consist of level of physical ability, self-concept, and orientation toward coping. Environmental factors consist of family functioning and social support. The goal of the analysis is to determine whether physicians are perceived as a positive or negative influence in the coping process and the antecedent conditions associated with each view.

The analysis proceeds in several steps. Following an initial discussion of the instruments used to measure personal and environmental factors associated with coping, cluster analysis is used to discover the shared mental images that define subject orientations toward each of the personal and environmental factors. Object typing is then used to determine shared subject orientations toward coping and health-care providers.

Personal Factors That Influence Adaptation

Physical Disability. Level of physical ability is the primary indicator of the challenge a person faces in attempting to meet the demands of daily living. A mild form of disability will impose fewer disruptions and make fewer demands on an individual than will a more severe form of disability. Disability was measured by revising the Kurtzke Disability Scale to include 14 rankings that correspond to four categories of impairment: minimal to moderate mobility impairment (24% of subjects), severe mobility impairment (59%), restricted mobility (15%), and nonmobile (2%).

Self-Image. Individuals with a disability can experience a crisis of identity as conflict emerges between their image of a normal self and the reality of what is happening to them. A loss of self-worth and esteem can occur when people are faced with an inability to perform in a way that has come to be expected. Successful adaptation to chronic illness implies the maintenance or restoration of a sense of control to the degree possible over their own personal life. The Rosenberg Self-Esteem Scale (1965) was used to assess personal coping resources. The instrument was converted to a five-step agreement/ neutrality/disagreement scale.

Orientation Toward Coping. Physical disability is an indication of the severity of the challenge faced by a person with MS, but it is far from an absolute indicator of the ability of a person to cope with chronic illness. Some people strive for autonomy and independence while others opt for some form of dependent relationship. Individuals rarely rely exclusively on a single mode of adaptation but can fluctuate among or emphasize one of three coping modes (Chodoff, 1959).

In one mode, characterized by denial, individuals can resist the temptation to engage in dependency, which consists of an unwillingness to accept the loss of ability they are experiencing. In another mode individuals can give in to the temptation to engage in dependency. There is a tendency to exaggerate the effects of disability in order to elicit the support and intervention of others. In still a third mode of adapting to MS, one characterized by insightful acceptance, there is acceptance of disability and a desire to move beyond the disease in the way one defines the meaning of one's life and life goals. There is positive engagement of the effects of the illness.

Subscales from a 50-item Q sort were used to assess orientation toward coping. (See the appendix for a complete list of subscales and some sample items.) The instrument was created by the author and a colleague after extensive consultation with health-care professionals and people with MS.

Environmental Factors That Influence Adaptation

Family Functioning and Social Support. Family, friends, and co-workers play a crucial role in the process of individual adaptation to chronic illness. Through their action or inaction they can influence the pattern of adaptation a person with MS will rely on. As with the person with MS, there is a need on their part to attain an attitude of insightful acceptance of the disease and of the changes the disease imposes on all concerned.

The APGAR was used to assess family support (Smilkstein, 1978). Question 11 of the Personal Resource Questionnaire (PRQ) was used to assess social as well as family support (Brandt & Weinert, 1981; Weinert, 1987; Weinert & Brandt, 1987). The APGAR and PRQ were converted to a five-step agreement/neutrality/disagreement scale.

Health-Care and Service Providers. Members of the health-care profession play a crucial role in the process of individual adaptation to MS. As with family, friends, and co-workers, health-care professionals must strive to achieve a balance between two modes of interacting with persons who have MS. Generally, there is a need for them to assume a traditional, goal-directed orientation toward patients with MS in the management of symptoms for which there is a recognized cure. This same mode of interacting can prove dysfunctional to the interests of the person if used by the provider to assert control over the entire disease process. The patient needs the opportunity to take the kind of initiatives on his or her own behalf that will lead to a sense of independence and control over the disease process. Orientation to health-care providers was assessed by several of the subscales in the previously mentioned 50-item instrument (appendix).

The Identification of the Shared Mental Images of Patients Toward Coping and Support Resources

The data from the self-concept, family and social support, and coping/ physician-orientation instruments were combined into a single matrix and

Table 8-3. Cluster Analysis of Items Defining the Shared Mental Images of People With MS Toward Coping and Support Resources

Loading	Item

Cluster 1: Positive family support

Loading	Item
.85 D	My family discusses things with me.
.84 D	My family expresses affection toward me.
.83 D	My family supports my initiatives.
.80 D	My family and I share time together.
.77 D	My family is available to help me when I need it.
.70	My family accepts and understands my condition.
.63	My family lets me know I'm important to family.
.58	There is someone who loves me and cares about me.
.56	People are available if I need help for a long period.

Cluster 2: Positive self-concept

Loading	Item
.79 D	I take a positive attitude toward myself.
.67 D	On the whole I am satisfied with myself.
.63 D	I spend time with others who have same interests as I do.*
.58 D	I am able to do things as well as others with my disability.
.49	I am able to encourage others to develop their interests.
.48	I have a number of good qualities.
.47	I can do just about anything I really set my mind to.
.46	All in all, I am inclined to feel that I am a failure.
.46	Sometimes I feel that I'm being pushed around in life.
.44	I often feel helpless dealing with problems of life.
.42	I have little control over the things that happen to me.

Cluster 3: Disability is a problem

Loading	Item
.76 D	This area needs an outreach program.
.61	MS society must inform more.
.59 D	Doctors need to refer more to available services.
.57	Physicians fear appearing incompetent.
.57 D	Doctors are frustrated by inability to do more.
.53 D	Physicians more comfortable treating symptoms of the disease than difficulties associated with disability.
.52	Doctors assume clients know more about MS than they do.
.50	The greatest trial is maintaining self-sufficiency.
.46	Doctors unable to discuss problems associated with illness.

Cluster 4: Positive social support

Loading	Item
.83 D	There is someone who is close who makes me feel secure.
.82 D	I have a close friend to whom I can turn for help.
.77 D	When I'm upset there is someone who lets me be myself.
.65	There is someone to help me with my problems.

Table 8-3. *Continued*

Loading	Item
	Cluster 4: Positive social support (*Cont.*)
.65 D	Among my group of friends we do favors for each other.
.63	I have people to share social and fun activities.
.60	I have a sense of being needed by another person.
−.60	There is no one to talk to about how I feel.
.58	I belong to a group in which I feel important.
.57	If I get sick there is someone to care for me.
.57	I'm satisfied with the support I receive from friends.
.54	I know others appreciate me as a person.
.52	Relatives and friends will help even if I can't pay back.
	Cluster 5: Positive physician support
.8129 D	Physician involved in search for workable solutions.
.7110 D	Physician visits are encouraging.
	Cluster 6: Positive coping
.77 D	I must strive to maintain normal lifestyle.
.65 D	Emotional support is crucial for coping.
.59	A fulfilling life is possible despite MS.
.50	I am responsible for quality of my own life.
.48	The effects of MS are not all disabling.
.40	Doctors are obligated to be straightforward.
	Cluster 7: Negative physician support
.74 D	Visiting a specialist makes me feel overwhelmed and uncertain about myself.
.68 D	I avoid visiting health care professionals.
.47	I have never had a satisfying visit with a doctor.
.42	The thought of dependency is uncomfortable.
.41	Doctors are uncomfortable around people with MS.
−.40	I am satisfied with the medical knowledge of doctors.

cluster analyzed (Anderberg, 1972). The clusters are presented in Table 8-3. Definers (labeled "D") are the key items, or "pivots," that the computer uses to construct each cluster. All definers are computer generated. The seven clusters constitute the shared mental images that subjects rely on to define coping and support resources.

With one exception (the third item in cluster 2, labeled with an asterisk), definers for each cluster come from the same instrument. All but two of the clusters have insignificant intercluster correlation scores. Clusters 1 and 4, both from the same social support scale, have an intercluster correlation of .55. Cluster independence is a sign that the subscales are valid measures of conceptually distinct dimensions (McCormick, Siegert, & Walkey, 1987).

The clusters in Table 8-3 portray support resources and the role of physicians in both a positive and negative light. Cluster 1 depicts a supportive family environment. Cluster 2 reflects a positive self-image. Cluster 4 depicts a supportive social environment. Cluster 5 depicts a positive orientation to physicians. Cluster 6 depicts a positive orientation to coping. Acknowledgment of the individual's responsibility to accept the challenge of disability is combined with an attitude of enlightened acceptance.

Two clusters describe aspects of coping that are problematic for the individual. Cluster 3 depicts a health-care community that is failing to meet its obligation to help the individual cope with disability. Services are lacking, doctors do not refer patients to services that are available, and doctors feel threatened or insecure about their inability to cure or do more for people with MS. Cluster 7 focuses directly on the doctor–patient relationship and finds it wanting. Not only are doctors unable to help patients, but patients actually feel worse about themselves than they did before their visit.

The Identification of Diverse Patient Orientations Toward Coping and Support Resources

In this section object typing is used to identify diverse patient orientations toward coping and support resources. Figures 8-4 through 8-6 identify five patient profiles. The TRYSYS1 computer program was utilized for carrying out the object typing.[5]

Figure 8-4 is comprised of two patient profiles that share a positive orientation toward coping, the high achieving copers (7% of subjects) and the active copers (50% of subjects). Family and social support are high, they have a positive self-image, and the physician is perceived as a positive source of support in relation to coping.

Figure 8-5 is comprised of two patient profiles whose members are struggling with disability, the active strugglers (23% of subjects) and the passive strugglers (13% of subjects). The most remarkable feature of the active struggler profile is the juxtaposition of positive support from family and friends on the one hand and the negative influence of health-care and service providers on the other. Its orientation to positive coping (cluster 6) is the key to explaining this juxtaposition.

---

[5] Profiles are based on a total of 102 subjects. One profile consisting of two people is not included for analysis in this study.

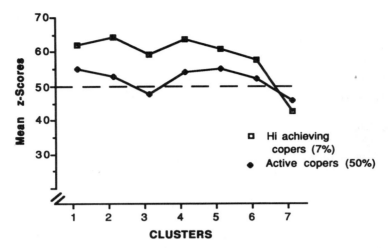

Figure 8-4. MS patient profile: active and high achieving copers. Clusters: 1, positve family support; 2, positive self-concept; 3, disability is a problem; 4, positive social support; 5, positive physician support; 6, positive coping; 7, negative physician support. (Hi = High.)

Active strugglers acknowledge the need to actively engage the coping process (cluster 6). From these data it is not possible to determine how well they perform in this regard, only that they acknowledge the struggle. A high level of social and family support indicates that they have achieved some coping success. This and the fact that they are in a support group indicate that they are working very hard to deal with their disability.

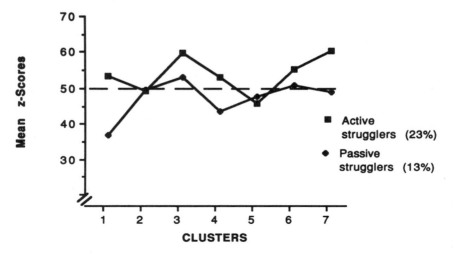

Figure 8-5. MS patient profile: active and passive strugglers.

Based on these factors it appears that active strugglers are expressing a legitimate complaint with the quality of care they receive from the health-care system. The health-care and service community are not addressing their needs. They appear to have the energy, desire, and capability to take a more active role in their own treatment process. With regard to the people represented by this profile, there seems to be room for improvement in the health-care delivery system.

The problem that passive strugglers experience with disability appears to require a nonmedical solution. They are ambivalent about the role of the physician as a facilitator in the coping process. The physician relationship is not the source of their problem. On the other hand, there is a profound deficit in the support they receive from family and friends. While not especially high in coping skills and self-image, there appears to be sufficient acknowledgment of their own role in the coping process to sustain a support network if these sources of support were available.

Figure 8-6 is comprised of individuals who appear to be psychologically depressed. There is a profound deficit in coping skills and family and friends are not available for support. Neither disability nor the quality of care they receive from health-care and service providers appears to be a factor in their depression. The medically appropriate response would appear to be psychological help for depression.

It is important to remember when analyzing these profiles that they are not based on a representative sample of people with MS. There is no clear instance of denial. This makes perfect sense when one considers that those involved in denial are probably the least likely to join a multiple sclerosis support group. The majority of people, some 80%, possess positive coping

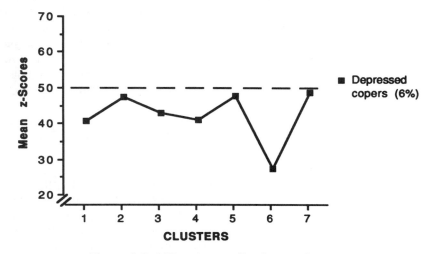

Figure 8-6. MS patient profile: depressed copers.

skills and receive positive social support from family and friends. These are people one would expect to find in a support group.

Conclusion

The doctor–patient relationship is especially problematic for the physician from the standpoint of his or her role as treatment provider. Standard tests such as the Minnesota Multiphasic Inventory are available for assessing the psychological status of patients, but very little is available for assessing the role of the health-care provider as a source of intervention. Physicians have only what they see before them as a means of assessing the needs of their patients in relation to themselves. An important source of stability and/or disruption to the patient is unavailable to the physician for systematic examination.

The doctor–patient relationship is problematic for the patient because the strong desire to be well can make it difficult to evaluate the legitimacy of demands made upon the health-care system. Patients have only their own experience and what they can learn from one another in passing as a frame of reference for distinguishing demands that are legitimate from those that are wish-driven. The doctor–patient exchange itself is geared almost exclusively to the discussion of symptomatology. In the absence of a structured format for evaluating the legitimacy of expectations of providers with those most in a position to make a difference (providers themselves), there is no knowledge-based solution for dealing with the disjuncture between expectation and performance. Feelings of dissatisfaction and resentment are left unresolved and may become a source of dysfunction.

A mental representation approach to problem-structuring can serve the needs of both patients and providers. It affords doctors a means to sort out those that are depressed from those struggling with symptomatology. With regard to the latter they can evaluate their own role as an instrument of treatment. It gives patients some control of their own treatment process. They can have a systematic and reality-based means of evaluating their own expectations in relation to others with similar experiences. They can make knowledge-based choices about the type of care that is best suited for them.

Implications of a Mental Representation Approach for Community Intervention

Community organization is increasingly used in public health efforts at prevention (Carlaw, Mittlemark, Bracht, & Luepker, 1984; Farquhar et al., 1985; Schwebel, Kershaw, Reeve, Harung, & Reeve, 1973). It is generally accepted among public health professionals that prevention must address the social and environmental context in which chronic health problems occur (Wallack, 1985). It is not enough to target individuals in the hope that this will lead to widespread behavioral change (Syme & Alcalay, 1982). Intervention must also target environmental influences that reinforce and encourage health-threatening behaviors.

Increasingly, community organization assumes that community ownership is a prerequisite to structural change. Communities are likely to be transformed only if individuals invest themselves in the process of change (Gruber & Trickett, 1987; Rappaport, 1987). Community ownership is often conceived in terms of individual involvement through participation in program activities and identification with program goals. Activation occurs through the mobilization of diverse community sectors, such as health care, social service, local business, and the media (Thompson & Kinne, 1990).

A presupposition of this approach is that identification will occur as a result of participation (Green, 1986; Rifkin, 1986). It is felt that widespread participation in sector-specific activities, combined with public education, will lead to increased awareness and identification with the values the intervention is trying to promote. Such participation will have a synergistic effect. Individuals in positions to influence the structure and flow of cues and messages that shape individual behavior will begin to act to implement change on behalf of these values.

This approach to community ownership may not be the most effective as a means of obtaining long-term structural change. Instead of relying exclusively on sectoral participation and public education to facilitate ownership, it may be more effective to combine this strategy with one that orients participation to individuals' core beliefs about the problem itself. A prerequisite of community ownership is identification with the problem, not with sectors per se.

Community organization efforts may also be undermined if intervention specialists bring their own definition of a problem to a community or if mobilization efforts result in the displacement of a definition of a problem by another. This is the basic criticism of Leventhal et al. (1980) of the Stanford Heart Disease Prevention Program. They argue that "the medical perspective of the project led the investigators to ignore a variety of issues that formed essential links for meeting their overall objectives and led them to confuse medical and behavior endpoints in evaluating their program" (p. 151). This is the main point of this analysis. The way problems are defined can play a crucial role in determining how mobilization efforts are received by those whose involvement is sought.

Conclusion

Mental representation provides a way to define problems in areas where the dimensions of a problem are not entirely understood. The most crucial stage in program development, problem-structuring, is often the least understood. It is widely believed that a definition of a problem that is compatible with the values and policy orientations of key participants will emerge spontaneously if the right combination of people are brought together to discuss a problem. Wallack and Wallerstein suggest that "the first step in identifying a problem is to convene a public meeting or series of meetings with the appropriate diversity of interests. This group will identify an initial formulation of the problem" (1987, p. 330).

This is far from self-evident. Often the sources of conflict that preclude effective program development—what Wallack and Wallerstein call "interests"—are far from apparent to those directly involved. The basis for mutual dialogue is not present. Mental representation provides policymakers with the means to objectively portray their own and each other's orientation to a problem. This is a first step in framing problems in ways that are compatible with the values and policy orientations of key participants.

Acknowledgments. I would like to thank the editors, Noel J. Chrisman, Dia S. Dissmore, Edward J. Fox, Arthur H. Ginsberg, Joan Gusa, Susan Kinne, Herman D. Lujan, Charles L. and Justine F. Nagel, Charles D. Treser, and Robert Walker for their substantive comments and/or help editing various parts or drafts of this chapter and also Gerard P. Duguay and Cynthia Lostoski for producing most of the statistics for the MS study. I also want to thank the people of the (unnamed) community described in this study and the people of the MS support groups whose participation made this study possible. William J. Gore taught me much of what I know about the scientific foundations of a mental representation approach to policy analysis.

References

Advani, M. (1973). Observing doctor–patient interaction in a small community general hospital. *Manas, 20,* 9–19.

Allison, G. (1969). Conceptual models and the Cuban missile crisis. *American Political Science Review, 63,* 689–718.

Anderberg, M. R. (1972). *Cluster analysis for applications.* New York: Academic Press.

Brandt, P., & Weinert, C. (1981). The PRQ: A social support measure. *Nursing Research, 30,* 277–280.

Brown, S. R. (1980). *Political subjectivity: Applications of Q methodology in political science.* New Haven, CT: Yale University Press.

Carlaw, R. W., Mittlemark, M. B., Bracht, N., & Luepker, R. (1984). Organization for a community cardiovascular health program: Experiences from the Minnesota Heart Health Program. *Health Education Quarterly, 11,* 243–252.

Carter, W. B., Inui, T. S., Kukull, W. A., & Haigh, V. H. (1982). Outcome-based doctor–patient interaction analysis. II. Identifying effective provider and patient behavior. *Medical Care, 20,* 550–566.

Chodoff, P. (1959). Adjustment to disability: Some observations on patients with multiple sclerosis. *Journal of Chronic Disease, 9,* 653–670.

Cobb, R. W., & Elder, C. D. (1971). The politics of agenda-building: An alternative perspective for modern democratic theory. *Journal of Politics, 33,* 892–915.

Cobb, R. W., & Elder, C. D. (1983). *Participation in American politics: The dynamics of agenda-building*. Baltimore: Johns Hopkins University Press.

Collins, R. (1973). A comparative approach to political sociology. In R. Bendix (Ed.), *State and society* (42–67). Los Angeles: University of California Press.

DiMatteo, M. R., & Rodin, M. (1980). Predicting patient satisfaction from physicians' nonverbal communication skills. *Medical Care, 18*, 376–387.

Dunn, W. N. (1981). *Public policy analysis*. Englewood Cliffs, NJ: Prentice-Hall.

Edelman, M. (1972). *The symbolic uses of politics*. Urbana: University of Illinois Press.

Elmore, R. F. (1978). Organizational models of social program implementation. *Public Policy, 26*, 188–228.

Elster, J. (1985). *Explaining technical change*. Cambridge: Cambridge University Press.

Farquhar, J. W. (1978). The community-based model of life style intervention trials. *American Journal of Epidemiology, 108*, 103–111.

Farquhar, J. W., Fortmann, S. P., Maccoby, N., Haskell, W. L., Williams, P. T., Flora, J. A., Taylor, C. B., Brown, B. W., Solomon, D. S., & Hulley, S. B. (1985). The Stanford five-city project: Design and methods. *American Journal of Epidemiology, 122*, 323–334.

Gesten E. L., & Jason, L. A. (1987). Social and community interventions. *Annual Review in Psychology, 38*, 427–460.

Gore, W. J., & Leek, K. M. (1987). Negative implications of fragmented public perspectives toward local alcohol programs. *American Journal of Community Psychology, 15*, 445–458.

Green, L. W. (1986). The theory of participation: A qualitative analysis of its expression in national and international health politics. In *Advances in Health Education and Promotion* (Vol. 1, pp. 211–236). Greenwich, CT: JAI Press.

Green, L. W., & McAlister, A. L. (1984). Macro-intervention to support health behavior: Some theoretical perspectives and practical reflections. *Health Education Quarterly, 11*, 322–339.

Gruber, J., & Trickett, E. J. (1987). Can we empower others? The paradox of empowerment in the governing of an alternative public school. *American Journal of Community Psychology, 15*, 353–371.

Hjern, B., & Porter, D. O. (1981). Implementation structures: A new unit of administrative analysis. *Organization Studies, 2*, 211–227.

Inglehart, R. (1977). *The silent revolution: Changing values and political styles among western democracies*. Princeton, NJ: Princeton University Press.

Inui, T. S., & Carter, W. B. (1985). Problems and prospects for health services research on provider–patient communication. *Medical Care, 23*, 521–538.

Inui, T. S., Carter, W. B., Kukull, W. A., & Haigh, V. H. (1982). Outcome-based doctor–patient interaction analysis: I. Comparison of techniques. *Medical Care, 20*, 535–549.

Kelly, J. G., Snowden, L. R., & Ricardo, M. F. (1977). Social and community interventions. *Annual Review in Psychology, 28*, 323–361.

Kessel, J. H. (1983, August). Structures of the Carter White House. *American Journal of Political Science, 27*, 430–463.

Leek, K. M. (1982). *The cognitive orientations of political leaders and followers in a small rural community*. Unpublished master's Thesis, Johns Hopkins University, Baltimore, MD.

Leventhal, J., Cleary, P. D., Safer, M. A., & Gutmann, M. (1980). Cardiovascular risk modification by community-based programs for life-style change: Comments on the Stanford study. *Journal of Consulting and Clinical Psychology, 48,* 150–158.

Lindblom, C. E. (1965). *The intelligence of democracy.* New York: Free Press.

Majone, G. (1976). Choice among policy instruments for pollution control. *Policy Analysis, 2,* 589–613.

May, P. J. (1989). *Reconsidering policy design: Policies with and without publics.* Paper prepared for presentation at the Eleventh Annual Research Conference of the Association for Public Policy Analysis and Management, November 2–4, 1989, Arlington, VA.

McCormick, I. A., Siegert, R. J., & Walkey, F. H. (1987). Dimensions of social support: A factorial confirmation. *American Journal of Community Psychology, 15,* 73–77.

Moskowitz, E. S. (1978). Neighborhood preservation: An analysis of policy maps and policy options. In J. V. May & A. B. Wildavsky (Eds.), *The policy cycle* (pp. 65–87). Beverly Hills: Sage Publications.

Rappaport, J. (1987). Terms of empowerment—Exemplars of prevention: Toward a theory for community psychology. *American Journal of Community Psychology, 15,* 121–148.

Rein, M. (1976). *Social sciences and public policy.* New York: Penguin Books.

Richardson, J., Gustafsson, G., & Jordan, G. (1982). The concept of policy style. In J. Richardson (Ed.), *Policy styles in western Europe* (pp. 1–16). London: George Allen and Urwin.

Rifkin, S. B. (1986). Health planning and community participation. *World Health Forum, 7,* 156–162.

Rosenberg, M. (1965). *Society and the adolescent self-image.* Princeton, NJ: Princeton University Press.

Rothman, J. (1972). Three models of community organization practice. In F. M. Cox, J. L. Erlich, J. Rothman, & J. E. Tropman (Eds.), *Strategies of community organization* (pp. 20–36). Itasca, IL: F. E. Peacock.

Sabatier, P. A., (1987). Knowledge, policy-oriented learning, and policy change. *Knowledge: Creation, Diffusion, Utilization, 8,* 649–692.

Sabatier, P. A., & Hunter, S., (1989). The incorporation of causal perceptions into models of elite belief systems. *Western Political Quarterly, 42,* 229–261.

Schwebel, A. I., Kershaw R., Reeve, S., Harung, J. F., & Reeve, W. (1973). A community organization approach to implementation of comprehensive health planning. *American Journal of Public Health, 63,* 451–474.

Smilkstein, G. (1978). The family APGAR: A proposal for a Family Function Test and its use by physicians. *Journal of Family Practice, 6,* 1231–1240.

Snyder, D., Lynch, J., & Gruss L. (1976). Doctor–patient communication in a private family practice. *Journal of Family Practice, 3,* 271–277.

Stephenson, W. (1957). *The study of behavior: Q technique and its methodology.* Chicago: University of Chicago Press.

Syme, L. S., & Alcalay, R. (1982). Control of cigarette smoking from a social perspective. *Annual Review of Public Health, 3,* 179–199.

Thompson, B., & Kinne, S., (1990). Social change theory: Applications to community health. In N. Bracht (Ed.), *Health promotion at the community level.* Newbury Park, CA: Sage.

Thrasher, M. T. (1983). Exchange networks and implementation. *Policy and Politics, 11,* 375–391.

Walker, J. L. (1983). The origins and maintenance of interest groups in America.

American Political Science Review, 77, 390–406.

Wallack, L. (1985). A community approach to the prevention of alcohol-related problems: The San Francisco experience. *International Quarterly of Community Health Education, 5,* 85–102.

Wallack, L., & Wallerstein, N. (1987). Health education and prevention: Designing community initiatives. *International Quarterly of Community Health Education, 7,* 319–342.

Wasserman, R. C., & Inui, T. S. (1983). Systematic Analysis of Clinician-Patient Interactions: A Critique of Recent Approaches With Suggestions for Future Research. *Medical Care, 21,* 279–293.

Wasserman, R. C., Inui, T. S., Barriatua, R. D., Carter, W. B., & Lippincott, P. (1983). Responsiveness to maternal concern in preventive child health visits: An analysis of clinician–parent interactions. *Development and Behavioral Pediatrics, 4,* 171–176.

Wasserman, R. C., Inui, T. S., Barriatua, R. D., Carter, W. B., & Lippincott, P. (1984). Pediatric clinicians' support for parents makes a difference: An outcome-based analysis of clinician-parent interaction, *Pediatrics, 74,* 1047–1053.

Weinert, C. (1987). A social support measure: PRQ85. *Nursing Research, 36,* 273–277.

Weinert, C., & Brandt, P. (1987). Measuring social support with the PRQ. *Western Journal of Nursing Research, 9,* 589–602.

Williams, D., Gore, W., Broches, C., & Lostoski, C. (1987). One faculty's perceptions of its governance role. *Journal of Higher Education, 58,* 629–657.

Appendix. Patient Coping/Physician Orientation Instrument: Subscales and Sample Items

Orientation to Coping (Four Subscales)

1. Dependency/Victim/Denial (eight items)

   There are times when I find that I expect and want more help from others than I may actually require.

   There are times when I feel anger toward those upon whom I am dependent because of MS.

   The thought of being dependent upon others makes me feel very uncomfortable.

2. Enlightened Acceptance (three items)

   Even though my medical condition may not improve I can still have a fulfilling life.

   The effects of MS are not all destructive since an increase in human sensitivity and insight, patience, and understanding can result from it as well.

3. Acceptance of Personal Role in Maintaining Social and Psychological Equilibrium (seven items)

   Persons with MS often experience a loss of self-worth and esteem when confronted with their inability to contribute to the family unit in a way that they have come to expect of themselves.

   Individuals with MS must struggle to balance the constant slipping away of independence on the one hand with the need to maintain or regain self-direction on the other.

Orientation to Coping (Continued)

4. Family Role in Coping (four items)
   My family accepts my situation and understands what I am going through.
   I find that I receive a lot of resistance from my family when it comes to accepting
   the lifestyle changes that MS imposes upon us.

Patient–Physician Relationship (Four Subscales)

5. Client Orientation to Provider (nine items)
   I have been satisfied with the medical knowledge of most of the physicians I have
   consulted about MS.
   My faith in the ability of the medical community to help me deal with MS is so low
   that I avoid visiting health care professionals as much as possible.
6. Orientation of Providers Toward Persons With MS (nine items)
   My physician involves himself or herself with me in searching for workable
   solutions to the difficulties brought about by MS.
   Doctors are often unprepared or unable to discuss many of the problems, such as
   sexual dysfunction, which confront people with MS.
7. Effect of Provider–Patient Interaction on Ability to Cope With Disability (four
   items)
   I find my visits with physicians to be a source of encouragement in meeting the
   challenges I face because of MS.
   After visiting a medical specialist about MS I often feel overwhelmed and
   uncertain about myself and my ability to deal with the disease.
8. Patient/Client Concerns About the Availability of Services (six items)
   The National MS Society provides a useful information and referral service.
   What is really needed is a comprehensive outreach program staffed by
   professionals who are responsive to the needs of people who have MS.

9
Assessing Illness Schemata in Patient Populations

J. Michael Lacroix

There is often considerable discrepancy between the symptoms which patients present and the underlying pathology (Mechanic, 1962; Skelton, this volume). Several studies suggest that as many as 60% of visits to general practioners have no medical basis (Cummings, 1986), while substantial proportions of patients with clinically significant symptoms fail to consult a medical doctor (White, Williams, & Greenberg, 1961). As a consequence, a distinction is made with increasing frequency between disease and illness, with the former referring to strictly pathological conditions evident in a particular patient and the latter referring to the entire cluster of symptoms which he or she presents, regardless of origin (Cott & Pavloski, 1985). As the illness, by definition, has broader behavioral consequences than the disease, and as patients determine their degree of disability and their compliance with treatment regimens on the basis of their illness rather than their disease, it behooves us to understand the origin of patients' symptomatic complaints. It is evident that understanding of the nondisease component of patients' illnesses is fundamentally a psychological problem.

In keeping with the thrust of this book, this chapter takes the view that the nondisease component of patients' illnesses may best be studied through a cognitive approach, by seeking to understand the models or schemata that patients hold about their illness. We have developed a psychological instrument that allows us to record patients' schemata of their symptoms and that focuses on the accuracy of this understanding with respect to objective

This chapter was supported by Grant A0679 from the Natural Sciences and Engineering Research Council of Canada. Some of the research described was also supported by funds from the Academic Enrichment Fund, Division of Orthopaedics, Department of Surgery, Toronto Western Hospital, and by the Workers' Compensation Board of Ontario (to G. J. Lloyd).

medical and psychological evidence. This Schema Assessment Instrument (SAI) has been used in a number of studies, which have shown it to have good reliability and internal consistency and to serve as an excellent predictor of powerful "real-life" variables such as return to work and level of adaptive functioning.

The bulk of this chapter reviews our published research as well as our research in progress with the SAI. In the process, I also provide a discussion of the construct of schema as it has been applied to this area of investigation, and I touch on the implications of our work. However, let me begin by providing a rationale for the schema approach.

Why a Schema Approach?

Why seek to understand patients' models or schemata of their illness? We do this not only for the intrinsic value of such an undertaking but because alternative approaches to prediction and control of illness (and health) behavior have had such limited success. For example, let us consider the patient population that served as the basis for our initial studies with the SAI, low back pain patients. This is a population of enormous proportions and the costs of illness behavior in this population alone are staggering. Thus in Ontario, which numbers 8.5 millon people, 17% of the 426,800 Workers' Compensation Board claims registered in 1985 were for problems associated with low back pain, and 10% of these cases may be expected to go on to chronicity and become "problem cases" (Doxey, Dzioba, Mitson, & Lacroix, 1988). More generally, U.S. estimates are that 1.25 million Americans sustain back injuries each year, that on any given day 7 million Americans are undergoing treatment for back pain, and that approximately 65,000 become permanently disabled each year (Southwick & White, 1983).

Historically, of course, the first approach to the treatment of these patients and to predicting therapeutic success has been of a medical nature. Yet the organic treatment par excellence (surgery) is unsuccessful in 10–15% of cases (Waddell, 1982), and a large proportion of these failures remains unexplained in terms of traditional medical variables. Indeed, in a recent authoritative medical review, Waddell, Main, Morris, DiPaola, and Gray (1984) concluded that physical impairment accounts for less than half of the total disability of low back pain patients. They further suggested that account must be taken of the patients' psychological distress and illness behavior in order to understand the disability of low back pain.

There is now a substantial literature on putative psychological predictors of nonorganic, or "functional," involvement in low back pain ("functional" being operationalized in terms of the absence of appropriate medical findings). The focus of this literature has been on psychopathology as a predictor either of functional involvement or of treatment outcome. A recent review of this literature (Doxey et al., 1988) suggests that most psychological tests are not useful in this context, but it points to elevations on the neurotic triad on the Minnesota Multiphasic Personality Inventory (and particularly scales 1 and 3, the hypochondriasis and hysteria scales) as significant predictors of both nonorganicity and poor treatment outcome.[1] However, even these seemingly positive relationships should be considered weak, since not all studies have yielded positive evidence (e.g., Hamburger, Jennings, Maruta, & Swanson, 1985), and indeed, a number of investigators have noted that a substantial proportion of low back pain patients with no diagnosable organic disease show no evident psychological disturbances whatsoever (Ahles, Yunus, Gaulier, Riley, & Masi, 1986; Leavitt & Garron, 1979). Moreover, even where relationships have been obtained, the magnitude of the correlations has typically been modest. Thus in a recent study of predictors of outcome in back surgery candidates (Doxey et al., 1988), only 4 of 12 possible correlations between the MMPI neurotic triad scales and outcome measures were statistically significant, and the highest correlation involving these scales still accounted for only 23% of the variance in outcome.

In sum, although there are some statistically significant correlations here and there, measures of psychopathology do not allow much by way of prediction of low back pain patients' illness behavior, whether defined in terms of current (nonorganicity) or future presentation (treatment or rehabilitation outcome). But why look at cognitive variables? Why not simply look for better organic/physiological measures or for better measures of psychopathology or personality variables? Let us look at these questions in turn, and this will take us beyond the low back pain patient.

First, the answer may not lie simply in better physiological measures because of limits in the discriminability of physiological changes. Consider the biofeedback literature, which is concerned with bringing about control over (and changes in) well-defined physiological activity, often in the context of diagnostic entities for which the physiology is reasonably well understood. In general, biofeedback is effective as a treatment and results in changes in patients' symptom reports, yet there may be little relationship between the physiological changes and the changes in symptom reports. For example, Lacroix, Clarke, Bock, and Doxey (1986), working with muscle contraction headaches, observed significant effects on patients' headaches, but these were not accompanied by corresponding changes in frontalis EMG, which was the target response for biofeedback. Similarly, in analog (nonpatient)

---

[1] The MMPI is an "objective" personality test which consists of 566 self-reference true–false statements. It yields evaluation of the client in terms of 10 clinical scales and 3 so-called validity scales, which have clinical implications as well. It also yields scores on a number of special interest and research scales. Scales 1 and 3 are two of the basic clinical scales. Very broadly speaking, elevations on these scales are associated with physical complaints, a tendency to denial of emotional conflicts, and an associated tendency to "convert" emotional conflicts into physical complaints. Scale 2 (depression) is associated with depressive symptomatology and scales 1, 2, and 3 together are often referred to as the "neurotic triad."

studies, the physiological changes brought about through biofeedback training are not accompanied by correlated changes in subjects' awareness of these changes. For example, the ability to produce changes in heart rate or skin conductance following biofeedback training does not lead to or enhance an ability to discriminate changes in heart rate or skin conductance (response discrimination may be envisaged as an analog measure of symptom reports; Lacroix, 1981; Lacroix & Gowen, 1981). The relevance of this work in the present context is that, even with well-defined, discrete physiological responses (such as heart rate or EMG changes), there is often a discrepancy between physiological changes and symptomatic reports. It seems unreasonable to expect stronger relationships to emerge when the physiological responses are less well defined and their relationship to symptomatic complaints less well delineated.

If the answer is unlikely to lie in better physiological measures, it is also unlikely to lie simply in better measures of psychopathology or personality variables. There is a vast literature on the putative usefulness of psychological test data in predicting a whole array of diseases. It is not my intention here to review this voluminous literature. Nonetheless, I think it is fair to say that some investigators, sometimes, with some measures, and some diseases, have reported positive relationships, but that taken as a whole this literature is quite depressing (Pennebaker, 1982). Moreover, it is unlikely that different ("new and improved") psychometric measures will lead to greener pastures, for a very simple reason. While both psychological and medical variables may be expected to contribute to symptom presentation, the medical variables (viruses, bacteria, trauma, etc.) happen both to psychopathological and to nonpsychopathological individuals, to introverts as well as extraverts, to Type A's as well as Type B's, and so on. Thus any measure of psychopathology or personality variable, at best, might be expected to account for only a small proportion of the variance in symptom reports. Indeed, this is exactly what was found in the literature on low back pain referred to earlier, and this continues to be the case with newer measures, newer diseases (Lacroix & Offutt, 1988), and more sophisticated methodologies (Offutt & Lacroix, 1988). In contrast, cognitive variables have the distinct a priori advantage of universality in that all patients think. It makes sense, therefore, to consider these variables as possible modulators of symptom experiences and symptom reports.

If we agree that cognitive variables are worthy of attention, where do we begin? Fortunately, a good deal of groundwork has already been laid in Pennebaker's book (1982) *The Psychology of Physical Symptoms*, where he provided a theoretical analysis of the psychology of physical symptoms and proposed a theory of symptom perception that emphasizes patients' cognitive models, or "schemata," of their medical condition. He argued that symptom perception is typically the result of an active symptom-seeking process which is not random, but rather is in keeping with the schemata that patients hold about their symptoms. Support for the theory has come primarily from a broad range of analog studies with university students in which schemata imposed by means of instructional manipulations were found to lead to predicted changes in symptom reports, ascertained by symptom checklists. It emerges from Pennebaker's work that the construct of schema may be central to our understanding of how patients come to present symptoms that are widely at variance with their pathology.

Other investigators, coming from different perspectives, have also pointed to the importance of patients' schemata of their illness for understanding their seeking and use of medical treatment. For example, Leventhal and colleagues (Baumann & Leventhal, 1985; Leventhal, Meyer, & Nerenz, 1980; Meyer, Leventhal, & Gutmann, 1985) explored the implicit "models or beliefs" that hypertensive, cancer, and cardiac patients hold about their illness through a structured interview technique. Their work, buttressed by that of Lau and Hartmann (1983), suggests that schemata of illness include five basic components in addition to the reported symptoms: label, consequences, timeline, cause, and cure. The invariance of these components has further been demonstrated in a historical analysis by Schober and Lacroix (this volume), who showed that the same components characterized the illness schemata of patients from the 17th and 18th centuries. Bishop and colleagues (Bishop, this volume; Bishop & Converse, 1986) recently studied what they call "disease prototypes" in the process of self-diagnosis. Moreover, scattered throughout the medical literature are to be found references to the importance of what patients think is wrong with them, for treatment and rehabilitation (e.g., Kleinman, Eisenberg, & Good, 1978; Roberts et al., 1984). It is clear that these different investigators are all concerned with patients' illness schemata, although there are important differences between them in terms of emphasis and methodology, which are highlighted by the use of different terminologies. Thus, before proceeding further, it might be wise to deal with the question of what I mean by schema.

The Construct of Schema

Fiske and Linville (1980) define schemata generically as referring to "cognitive structures of organized prior knowledge, abstracted from experience with specific instances; [schemata] guide the processing of new information and the retrieval of stored information" (p. 543). For present purposes, we define a schema as a distinct, meaningfully integrated cognitive structure that encompasses (1) a belief in the relatedness of a variety of physiological and psychological functions, which may or may not be objectively accurate; (2) a cluster of sensations, symptoms, emotions, and physical limitations in keeping with that belief; (3) a naive theory about the mechanisms that underlie the relatedness of the elements identified in (2); and (4) implicit or explicit prescriptions for corrective action. I surmise with Pennebaker that a patient's schema serves not only as a cognitive structure for organizing the symptoms and the emotions and beliefs that are held in order to understand his or her medical condition, but also that the schema serves a guiding function in that it directs the patient to carry out active searches for symptoms in the relevant body systems and in that it monitors on a continuous basis both the symptoms and the putative causes for these symptoms. With Pennebaker also, I surmise that the schema follows inferential analysis processes in treating ambiguous information as though it were relevant to itself. Thus the patient's schema is conceptualized as the link between disease and illness; and if the focus is shifted from diagnosis to prognosis, the schema may be conceptualized as the link between medical pathology and disability.

Investigations of the relationship between illness schemata and disease could follow one of two general methodological strategies. First, schemata could be manipulated as independent variables by varying the nature of the information given to subjects and examining the effects of these manipulations on symptom reports (Pennebaker, 1982) or other aspects of the schema (Bishop, Briede, Cavazoz, Grotzinger, & McMahon, 1987). This strategy provides for interesting demonstrations of the viability of the construct, but it tells us little about the role of schemata in "real" diseases because ethical constraints preclude any but the most innocuous manipulations.

Second, patients' schemata could be measured as dependent variables. Measuring how patients conceptualize what is wrong with them is methodologically much more difficult to do than is telling one group of subjects that this is the time of year for colds and withholding that information from another group. The investigators who have attempted to measure patients' schemata have typically done so on rather homogeneous groups of patients suffering from the same disease entity (e.g., Meyer et al., 1985). While this general approach has more "ecological" validity, it is nonetheless limited by virtue of the fact that the subjects all suffer from a single diagnosed entity which is followed over an extensive period of time. In contrast, in the "real world" which exists outside of well-controlled studies, the patient must first diagnose himself or herself as sufficiently ill to take the trouble to consult a physician and obtain a diagnosis, patients may suffer from more than one disease at a time, and follow-ups (and the information derived therefrom) vary considerably.

In the present research we were concerned initially with illness schemata in chronic workers' compensation patients suffering from a wide range of symptoms stemming from a variety of causes. We were also concerned with a particular aspect of illness schemata, schema accuracy. Specifically, we were interested in the implications of patients holding illness schemata that are significantly at variance with the views of their treatment specialists. Our interest in this aspect of illness schemata stemmed from observations of negative correlations between medical improvement on the one hand and English proficiency and education on the other (Doxey et al., 1988). The latter factors may be conceptualized as barriers to communication with physicians. We hypothesized that where such communication problems exist, they may inadvertently lead these patients to develop schemata about their medical condition which are rather removed from objective findings, and that the inability to "test" these schemata by discussing them with physicians may then lead to symptom presentations that become progressively more divergent with time from medical findings.

Our first task was to develop a metric by means of which we could assess patients' illness schemata. The literature indicates that attempts to measure schemata as dependent variables have typically made use of questionnaires from which putatively relevant schema dimensions are abstracted (e.g., Turk & Salovey, 1985). We tried this approach initially but quickly abandoned it because the questionnaire technique did not do justice to the diversity of symptoms presented by our patients. This approach also suffers from a major conceptual limitation. By the very nature of the questionnaire strategy, the approach can yield only a static picture of the patient's illness schemata, which resides in dimensional descriptions; it cannot provide a model of how the descriptors of the schemata interact dynamically with the symptoms which constitute the content of the schemata. Thus we sought to develop an alternative that would take account of the dynamic component of patients' symptom schemata and that would be generic in the sense that it could be applied to any cluster of symptoms and not be restricted to those with a particular disease entity. We eventually opted for a protocol based on open-ended interview questions, similar in part to that used previously by Meyer et al. (1985).

The protocol is as follows. Included in the interview, which is part of the psychological assessment, are specific stepwise probings for information about (1) the patient's presenting physical and psychological symptoms and how these may be related to one another; (2) the patient's understanding of his or her medical condition(s) and prognosis; and (3) the patient's understanding of the relationship between his or her medical condition and the presenting symptoms. On the basis of this information the symptomatic content and the patient's understanding of the medical bases for these symptoms are entered as "assessed" schemata on the SAI. An alternative structure of "expected" schemata is then constructed, which reorganizes the patient's symptoms in terms of the groupings that would be expected on the basis strictly of the results of medical, orthopedic, psychological, and other available assessments.

Having thus constructed models both of the way in which the patient clusters symptoms and of the way the symptoms should optimally have been clustered, rating are then obtained on a number of dimensions, scored in terms of seven-point scales. First, the severity of the patient's condition and the prognosis are rated strictly on the medical evidence (Table 9-1). Then the assessed and expected clusters are compared with respect to (1) the degree to which overall symptom groupings concur (differentiation); (2) the degree to which the content of each of the assessed clusters concurs with the

Table 9-1. Rated Dimensions on the SAI

Based on the medical file only
  Severity
  Prognosis
Based on a comparison of assessed and expected clusters
  Differentiation
  Content (for each cluster)
  Etiology (for each cluster)
  Global

---

medical/psychological evidence; (3) the degree to which the patient's understanding of the causes for each assessed cluster accurately represents the medical/psychological evidence (etiology); and (4) an overall (global) rating of the patient's understanding of the condition, which takes into account the number of clusters, the composition of each cluster, the putative etiology for each cluster, and the importance of the various clusters to the patient's presenting symptomatology. These last four scales, and particularly the Global comparison scale, constitute the heart of what the instrument seeks to measure: the accuracy of the patient's schemata.[2] The version of the SAI employed with our first group of patients is given in the appendix.

Research Findings

This section begins with two initial studies which examined some psychometric properties of the SAI. I then report on four further studies which examined whether schema accuracy may be related to rehabilitation outcome and other "real-life" variables, in three separate populations: low back pain patients, nonpatients, and patients with respiratory disease.

Reliability Studies

The purpose of these studies was to examine interrater reliability of the SAI and the statistical relationship between the SAI scales. This was done on two separate samples in order to assess replicability of the findings (Bacal & Lacroix, 1987).

---

[2] Ratings on the Global scale are not simply the sum of the scores on the other scales. Rather, I like to think of the other scales as serving the purpose of forcing the clinician to consider the relevant areas of difference and similarity between assessed and expected clusters before making his or her overall (Global) rating, so as to make sure that the Global rating is informed of all the relevant considerations.

Method

Participants were inpatients at the Downsview Rehabilitation Center. This facility is used exclusively in the assessment and treatment of individuals who have undergone industrial accidents in Ontario. Referral to the Center was at the request either of the treating physician or of the Workers' Compensation Board, for purposes of assessment, and the patients had then been referred for a psychological assessment by their attending physician at the Center. In study 1 the patients consisted of 8 men and 6 women; they averaged 42.4 years of age, had suffered their compensable injury a mean of 37.6 months previously, and in 10 of the cases this injury had been to the back. Study 2 comprised 12 men and 3 women; they averaged 37.1 years of age, had been injured a mean of 30.8 months previously, and in 12 of the cases the compensable injury had been to the back. Specific medical diagnoses varied widely in both samples. Exclusion criteria included lack of proficiency in English of such magnitude as to require the assistance of an interpreter, unwillingness to undergo a psychological assessment, and unwillingness to participate.

Information critical to the SAI (symptoms, symptom clusters, etc.) was obtained from the participants in the context of the psychological assessment by the examining psychologist. On the basis both of this information and of the information provided in the various assessments on the patient, assessed and expected schemata (*not* ratings on the SAI scales) were then constructed by two psychologists, with differences in opinion resolved by discussion. The two psychologists subsequently carried out the ratings on the various SAI scales independently, and these ratings formed the basis for interrater comparisons. Differences in these ratings were subsequently resolved again by discussion, and the consensual ratings were used to correlate the SAI scales with one another.

Results

Table 9-2 addresses the issue of reliability and presents interrater correlations between the two psychologists' ratings on the various SAI scales. These correlations were quite impressive and highly significant in both studies.

Table 9-2. Inter-Rater Correlations (Pearson r)

Scale	Study 1	Study 2
Severity	.78	.72
Prognosis	.79	.91
Differentiation	.88	.96
Content	.92	.99
Etiology	.83	.85
Global	.93	.75

Table 9-3. Interscale Correlations (Pearson r)

Scale	A	B	C	D	E
			Study 1		
Severity (A)					
Prognosis (B)	.87***				
Differentiation (C)	−.09	−.05			
Content (D)	−.44	−.43	.73**		
Etiology (E)	−.10	.08	.30	.28	
Global (F)	−.32	.05	.72**	.53*	.67**
			Study 2		
Severity (A)					
Prognosis (B)	.90***				
Differentiation (C)	−.44	−.37			
Content (D)	−.53*	−.42	.93***		
Etiology (E)	−.55*	−.43	.22	.30	
Global (F)	−.50*	−.33	.60**	.58*	.80***

$*p < .05; **p < .01; ***p < .001$

Table 9-3 addresses the question of internal consistency and presents the interscale correlations obtained in the two studies. It can be seen that two SAI scales measuring severity of medical condition and prognosis were highly correlated in both studies ($r = .87$ and $.90$), but that these correlated poorly or negatively with the more properly psychological dimensions of the SAI, which in turn generally correlated positively. It is notable that in both studies the differentiation, content, and etiology scales all correlated with (and presumably contributed to) the Global mesure of schema accuracy.

Discussion

The SAI was designed to be administered to patients varying widely in symptoms and medical condition. The results of these initial studies suggest that despite the variance in presenting problems, the SAI can be reliably scored, with respect to both disease aspects (medical severity and prognosis) and schema accuracy. Moreover, the lack of relationship between the medical severity and prognosis scales and the other scales of the SAI suggests that our metric of illness schema accuracy does not simply reflect severity of medical condition, but rather is orthogonal to these disease aspects.

The Retrospective Studies

Having established the reliability of the SAI we proceeded with two studies in which we evaluated retrospectively the usefulness of the instrument in predicting return to work in a group of low back pain Workers' Compensation patients (Lacroix, Doxey, Powell, Mitson, & Lloyd, 1988; Lacroix et al., 1990). In addition, the predictive value of the SAI was compared with more traditional orthopedic assessments (number of nonorganic physical signs), demographic data (age, education, English proficiency), and psychological predictors (MMPI scales 1 and 3).

Method

Two separate studies were undertaken, on two independent samples. This strategy was employed in order to assess replicability of the findings. Two samples of 50 patients each were drawn randomly from an initial cohort of 197 consecutive patients who had been referred to the Downsview Rehabilitation Center and who satisfied the following criteria: all had suffered a work-related injury involving the low back, without prior history of low back pain; the work-related injury had occurred in the previous 3–6 months; the pain was such as to prevent a return to work; and all patients were aged between 18 and 65. There were 39 men and 11 women in sample 1 and 38 men and 12 women in sample 2. The patients were seen within 3–6 months of their initial injury, at which time they underwent a detailed history and orthopedic examination as well as a psychological assessment. The orthopedic examination was repeated at 6–24 months postinjury (mean = 13.7 months), at which time work status was assessed.

For present purposes, SAI ratings were obtained retrospectively on the basis of the information in the files. The medical scales of the SAI (severity and prognosis) were rated by an orthopedic clinical fellow on the basis of the information available from the first clinical assessment. The other scales of the SAI were rated in a conference between the orthopedic clinical fellow and the psychologist who had seen the patient and carried out the psychological assessment initially, again on the basis of information obtained on the first assessment (information from the second assessment was purposely not made available at that time).

Predictors other than the SAI included MMPI scales 1 and 3. In addition, the number of nonorganic physical signs (N-OPS) was determined at the first orthopedic examination, as described by Waddell, McCulloch, Kummel, and Venner (1980). Demographic variables of interest included age, number of years of education, and proficiency in the English language (1 = nil; 2 = poor; 3 = fair; 4 = good).

Return to work measures were of two types. First, with respect to work status, patients were given a rating of 0 if they were still not working by the time of the second assessment, a rating of 1 if they had returned to work but were on lighter duties than prior to the accident, and a rating of 2 if they had returned to work in a full capacity. Second, for those patients who had returned to work, the total number of weeks off work was recorded.

The initial analyses for both samples focused on the predictive value of the SAI. The patients were divided into approximate thirds on the basis of their score on the Global scale of the SAI, reflecting groups of patients with a very poor understanding of their condition (global scale ≤2); those with some partial understanding of their condition (global scale = 3 or 4); and those with a good or very good understanding of their condition (global scale ≥5). One-way analysis of variance tests (ANOVAs) compared these groups in both studies with respect to the return to work variables. In addition, product–moment correlations were computed between the work status variable as the criterion and the Global SAI scores, MMPI scale 1, MMPI scale 3, SAI medical severity and prognosis ratings, initial N-OPS, age, education, and level of English proficiency, as predictors.

Results

Figures 9-1 and 9-2 present the major results of the investigation separately for the two studies. In both cases the sample has been divided into three groups, with a poor, mediocre, and good understanding of their condition. The lower half of each figure depicts the mean severity and prognosis ratings as determined strictly on the basis of the initial orthopedic assessment. It is clear that the three groups were well matched on the basis of their orthopedic

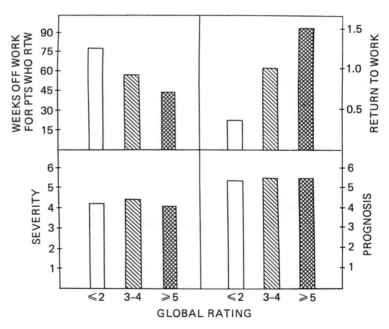

Figure 9-1. Upper panels: mean number of weeks off work for patients who returned to work and work status; lower panels: orthopedic assessments of severity and prognosis of medical condition; in patients with poor (Global ≤2), mediocre (Global = 3 or 4), and good (Global ≥ 5) schemata in study 1.

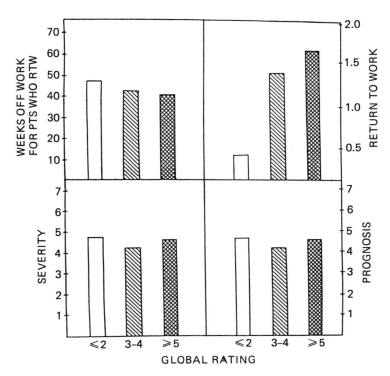

Figure 9-2. Upper panels: mean number of weeks off work for patients who returned to work and work status; lower panels: orthopedic assessments of severity and prognosis of medical condition; in patients with poor (Global ≤2), mediocre (Global = 3 or 4), and good (Global ≥ 5) schemata in study 2.

conditions in both studies, in that none of the group differences in medical severity or prognosis approached statistical significance.

The upper panels in each figure present return to work statistics. The top right-hand panels depict mean ratings on the work status scale. There were evident and large differences in the predicted direction. These were statistically significant in both studies [$F(2/47) = 10.39$, $p < .0002$ for study 1; $F(2/47) = 17.48$, $p < .0001$ for study 2]. Of the patients with a poor understanding of their condition, only 6 of 15 in study 1 and 5 of 18 in study 2 returned to work at all, and of the total of 11 who did return to work, only 2 did so in a full capacity. On the other hand, the return to work figures were excellent for those patients with a good understanding of their condition, with 18 of 20 and 16 of 16 returning to work in studies 1 and 2, respectively, and among those 34 were 23 who returned to work in a full capacity. The patients with a mediocre understanding of their condition fell between the other groups, with 10 of 15 and 13 of 16 returning to work in studies 1 and 2,

Table 9-4. Cross-Correlations Between Variables (Sample 1)

	Work Status	Global	MMPI-1	MMPI-3	Severity	Prognosis	N-OPS	Age	Education
Work status									
Global	.60***								
MMPI-1	−.40**	−.28							
MMPI-3	−.38*	−.25	.77***						
Severity	.26	−.06	−.05	−.04					
Prognosis	.41**	.04	−.21	−.23	.83***				
N-OPS	−.40**	−.49***	.19	.10	−.19	−.19			
Age	−.30	−.05	.08	.11	−.70***	−.76***	.04		
Education	.50	.41	−.60*	−.47	−.06	.08	−.14	−.33	
English proficiency	.24	.40**	−.17	−.01	−.32*	.29*	−.36*	−.34*	.66**

$*p < .05; **p < .01; ***p < .001$

respectively, and among those 23 were 15 who returned to their previous duties.

The upper left-hand panel in each figure shows the number of weeks off work for the patients who did eventually return to work. Again, group differences are apparent, in the predicted direction, although these are more marked in study 1. The patients with a poor understanding of their condition, by the large, took longer to return to work, when they did return to work, than those with a better understanding of their condition. The group differences were significant in study 1 [$F(2/29) = 3.18$, $p = .05$] but not in study 2 ($F < 1$).

Tables 9-4 and 9-5 present the correlations between the variables relevant to this investigation, separately for studies 1 and 2; those correlation coefficients which met the .05 level of significance in both studies appear in bold type. The only variable to predict work status in both studies was the Global SAI scale. The more traditional variables were less consistent. In addition, the two MMPI scales were consistently correlated with each other, as were the medical severity and prognosis ratings of the SAI. Finally, English proficiency emerged as a consistent predictor of ratings on the global SAI scale, N-OPS, age, and education.

One set of nonsignificant correlations is worth noting. In neither study did the correlations between the Global SAI scale and medical severity of prognosis approach significance. Thus it is clearly not the case that patients with a good understanding of their condition were simply those with less complicated medical problems.

Discussion

The present data make a powerful argument for the SAI as a useful clinical instrument. Insofar as the SAI provides a measure of the accuracy of patients' understanding of their condition, these data point to the importance of patients' schemata for their prognosis. The Global scale of the SAI was a very significant predictor of return to work statistics with these low back pain Workers' Compensation patients. Indeed, it was the only variable to predict work status significantly in both studies, and it was successful in doing so to a surprising (and gratifying) extent. Moreover, our use of a replication design here is particularly valuable in that it validates the results. Furthermore, the correlational data make it clear that patients' understanding of their condition is orthogonal to the severity of their diagnoses and prognoses. Finally, the SAI proved superior to more commonly used predictors of return to work, including orthopedic assessments of severity and prognosis, N-OPS, and MMPI scales 1 and 3.

A couple of subsidiary aspects of the data are also worth noting. First, the absence of correlations between MMPI variables and Global SAI ratings buttresses the earlier suggestion that these cognitive factors do not simply reflect psychopathology. And second, the consistent correlations between

Table 9-5. Cross-Correlations Between Variables (Sample 2)

	Work Status	Global	MMPI-1	MMPI-3	Severity	Prognosis	N-OPS	Age	Education
Work status									
Global	.54**								
MMPI-1	-.22	-.11							
MMPI-3	-.09	-.04	.73***						
Severity	.14	-.04	.00	-.01					
Prognosis	.24	.01	-.06	-.11	.93***				
N-OPS	-.29	-.30	.25	.26	.28	.17			
Age	-.19	-.28*	-.20	-.25	-.23	-.29	.16		
Education	.40	.22	.11	-.11	-.02	.05	-.36	.19	
English proficiency	.49***	.37*	-.27	-.23	.02	-.23	-.51***	-.36**	.77***

*$p < .05$; **$p < .01$; ***$p < .001$

English proficiency and the Global scale of the SAI, N-OPS, age, and education are also interesting. The correlations with age, education, and nonorganic signs replicate those mentioned earlier. To reiterate, our interpretation of these relationships is in terms of the difficulties that patients with poor English skills, who also tend to be poorly educated, may experience in communicating with their physicians. Because of these communication problems, these patients may be more likely to develop naive schemata about their medical condition which are quite removed from objective findings. The inability to "test" these theories by discussing them with physicians may then lead to their symptom presentations becoming progressively more divergent with time from medical findings.

A Study With Nonpatients

I mentioned earlier that when we developed the SAI we sought to develop an instrument that would be "generic" in the sense that it could be applied to any cluster of symptoms and not be restricted to a particular disease entity. While most of our work thus far has focused on low back pain Workers' Compensation patients, we have also gone beyond this population. All of us experience symptoms at some point, and seemingly the same symptoms that some of us simply grumble about cause others to miss work and curtail leisure and social activities.

In an as yet unpublished study, Brenda Martin and I examined the ability of the SAI to predict level of functioning in the occupational, social, and leisure areas. (For the purpose of this study, the anchor points on the medical severity and prognosis scales were modified somewhat from the anchor points used with the low back patients.) Twenty-five individuals were selected from the university campus and from an office environment on the basis that they were willing to spend some time discussing their lives in general and their symptoms in particular. Their symptom reports and medical history were sufficiently detailed to allow for an estimate of the severity of their medical condition and of their medical prognosis and to use the SAI to estimate schema accuracy. The subjects' level of occupational, social, and leisure functioning was then rated separately (and blindly) in terms of the criteria for Axis V of DSM-III. This scale provides a rating (on a seven-point scale) of the person's level of adaptive functioning, according to criteria outlined in the *Diagnostic and Statistical Manual of the American Psychiatric Association* (3rd ed.). This study yielded a correlation of $-.77$ ($p < .01$) between the Global scale of the SAI and Scale V of DSM-III: subjects with a more accurate understanding of their symptomatology were found to function at a higher level in the broader aspects of their lives than subjects with inaccurate schemata.

These data make a number of points. First, they reinforce the finding that the SAI is a useful instrument in that the accuracy of symptom schemata is related to powerful real-life variables. Presumably, those individuals with more accurate schemata are better able to keep their symptoms in perspective (i.e., they do not make mountains out of molehills). In addition, they may make proper allowances for the more severe conditions that they do suffer, for example, by restructuring rather than eliminating work and leisure activities when the symptoms become manifest. Second, the proportion of the variance in adaptive functioning that is accounted for by the SAI (almost 60%!) points to the tremendous importance that our medical conditions play in our lives, even when there is no major disease. And finally, these data tie in rather nicely with the literature on symptom reporters. This literature suggests a positive link between symptom reports and such factors as living alone, being unmarried, and being unemployed (cf. Pennebaker, 1982) — factors that may be "macroindicators" of the social adjustment measure which we employed here.

Patients With Respiratory Disease

We have carried out another study, in the Respiratory Disease Unit of West Park Hospital, a chronic care facility in Toronto (Lacroix, Martin, Avendano, & Goldstein, in press). Patients in this unit have in common the fact that they all suffer from significant respiratory conditions. However, there is considerable range among them in terms of disease severity and diagnoses. Thus some patients (e.g., those with advanced cases of chronic obstructive pulmonary disease or with C-1 quadriplegia) require permanent artificial ventilation and reside at the hospital, while others (e.g., those with emphysema) are there for a few weeks, primarily for purposes of diagnosis and education. In addition, many of these patients suffer from diagnoses stemming from their respiratory conditions (e.g., cor pulmonale) and from other, unrelated, diseases. Thus many of these patients are medically in a much more severe condition than our low back pain patients, and they constitute an even more varied group in terms of diagnosis.

Thirty-one of these patients were included in the study, on the basis that they were fluent in English and were willing to participate. As with our study with nonpatients, the anchor points on the medical severity and prognosis scales again had to be modified somewhat from the anchor points used with the low back pain patients. The study also followed in the footsteps of our study with nonpatients in examining whether the SAI could predict level of functioning. However, level of functioning was operationalized here slightly differently, in terms of a 100-point Global Assessment Scale (GAS) (Newman, 1983) designed to measure a person's most recent level of physical, social, and psychological adjustment. Ratings on this scale were obtained from the Nursing Unit managers, who are in daily contact with the patients and are well aware of their level of participation in social, leisure, and work activities.

Apart from the fact that this study focused on a different group, it is also important in that I chose not to be involved in any part of the investigation

Table 9-6. Relationship Between Accuracy of Patients' Schemata, Medical
Condition, and Level of Functioning (GAS)

	Poor Global ≤ 3 ($N = 12$)	Mediocre Global $= 4$ ($N = 12$)	Good Global ≥ 5 ($N = 7$)
Severity ($\bar{x}$)	2.92	2.19	2.71
Prognosis ($\bar{x}$)	2.42	2.58	2.43
Level of functioning ($\bar{x}$)	63.00	76.10	78.60

other than its planning: I had no role in collecting the data (which was done
by B. Martin), in constructing the assessed or expected schemata or
providing ratings on the SAI (which was done by M. Avendano, M.D.), or in
rating the patients' level of adaptive functioning (which was done by the
Nursing Unit managers). Thus whereas I had a concrete role in all of our
prior investigations, which leaves open the possibility that I might have
inadvertently biased the results in favor of the research hypotheses, every
aspect of this study was done blind.

Results and Discussion

The major results replicated very nicely our earlier findings with other
populations in every respect. Table 9-6 presents the major results of the
study for groups with a poor, mediocre, and good understanding of their
condition. Examination of the table makes it clear that there was again no
relationship between medical severity or prognosis on the one hand and
schema accuracy on the other [$F(2/28) = 1.13$ for severity, and $F < 1$ for
prognosis]. The medical severity and prognosis ratings were lower here than
with our low back pain patients, but, as indicated, these patients had more
serious medical problems.

Moreover, the Global SAI scale again predicted adaptive functioning
[$F(2/28) = 3.34$, $p < .05$]. This was confirmed by an alternative correlational
analysis of those data, which yielded a Pearson $r = .50$ ($p < .01$).[3] Finally, the
pattern of correlations was again very similar to those obtained earlier:
medical severity and prognosis ratings correlated significantly with each
other ($r = .46$, $p < .01$) but not with any of the more properly psychological
dimensions of the SAI, all of which in turn correlated significantly with the
Global measure of schema accuracy.

These data provide further evidence that the SAI is a reliable instrument
that can be used with patients across a broad spectrum of disease entities.
They also point, again, to the usefulness of the instrument in predicting
real-life variables.

---

[3] This is probably an underestimate. If we remove one "outlier" from the analysis (and there are
powerful reasons for removing him), the Pearson r value changes to .63.

Implications

The major conclusions to be drawn from these studies are that (1) we have developed an instrument which reliably measures the accuracy of people's symptom schemata, and (2) the extent to which people understand their symptoms is related to very powerful real-life variables such as functional adjustment and return to work. The first of these points, of course, is important only as it bears on the second, and this section therefore focuses on the critical second point.

First, let us consider three possible confounding variables in our work. It might be argued that schema accuracy may be simply a correlate of some psychopathological factor, for example, that our low back pain patients with inaccurate schemata (and who failed to return to work) were simply more histrionic. Although this possibility cannot be completely eliminated, there is no support in our data for this view, in that MMPI variables were not systematically correlated with scores on the Global SAI scale. Furthermore, the one factor that emerged as most systematically correlated with schema accuracy was English proficiency, a factor tied strongly to education (and thereby presumably to understanding) and not to psychopathology. Thus to the extent that indicants of psychopathology may predict return to work in this population, these may be orthogonal to cognitive variables as measured by the SAI.

Second, the emphasis given here to English proficiency and education might suggest that it is not understanding but rather *ability to communicate* understanding which relates to return to work and adaptive functioning generally. In other words, the SAI might simply tap communication skills. There are two empirical arguments against this notion. First, English proficiency and education were much less systematically correlated with return to work in our low back pain patients than the Global SAI ratings. Yet if these are the key variables, they should be more closely related to the predicted variables than the putative "indirect" measure of communication skills provided by the SAI. And second, while English proficiency was a factor of relevance to our low back Workers' Compensation patients (for demographic reasons), it applied to a much lesser extent to our respiratory patients and not at all to our nonpatient population (which comprised university students and office workers).

A third possible confounding variable is motivation: some of my colleagues have suggested that those patients who failed to return to work may simply have been those who lacked in such motivation, and that they may also have lacked in the motivation to inform themselves about that was wrong with them. Similarly, in the studies with nonpatients and with respiratory patients, it might be that those individuals who were less well adapted functionally were simply "unmotivated" either to work or to play and used their symptoms as a convenient excuse. This is an impossible argument to refute because motivation invariably is simply inferred from behavior rather than operationalized in its own right. Thus instead of trying to refute the argument (which I could do only on the basis of unsystematic clinical observations), I will simply suggest the possibility that poor motivation may be a consequence rather than a cause of inaccurate schemata: Patients who misattribute relatively innocuous symptoms to a serious condition, or who do not understand anything at all of their medical condition, may be more likely to adopt a passive attitude toward treatment and "give up," thereby giving the appearance of lack of motivation. This alternative viewpoint has the advantage that it should be relatively easily testable. In principle, it should be easier to educate such patients than to raise their level of "motivation."

The issue of whether patients may be educated to develop more informed and accurate schemata, of course, begs the more fundamental question of how symptom schemata originate. The simple view is that schemata, as cognitive structures, have a cognitive origin, and thus are modifiable by introducing new cognitive "evidence," for example, through education. However, this view is unquestionably an oversimplification, since we are dealing here with cognitive structures that are used to summarize and make sense of a data base that is physiological in nature, at least in part. There are some interesting parallels here with the role of similar schemata which underlie the acquisition of response control in biofeedback (Lacroix, 1986), and these have been explored elsewhere (Lacroix, in press). Thus verbal and other cognitive channels of information certainly affect the development of symptom schemata [e.g., through readings or physicians' explanations, as well as life experiences ("my father died of a heart attack, and he always had headaches like these . . .")]. However, it is likely that schemata are also constructed, in part, from detectable physiological variables, although not necessarily from the obvious ones and not necessarily in a simple way.

For example, it is possible that schema accuracy may relate to subjects' ability to discriminate interoceptive events. Recent research suggests that, even for such "asymptomatic" disorders as hypertension, some symptoms are significantly correlated with physiological changes (Pennebaker & Watson, 1988). Thus it may be that subjects who can accurately discriminate their internal states are relatively unlikely to be misled into constructing inappropriate schemata. Another possibility is that schema accuracy may relate to resting levels of activity in psychophysiological systems. Pennebaker (1982) advanced the hypothesis that symptom perception relates to the ratio of information from internal and external sources: When there is relatively more information from internal sources, the subject is more likely to attend to (and to misinterpret) information from these sources. The ratio of internal to external information should be influenced by factors that affect selectively either the amount of internal or the amount of external information available to the subject. According to this view, subjects with high levels of resting psychophysiological activity should have more symptom information available for processing than subjects with low resting levels of activity; the former should therefore perceive more symptoms and might be more likely to construct elaborate (and inaccurate) schemata to incorporate these symptoms. These hypotheses are readily testable.

There are other questions also worthy of attention. For example, is schema accuracy primarily a function of the subject or of the subject matter: Do subjects with accurate illness schemata differ from those with poor schemata with respect to reasoning skills generally? Do the latter tend to be overinclusive (or underinclusive) in tasks requiring categorizing? Are there group differences with respect to general intelligence? Moreover, schema characteristics in addition to accuracy need to be examined. How stable are these schemata over time—say, over a year? Are they affected by intervening major illnesses? These questions are only beginning to be raised in the literature (notably by the authors in this volume), but much more work remains to be done.

I would like to make one final comment. I indicated from the outset that my interest here is with respect to symptom schemata as they apply to "real" patients with "real" diseases. However, it is entirely possible to study the development of schemata by means of analog studies with nonpatient populations. Pennebaker, Bishop, Skelton, and their respective colleagues, have done so with great success. However, there is one potentially very useful experimental strategy that has received almost no attention in the literature. This strategy involves developing a "laboratory model" of the development of physical symptoms. This can be done by inducing symptoms in the laboratory and then teasing apart the factors that contribute to symptom development. This is a strategy that we have begun to employ, with headache as the target symptom (Lacroix & Corbett, 1990), and which, in my view, holds great promise.

Acknowledgments.   Thanks are due to S. Bacal, P. Voorneveld, B. Martin, N. Doxey, L. Mitson, J. Powell, G. Lloyd, A. Garland, and M. Avendano for their contributions to the studies described here.

References

Ahles, T. A., Yunus, M. B., Gaulier, B., Riley, S. D., & Masi, A. T. (1986). The use of contemporary MMPI norms in the study of chronic pain patients. *Pain, 24,* 159–163.

Bacal, S., & Lacroix, J. M. (1987). Illness schemata in multi-symptomatic patients. *Canadian Psychology, 28,* 2a, 17.

Baumann, L. J., & Leventhal, H. (1985). "I can tell when my blood pressure is up, can't I?" *Health Psychology, 4,* 203–218.

Bishop, G. D., & Converse, S. A. (1966). Illness representations: A prototype approach. *Health Psychology, 9,* 95–114.

Bishop, G. D., Briede, C., Cavazos, L., Grotzinger, R., & McMahon, S. (1987). Processing illness information: The role of disease prototypes. *Basic and Applied Social Psychology, 8,* 21–43.

Cott, A., & Pavloski, R. P. (1985). Behavioural medicine: A process for managing performance problems. *Canadian Psychology, 26,* 160–167.

Cummings, N. (1986). The dismantling of our health system: Strategies for the survival of psychological practice. *American Psychologist, 41*, 426–431.

Doxey, N. C. S., Dzioba, R. B., Mitson, G. L., & Lacroix, J. M. (1988). Predictors of outcome in back surgery candidates. *Journal of Clinical Psychology, 44*, 611–622.

Fiske, S. T., & Linville, P. W. (1980). What does the schema concept buy us? *Personality and Social Psychology Bulletin, 6*, 543–557.

Hamberger, M. E., Jennings, C. A., Maruta, T., & Swanson, D. W. (1985). Failure of a predictive scale in identifying patients who may benefit from a pain management programme: Follow-up data. *Pain, 23*, 253–258.

Kleinman, A., Eisenberg, L., & Good, B. (1978). Culture, illness, and care: Clinical lessons from anthropological and cross-cultural research. *Annals of Internal Medicine, 88*, 251–258.

Lacroix, J. M. (1981). The acquisition of autonomic control through biofeedback: The case against an afferent process and a two-process alternative. *Psychophysiology, 18*, 573–587.

Lacroix, J. M. (1986). Mechanisms of biofeedback control: On the importance of verbal (conscious) processing. In R. J. Davidson, G. E. Schwartz, & D. Shapiro (Eds), *Consciousness and self-regulation: Advances in research* (Vol. 4, pp. 137–162). New York: Plenum Press.

Lacroix, J. M. (in press). Psychophysiology, biofeedback, and psychosomatic medicine. In A. Baudot (Ed.), *Vingt ans, et après? Mélange en l'honneur de John Bruckman*. Toronto: Les Editions du GREF.

Lacroix, J. M., Clarke, M. A., Bock, J. C., & Doxey, N. C. S. (1986). Physiological changes after biofeedback and relaxation training for multiple-pain tension-headache patients. *Perceptual and Motor Skills, 63*, 139–153.

Lacroix, J. M., & Corbett, L. (1990). An experimental test of the muscle tension hypothesis of tension-type headache. *International Journal of Psychophysiology, 10*, 47–51.

Lacroix, J. M., Doxey, N. C. S., Powell, J., Mitson, G. L., & Lloyd, G. (1988). Patients' illness schemata as predictors of return to work in injured WCB patients. *Canadian Psychology, 29*, 2a, 433. (Abs.).

Lacroix, J. M., & Gowen, A. (1981). The acquisition of automatic control through biofeedback: Some tests of discrimination theory. *Psychophysiology, 18*, 559–572.

Lacroix, J. M., Martin, B., Avendano, M., & Goldstein, R. (in press). Symptom schemata in chronic respiratory patients. *Health Psychology*.

Lacroix, J. M., & Offutt, C. (1988). Genital herpes and Type A behavior. *Journal of Psychosomatic Research, 32*, 207–212.

Lacroix, J. M., Powell, J., Lloyd, G. J., Doxey, N. C. S., Mitson, G. L., & Aldam, C. F. (1990). Low back pain: Factors of value in predicting outcome. *Spine, 15*, 495–499.

Lau, R. R., & Hartman, K. A. (1983). Common sense representations of common illness. *Health Psychology, 2*, 167–185.

Leavitt, F., & Garron, D. C. (1979). Psychological disturbance and pain report differences in both organic and non-organic low back pain patients. *Pain, 7*, 187–195.

Leventhal, H., Meyer, D., & Nerenz, D. (1980). The common sense representation of illness danger. In S. Rachman (Ed.), *Contributions to medical psychology* (Vol. 2, pp. 7–30). Oxford: Pergamon Press.

Mechanic, D. (1962). The concept of illness behavior. *Journal of Chronic Disease, 15*, 189–194.

Meyer, D., Leventhal, H., & Gutmann, M. (1985). Common-sense models of illness: The example of hypertension. *Health Psychology*, *4*, 115–135.

Newman, F. (1983). Level of Functioning scales: Their use in clinical practice. In P. Keller & L. Ritt (Eds), *Innovations in clinical practice: A sourcebook*. Sarasota, FL: Professional Resource Exchange.

Offutt, C., & Lacroix, J. M. (1988). Type A behavior pattern and symptom reports: A prospective investigation. *Journal of Behavioral Medicine*, *11*, 227–237.

Pennebaker, J. (1982). *The psychology of physical symptoms*. New York: Springer-Verlag.

Pennebaker, J., & Watson, D. (1988). Blood pressure estimation and beliefs among normotensives and hypertensives. *Health Psychology*, *7*, 309–328.

Roberts, N., Smith, R., Bennett, S., Cape, J., Norton, R., & Kilburn, P. (1984). Health beliefs and rehabilitation after lumbar disc surgery. *Journal of Psychosomatic Research*, *28*, 139–144.

Southwick, S. M., & White A. A. (1983). The use of psychological tests in the evaluation of low-back pain *Journal of Bone and Joint Surgery*, *65A*, 560–565.

Turk, D. C., & Salovey, P. (1985). Cognitive structure, cognitive processes, and cognitive-behavior modification: I. Client issues. *Cognitive Therapy and Research*, *9*, 1–17.

Waddell, G. (1982). An approach to backache. *British Journal of Hospital Medicine*, *28*, 187–219.

Waddell, G., Main, C. J., Morris, E. W., DiPaola, M., & Gray, I. C. (1984). Chronic low-back pain, psychologic distress, and illness behavior. *Spine*, *9*, 209–213.

Waddell, G., McCulloch, J. A., Kummel, E., & Venner, R. M. (1980). Nonorganic physical signs in low-back pain. *Spine*, *5*, 117–125.

White, K. L., Williams, T. F., & Greenberg, B. G. (1961). The ecology of medical care. *New England Journal of Medicine*, *265*, 885–892.

Appendix. Schema Assessment Instrument

Name: _____

Date: _____

Severity of Medical Condition

On strictly organic criteria, how severe is the patient's medical condition?

1	2	3	4	5	6	7
Extreme	Very severe	Severe	Moderate	Minor	Very minor	No condition

where 1 = numerous major physical findings (in excess of no. 2)
      2 = very advanced, multilevel degenerative disc disease (DDD), 2 or more discs protruding
      3 = advanced DDD, acute/chronic nerve irritation, herniated disc
      4 = some DDD, moderate mechanical pain, facet pain
      5 = major soft tissue injury, bad sprain/strain
      6 = minor soft tissue injury, pulled muscle
      7 = some spasm, tender points

Functional Prognosis

On the basis of physical findings only, what is the prognosis for the patient's condition?

1	2	3	4	5	6	7
Extreme	Very poor	Poor	Moderate	Good	Very good	Excellent

where 1 = unable to work, receives permanent total disability pension
   2 = sedentary, part-time work, receives permanent partial (PP) disability pension
   3 = permanent modified work, numerous restrictions, receives PP
   4 = permanent modified work, few restrictions, PP disability pension
   5 = should eventually resume regular work after temporary modified work
   6 = discharged to regular duties, little difficulty expected
   7 = discharged to regular duties, no difficulty expected

Symptom List	Patient's Clusters
1. _____	1. _____
2. _____	2. _____
3. _____	3. _____
4. _____	4. _____
5. _____	5. _____
6. _____	6. _____
7. _____	
8. _____	
9. _____	
10. _____	

Inquiry

Specify the Assessed Clusters (AC)

Specify the clusters provided by the patient (assessed clusters).
1. _____
2. _____
3. _____
4. _____
5. _____
6. _____

Specify the Expected Clusters (EC)

Specify the way in which the patient should have clustered according to the available medical/psychological information.
1. _____
2. _____
3. _____

4. _____

5. _____

6. _____

AC–EC Differentiation

In comparing the assessed and expected clusters, to what extent does the patient's differentiation of symptoms into clusters concur with the expected clusters?

1	2	3	4	5	6	7

No differentiation at all;   Perfect differentiation;
purely arbitrary   fully in keeping
                                with the medical/psychological evidence

AC–EC Congruency: Cluster Content

In comparing the assessed and expected clusters, to what extent do the symptoms in each assessed cluster concur with the medical/psychological evidence? In terms of percent agreement:

1	2	3	4	5	6	7
<14%	14–28%	28–42%	42–56%	56–72%	72–86%	>86%
None	Very poor	Poor	Moderate	Good	Very good	Perfect

Cluster 1

1	2	3	4	5	6	7

Cluster 2

1	2	3	4	5	6	7

Cluster 3

1	2	3	4	5	6	7

Cluster 4

1	2	3	4	5	6	7

Cluster 5

1	2	3	4	5	6	7

Cluster 6

1	2	3	4	5	6	7

AC–EC Congruency: Symptom Etiology

With respect to each assessed cluster, to what extent does the patient's understanding of the causes of the symptoms grouped together in each cluster accurately represent the medical/psychological evidence?

1	2	3	4	5	6	7
None	Very poor	Poor	Moderate	Good	Very good	Perfect
Not at all, no understanding of medical/psychological conceptions whatsoever			Some approximation of understanding for some symptoms (half) but very poor for others			

Cluster 1

1	2	3	4	5	6	7

Cluster 2

1	2	3	4	5	6	7

Cluster 3

1	2	3	4	5	6	7

Cluster 4

1	2	3	4	5	6	7

Cluster 5

1	2	3	4	5	6	7

Cluster 6

1	2	3	4	5	6	7

Global Rating

Overall, taking into consideration the number of clusters, the composition of each cluster, the putative etiology for each cluster, and the importance of the various clusters to the patient's presenting symptomatology, how appropriate is the patient's understanding of his/her condition?

1	2	3	4	5	6	7
Completely inappropriate; purely arbitrary			Moderate			Perfect

Subjective Disability Rating

What is the patient's subjective perception of his/her disability on a percentage scale of increasing disability?

0	10	20	30	40	50	60	70	80	90	100
No disability										Bedridden

10

Symptom Perception, Symptom Beliefs, and Blood Glucose Discrimination in the Self-Treatment of Insulin-Dependent Diabetes

Linda A. Gonder-Frederick and Daniel J. Cox

From a pragmatic perspective, one of the most important types of illness representations people use to understand and regulate their own health status is subjectively perceived symptoms. Recognition and interpretation of physical symptoms influence behavior in nearly every illness experience— guiding self-diagnosis, medical help-seeking, health-care decision making, and self-treatment processes. Perceived symptoms and the inferences made about those symptoms play an especially important role in the day-to-day management of chronic diseases in which patients are required to monitor and regulate their own health status. In this chapter, we summarize findings from a nine-year investigation of subjectively perceived symptoms, symptom beliefs, and ability to estimate blood glucose levels in patients with insulin-dependent diabetes mellitus (IDDM).

Our interest and research in this area are both theoretically and pragmatically oriented. The IDDM patient offers a unique opportunity to investigate the influence of subjective symptom representations on self-regulatory health behaviors. IDDM treatment requires patients to behaviorally self-regulate their own blood glucose (BG) levels using insulin, diet, and exercise therapy. This self-regulatory process requires the patient to monitor information about changing BG levels, including perceived symptoms that signal unacceptable or dangerous levels. As our findings demonstrate, these subjective symptom and BG representations have a

This chapter was supported, in part, by National Institutes of Health grants DK28288, DK22125, and RR00847.

significant impact on patients' self-treatment decisions and ability to control their diabetes.

Of primary importance, then, is the degree to which patients can accurately recognize symptoms that reliably covary with extremely low and high BG levels. Because this is determined largely by the types of symptoms available to subjective awareness, we have investigated the etiology and nature of BG symptomatology in IDDM patients. One of the major questions addressed by these studies is, To what extent do subjective symptoms reliably covary with BG fluctuations? In addition, a number of studies have focused on the types of errors IDDM patients make in BG discrimination, inferences, and beliefs. These findings tell us a great deal about how IDDM patients process symptom cues and other subjective BG information. On the basis of all these studies, we have developed and tested an intervention specifically designed to improve ability to recognize and respond to subjective symptom information.

Our approach to diabetes management, with its emphasis on subjective symptom representations and self-regulation of BG, deviates from more traditional approaches to treatment and adherence. For this reason, a brief summary of other medical and psychological models of diabetes management is presented, describing educational, personality, and cognitive-behavioral approaches. However, because diabetes and its treatment are quite complex, we begin with a brief overview of the causes and ramifications of IDDM, including a description of the treatment regimen. Some knowledge about IDDM is a prerequisite to understanding the behavioral task of the patient, the self-regulatory model of treatment, and the potential influence of subjective symptom representations on clinical outcome.

Insulin-Dependent Diabetes Mellitus: Consequences and Treatment

Glucose is the metabolic fuel used to provide energy for many types of body cells including fat, muscle, and brain cells. Consequently, regulation of the amount of glucose available in the circulating bloodstream is necessary for normal body functions. In the nondiabetic person, BG levels are maintained in a relatively narrow range between 60 and 150 mg/dl, depending on recent food intake and energy expenditure. Normal BG regulation depends primarily on the pancreatic hormone insulin, which plays a critical role in glucose utilization and storage. Diabetes is characterized by abnormalities in glucose metabolism due to deficiencies in insulin production and/or utilization (see Cox, Gonder-Frederick, Pohl, & Pennebaker, 1986).

Type I diabetes is caused by a combination of genetic and autoimmunological processes that destroy insulin-producing pancreatic beta cells. Type II, or non–insulin-dependent diabetes, appears to be related to insulin resistance, often associated with obesity. With the onset of diabetes, body cells cannot use the glucose circulating in the bloodstream, leading to abnormally high BG levels (hyperglycemia), which are associated with both acute and long-term pathology. Acute effects include polyuria and polydipsia, reflecting the body's attempt to eliminate excess glucose from the system. Excessive appetite accompanied by weight loss and blurred vision may also occur. If hyperglycemia is not detected and treated, accumulation of ketones in the bloodstream caused by the breakdown of body fat can lead to ketoacidotic coma and death.

To survive, the IDDM patient must take insulin injections to utilize glucose in the bloodstream and to lower BG levels. Unfortunately, insulin therapy usually does not completely normalize glucose levels. Even with insulin therapy, the majority of patients are chronically hyperglycemic, which contributes to the serious long-term complications of diabetes, including heart disease, kidney disease, retinopathy, and neuropathy.

An important complication resulting from insulin therapy itself is abnormally low BG, or hypoglycemia. Often called "insulin reactions," hypoglycemic episodes are a significant problem for IDDM patients. Glucose is the brain's primary source of metabolic energy and, because the brain does not store glucose, it is completely dependent on glucose from the circulating bloodstream. Consequently, hypoglycemia disrupts central nervous system as well as neurobehavioral function. Moderate hypoglycemia (45–60 mg/dl) can cause mental confusion, slurred speech, poor motor coordination, and mood changes. Severe hypoglycemia (< 35 mg/dl) can result in fainting, seizures, coma, and even death. Hypoglycemic episodes can be unpredictable, with sudden onset. For the patient, hypoglycemia is frightening, physically unpleasant, socially embarrassing, and potentially dangerous.

The goal of IDDM treatment is to maintain BG in as close to a normal range as possible while avoiding hyperglycemia and hypoglycemia. Treatment regimens have four major components: daily insulin injections, dietary modification, exercise therapy, and self-testing of blood and/or urine samples. Although treatment always involves these components, the precise regimen varies greatly across patients. For example, some patients follow traditional insulin regimens that might include only one or two daily injections, with a fixed dose prescribed by the physician. Typically, however, this regimen will not provide good diabetes control. To normalize BG levels, patients must use an intensive insulin regimen that involves multiple daily injections with self-ajusted doses based on self-tests, food intake, and physical activity. The most intensive such regimen is insulin pump therapy, in which a low basal dose of insulin is continuously infused, supplemented by self-adjusted bolus doses before food intake or when BG is too high.

Problems in Self-Treatment of IDDM

As the technology and knowledge necessary to control diabetes have become available, it has become increasingly apparent that the greatest barriers to treatment often lie in the psychological and behavioral domains (Rosenstock,

1985). Adherence problems are not unique to IDDM, but the diabetic regimen has many characteristics that are predictive of difficulties in self-treatment. Self-care is complex, demanding, constant, and long-lasting (Epstein & Cluss, 1982; Haynes, Taylor, & Sackett, 1979). IDDM patients are also completely responsible for their own day-to-day diabetes management, requiring a unique level of active involvement on the part of the patient. The currently recommended intensive regimens are even more complex and demanding.

It is therefore not surprising that problems with adherence have been called the "most serious obstacle to effective management of diabetes" (Rosenstock, 1985, p. 610). It is also not surprising that adherence is an area of considerable interest and effort in clinical diabetes research. Traditional medical models of self-treatment have been relatively simplistic, emphasizing the role of patient characteristics such as knowledge and personality factors. More recent psychological models have taken a more complex cognitive-behavioral approach to self-care, with increased emphasis on motivation, environmental contingencies, health beliefs, and social learning processes. The next section briefly reviews these approaches to self-treatment of IDDM.

Educational models have received much attention because few illnesses require the patient to acquire as much information and many new skills as does IDDM. In fact, the IDDM patient is ideally a lay expert on glucose metabolism, with a vast knowledge of nutrition, insulin kinetics, and BG fluctuations. Advances and changes in treatment and technology also make continuing education and training critical for state-of-the-art diabetes management. Education is so uniquely important to diabetes management that the American Diabetes Association includes it as part of the recommended medical regimen. Unfortunately, diabetes knowledge remains disturbingly inadequate in many patients (Miller, Goldstein, & Nicholaison, 1978; Sanazaro, 1985; Stone, 1964).

Educational intervention, however, does not always result in improved self-treatment and diabetes control (Cox et al., 1986; Williams, Martin, Hogan, Watkins, & Ellis, 1967) or may produce short-term benefits that quickly disappear. Some types of intervention do appear to be more beneficial than others; for example, skill-based programs produce more positive results than didactic educational intervention (see Mazzuca et al., 1986). Even though education is a necessary prerequisite to adequate self-treatment, it is not sufficient to improve self-care and control. Education is thus considered to be a critical factor in models of IDDM self-treatment, but its ultimate impact on clinical outcome is mediated by a other variables, such as individual characteristics and environmental factors.

Personality-based models traditionally have been based on the premise that patients do not adhere to regimens or achieve good metabolic control because of personality deficits and/or psychological problems. This approach enjoyed much popularity throughout the 1970s with a number of studies attempting to identify personality variables that discriminated "good" from "bad" patients (e.g., Simonds, 1976–1977). In general, however, studies have failed to identify unique personality profiles predictive of poor outcome (Dunn & Turtle, 1981; Koch & Molnar, 1979). The intrinsic appeal of this model is obvious since it is congruent with the common belief that diabetic patients are often difficult, uncooperative, or self-destructive individuals who "cheat" on their regimens are "fabricate" self-reports of adherence. Not only is there no empirical justification for these negative attributions; they may also have detrimental effects on the practitioner–patient relationship (Bradley, 1982; Cox et al., 1986).

Although there is no reason to assume that poor outcome reflects personality pathology, this does not mean that individual differences in emotional stability and psychological coping do not influence self-treatment. Research has clearly shown that the presence of emotional disorders and other psychosocial problems can interfere with self-treatment. Consequently, depression, anxiety, and family or marital conflict are all associated with difficulties in diabetes management (Murawski, Chazan, Balodimos, & Ryan, 1979; Newbrough, Simpkins, & Maurer, 1985). Contemporary models of self-treatment of diabetes acknowledge that each individual patient is unique in personality, attitude, beliefs, experience, and resources—all of which play some role in guiding self-care decisions and behaviors.

Cognitive-behavioral models derive from a behavioral perspective: The IDDM patient should be highly motivated to adhere to daily insulin injections because severe hyperglycemia can be quite dangerous, even deadly. Unfortunately, the likelihood of adherence to other regimen requirements and the motivation to maintain tight glucose control are much lower than the likelihood of adherence to insulin (Surwit, Feinglos, & Scovern, 1983; Surwit, Scovern, & Feinglos, 1982). Many of the behavioral adaptations required to achieve tight control involve changing long-established daily habits, such as dietary and exercise routines. In addition, poor control has no immediate negative consequences. Long-term diabetic complications may take years to manifest, even though the degenerative processes leading to eventual heart, retinal, or kidney disease appear to begin soon after onset. The patient's behavioral task, therefore, is to follow a difficult and demanding daily regimen in order to avoid negative consequences that may or may not occur in the distant future—a poor formula for long-term maintenance of desired behaviors.

The likelihood of achieving optimal diabetes control can be even further reduced by motivation to avoid hypoglycemia, which occurs more frequently when patients attempt to normalize BG. Unlike hyperglycemia, the negative consequences of hypoglycemic episodes are immediate and very aversive, including unpleasant symptoms, embarrassment, and potential accidents. Motivation to avoid these episodes cause some patients to refuse intensive regimens and even to maintain hyperglycemic BG levels. Cox, Gonder-Frederick, Pohl, and Pennebaker (1986) as well as Weiner and Skipper (1979) have suggested that fear of hypoglycemia is a major psychological barrier to diabetes control. In support of this conclusion, we have found that the Hypoglycemic Fear Survey, a measure of behaviors and worries associated with avoidance of hypoglycemia, is predictive of poor metabolic control (Cox, Irvine, Gonder-Frederick, & Nowacek, 1987).

In view of these poor naturalistic contingencies, behavioral interventions have been used to increase motivation and adherence (Epstein & Cluss, 1982; Wing, Epstein, Nowalk, & Lamparski, 1986). Contingency-management programs, such as token economy systems, have yielded positive results with adolescent patients (Carney, Schechter, & Davis, 1983; Epstein, et al., 1981). Even without rewards, behavioral interventions such as goal-setting and contracting may improve self-care habits (Schafer, Glasgow, & McCaul, 1982). Although preliminary studies show some promise, they have not led to extensive research or application. Both the specific mechanisms contributing to improvements and the long-term stability of positive effects remain unclear. At present, behavioral interventions are most often used in clinical settings with patients exhibiting severe adherence problems.

In addition to motivation, the cognitive-behavioral approach takes into consideration patients' perceptions of their regimen and illness. Glasgow, McCaul, Shafer, and their associates have demonstrated the importance of patient-perceived environmental and social barriers to adherence, such as expense, embarrassment, time limitations, or poor family support. High levels of perceived barriers are associated with poor levels of self-reported adherence and metabolic control in adults and adolescents with IDDM (Glasgow, McCaul, & Schafer, 1986; Schafer, Glawgow, & McCaul, 1983). Health beliefs concerning vulnerability to complications, severity of IDDM, perceived cost of adherence, and ability to succeed also mediate self-treatment (Rosenstock, 1985). Both perceived barriers and diabetes health beliefs appear to be valid predictors of self-treatment behavior, but these constructs have not yet been translated into possible interventions designed to alter perception of barriers, actual barriers, or health beliefs.

A Self-Regulation Model of Diabetes Management

In our research and work with IDDM patients, diabetes management is viewed as a process of self-regulation (Gonder-Frederick & Cox, 1990; Hamera et al., 1988; Wing, et al., 1986). In fact, IDDM has been called the "ideal paradigm" for the study of behavioral self-regulation because the patient is required to duplicate behaviorally those functions usually performed automatically by the pancreas and other metabolic systems (Surwit et al., 1983): monitoring BG levels with self-tests, making insulin available with injections, and adjusting metabolic requirements and utilization with diet and exercise. A number of variables mediate this self-regulatory process, including those discussed in the previous section: knowledge, individual differences in personality and coping resources, environmental barriers, social support systems, health beliefs, and contingencies.

By definition, a self-regulating process depends on an accurate feedback system in order to maintain functions. In the self-regulation model of diabetes management, a feedback system to provide information about BG levels is needed that enables the patient to avoid hypoglycemic episodes and chronic hyperglycemia; make decisions about insulin, food, and exercise; assess the efficacy of self-treatment behaviors; and evaluate long-term diabetes control. IDDM patients have access to two primary types of information about BG levels, objective information from self-tests of urine or blood and subjective information from physical symptoms of hypoglycemia and hyperglycemia. Even though our interests focus primarily on subjective symptom feedback, objective measurement is essential to BG regulation and therefore is briefly described.

At the most minimal level, IDDM patients should perform daily urine tests for the presence of glucose or ketones, which indicates extreme hypeglycemia. The numerous problems with urine testing, including individual differences in renal threshold, have been discussed elsewhere (Hayford, Weydert, & Thompson, 1983). From our perspective, however, the greatest deficit of this self-testing regimen is that it yields minimal information for BG regulation. Urine testing provides no information about euglycemic, moderately hyperglycemic, or hypoglycemic fluctuations; thus its usefulness is limited to avoidance of severe hyperglycemia and ketoacidotic coma.

Technological advances in self-testing have vastly improved IDDM patients' ability to regulate BG levels. In fact, without self-measurement of BG (SMBG), which allows patients to monitor glucose fluctuations throughout the day, intensive insulin regimens and tighter glucose control would not be possible (Schiffrin & Belmonte, 1982). SMBG involves a small fingerprick to obtain one drop of whole blood, which is placed on a glucose oxidase–peroxidase reagent strip. After a brief "development" period, the blood is removed and the color change on the strip either visually interpreted or read by a reflectance meter. SMBG is recommended for all diabetic patients by the American Diabetes Association because it is absolutely essential for optimal control. The ideal regimen involves SMBG at least four times daily in combination with multiple self-adjusted insulin doses throughout the day. This might involve performing SMBG before breakfast and the first daily insulin dose, prior to lunch and insulin, mid-afternoon when hypoglycemia can occur due to peaks in insulin action, before dinner and insulin, and before bedtime to see if food or insulin is needed. Unfortunately, many patients find this regimen too time-consuming, inconvenient, aversive, and expensive (Gonder-Frederick, Cox, Pohl, & Carter, 1984).

The other important source of BG feedback, and the focus of this chapter, is subjectively perceived BG information, including physical symptoms, mood changes, and difficulties performing cognitive or motor tasks. As many authors have pointed out, symptoms are critical in any behavioral model of self-treatment (Nerenz & Leventhal, 1983; Pennebaker, 1982), providing immediate, free, and direct information about health status. People's past experiences with illness usually confirm that symptoms are reliable indicators of health status. It is not surprising, therefore, that the processes of perceiving and interpreting subjective symptoms play a prominent role in patients' mental representations of illnesses.

The extent to which people depend on and trust symptom information has been best illustrated in a series of studies with hypertensive patients (Leventhal, Meyer, & Nerenz, 1980; Nerenz & Leventhal, 1983). Even though these patients were told that hypertension is asymptomatic, they continued to monitor and rely on subjective symptoms which they believed indicated elevated blood pressure (BP) levels. Most importantly, these patients based self-treatment decisions on their perceived BP symptoms. There are mixed findings concerning the extent to which elevations in BP are subjectively symptomatic. Studies using a repeated-measures, within-subject design have found that symptoms do covary with BP levels, but studies using single-measure, between-subject designs find no covariation (e.g., Baumann & Leventhal, 1985; Pennebaker & Watson, 1988). For the purposes of this chapter, however, the most important conclusion is that symptom beliefs persist, even when patients are instructed not to monitor symptom information.

In contrast to hypertensive patients, IDDM patients are taught to monitor for certain symptoms indicative of BG extremes and to take action if these symptoms occur. Traditionally, medical practitioners have operated under the assumption that patients are able to recognize and respond appropriately to BG symptoms. For this reason, patients are typically encouraged to treat themselves on the basis of perceived symptoms, for example, to consume orange juice or some other fast-acting carbohydrate at the first signs of low BG. The extent to which medical practitioners trust patient ability to perceive BG symptoms accurately is sometimes surprising and even disconcerting. For example, the first author's diabetic father was once told by his physician that frequent SMBG was not necessary because he would supposedly be able to "feel it if it was too high."

Survey and interview studies conducted by our research team (Gonder-Frederick & Cox, 1986; Gonder-Frederick, Cox, Pennebaker, & Bobbitt, 1986) and others (O'Connell, Hamera, Schorfheide, & Guthrie, 1990) confirm that diabetic patients believe they can recognize BG symptoms, and they take action to correct their perceived glucose levels when symptoms occur. However, patients often report behavioral responses to symptoms that have no real effect on BG, such as lying down in response to weakness. Thus even if extremes in BG are accurately perceived, appropriate self-treatment behaviors do not necessarily follow (O'Connell et al., 1984). Surveys also demonstrate that patients have the highest level of confidence in their ability to recognize symptoms related to hypoglycemia as compared to hyper-glycemia. In fact, even patients who use SMBG tend to treat themselves for hypoglycemia on the basis of perceived symptoms without, or prior to, verifying actual low BG level with a self-test (Gonder-Frederick & Cox, 1986). Availability of objective BG measurements, therefore, does not eliminate reliance on subjective symptoms and BG perception. Reliance on subjective information is probably even greater in those patients who only use urine testing or very infrequent SMBG; unfortunately, this group is the majority of IDDM patients.

Blood Glucose Symptomatology

The ultimate impact of any feedback system on self-regulatory processes depends entirely on the accuracy and reliability of the information the system provides. Patients' tendency to rely on perceived symptoms for BG information and practitioners' encouragement to do so are based on the assumption that symptoms can provide reliable and accurate feedback about glucose fluctuations. However, when we began our investigation, there was no empirical documentation that perceived symptoms reliably covaried with BG levels in IDDM. Our first study, therefore, assessed the extent to which hypoglycemia and hyperglycemia are subjectively symptomatic (Pennebaker et al., 1981). Patients admitted to the University of Virginia Diabetes Inpatient Unit were asked to complete symptom checklists just prior to SMBG, which was performed 7 to 10 times daily during a one-week admission. This yielded approximately 60 concurrent measurements of perceived symptoms and BG level for each patient.

The results confirmed that both hypoglycemia and hyperglycemia can be symptomatic. In contrast to expectations, however, there were no specific symptoms that covaried with BG across patients. Rather, BG symptoms were highly idiosyncratic. This means that trembling and sweating may be the most reliable signs of hypoglycemia for one person, whereas these perceived symptoms would not occur for another person with low BG levels, but dizziness and confusion would. Some symptoms, such as weakness, can be related to hypoglycemia for some people and hyperglycemia for others.

The idiosyncrasy of BG symptomatology has been repeatedly observed in studies of IDDM adults (Cox, Gonder-Frederick, Pohl, & Pennebaker, 1983; Gonder-Frederick et al., 1986; Gonder-Frederick, Cox, Bobbitt, & Penne-baker, 1989; Moses & Bradley, 1985), adolescents, and children (Freund, Bennett-Johnson, Rosenbloom, Alexander, & Hansen, 1986; Gonder-Frederick, Snyder, & Clarke, 1991). Because of this inherent idiosyncrasy, identification of BG symptoms requires a within-subject research design in which repeated measurements are taken of perceived symptoms and concurrent BG levels. In addition to performing inpatient studies, we have investigated symptom–BG relationships on an outpatient basis, with subjects

Table 10-1. Symptoms and Moods Commonly Related to Blood Glucose in
IDDM Patients

Hypoglycemia	Hyperglycemia	Hypoglycemia and Hyperglycemia
Trembling	Dry mouth	Blurred vision
Sweating	Thirst	Fatigue
Pounding heart	Alert or energetic feeling	Weakness
Confusion	Sweet taste	Heavy breathing
Slurred speech	Tingling or pain in	Nausea
Hunger	extremities	Headache
Uncoordination	Frequent urination	Frustration
Anxiety	Stomach cramps	Irritation
		Dizziness

completing symptom checklists just prior to home SMBG. Additional studies have been conducted in a controlled hospital setting (Clarke et al., 1988; Cox, Antoun, et al., 1991) measuring perceived symptoms and concurrent BG while glucose was manipulated to low, normal, and high levels using an insulin/glucose infusion system that acts as an "artificial" pancreas (Biostator, Ames Company, Miles Laboratories, Elkhart, IN).

Table 10-1 summarizes the symptoms that most commonly occur with hypoglycemia and hyperglycemia in IDDM patients. For most patients, hypoglycemia appears to be more subjectively symptomatic than hyperglycemia. Low BG levels are typically associated with more symptoms and those symptoms are more severe in nature. Many of the hypoglycemic symptoms are actually related to hormonal counterregulatory responses and not to low BG per se. For example, epinephrine secretion, which causes the liver to release stored glycogen, can result in perceived trembling, heart palpitations, lightheadedness, and other adrenergic symptoms. Other symptoms are caused by depletions in brain glucose, resulting in mental confusion, slurred speech, lack of motor coordination, and other signs of neuroglycopenia.

The BG threshold for hypoglycemic symptoms varies greatly; some patients become noticeably symptomatic at 60 mg/dl whereas others remain asymptomatic until glucose falls to 45 mg/dl or lower (Cox, Antoun, et al., 1991). The traditional medical assumption has been that adrenergic symptoms occur first, providing "early warning" signs of impending hypoglycemia, and that neuroglycopenic symptoms occur later, when BG is severely low (Cryer & Gerich, 1985; Gerich, 1988). In contrast, we have found that adrenergic and neuroglycopenic symptoms can occur in any sequence, or even simultaneously (Cox, Antoun, et al., 1991). Both the sequence and the progression of hypoglycemic symptoms are quite idiosyncratic, and neuroglycopenic symptoms can occur at much more moderate levels of hypoglycemia than expected.

Much less is known about the etiology and progression of the hyperglycemic symptoms listed in Table 10-1. Some of the subjective responses,
such as thirst and frequent urination, reflect the body's attempts to eliminate
excess glucose. Hyperglycemia also appears to have immediate effects on the
peripheral nervous and microvascular systems, causing tingling, burning,
and painful sensations, especially in extremities. As Table 10-1 also shows,
many symptoms are related to hypoglycemia for some people and to
hyperglycemia for others. In fact, individual patients often report experiencing symptoms such as headache or fatigue with *both* low and high BG levels,
but these symptoms are qualitatively different for hypoglycemia and
hyperglycemia.

Both hypoglycemia and hyperglycemia also have affective consequences
(Gonder-Frederick et al., 1989; Moses & Bradley, 1985). In general,
hypoglycemia is associated with negative emotions, such as anxietylike states
and irritation. These negative mood changes are due partly to hypoglycemia-
induced epinephrine secretion. Numerous studies have demonstrated that
physiological arousal due to sympathetic nervous system activation can
produce or enhance emotional attributions (see Manstead & Wagner, 1981,
for a review of this literature). In addition, neuroglycopenia contributes to
hypoglycemia-related mood changes. Hyperglycemia can be associated with
negative moods but is more often related to positive affective states. Many
IDDM patients report feeling more alert, energetic, and cheerful when BG is
moderately high. The etiology of such positive mood relationships is
unknown but may reflect central nervous system adaptations to hyperglycemia, which increase the glucose concentration required for optimal
brain and behavioral functioning (Gjedde & Crone, 1981).

Accuracy of Symptom Perception and Beliefs

Both hypoglycemia and hyperglycemia are symptomatic, so the next
question of interest is, Do IDDM patients accurately recognize and label
subjective symptoms idiosyncratically related to their own BG? Following
the self-regulatory model, accurate perception of BG symptoms should
facilitate self-treatment, while errors in symptom perception could disrupt
self-treatment and diabetes control. For the patient who "feels" hypoglycemic symptoms at a BG level of 57 mg/dl, food intake to raise BG is an
appropriate response. However, the patient who mistakenly "feels" such
symptoms at a BG level of 160 mg/dl and consumes food is making an error
in self-treatment that will lead to hyperglycemia.

It might be argued that because symptoms reliably covary with BG, we
can safely assume that patients are generally accurate at detecting
hypoglycemia and hyperglycemia. Such a conclusion, however, is based on a
model of symptom perception that assumes a direct linear relationship

between physiological events and subjective perception of those events. Psychologists know better. The process of perceiving and making inferences about symptoms is, like all other human information processing, a complex phenomenon. Symptom perception is mediated by attentional, environmental, and attributional processes that often lead to perceptual and cognitive biases (Pennebaker, 1982). Consequently, people's beliefs and inferences about their physical symptoms may be erroneous (Nerenz & Leventhal, 1983; Pennebaker & Watson, 1988).

Perception of BG symptoms may be especially prone to such errors. As our research demonstrates, abnormal BG levels are associated with a variety of subjective sensations and symptoms. Many of these symptoms occur relatively frequently even in nondiabetic individuals—for example, trembling, weakness, hunger, anxiety, thirst, and headaches. Such symptoms occur in a variety of situations and have a number of possible causes. Appropriate labeling of these ambiguous and common symptoms requires no small amount of cognitive effort on the part of the patient who must always ask, "Is this symptom related to my BG?" Accurate recognition of hypoglycemic symptoms presents another unique problem. The cognitive dysfunction and subsequent poor judgment and decision making associated with hypoglycemic neuroglycopenia may severely compromise ability to recognize symptoms. A similar effect is seen in alcohol-intoxicated individuals who do not recognize their own symptomatology (slurred speech, lack of motor coordination, etc.) due to perceptual and cognitive dysfunction.

In addition to physical symptoms, accurate labeling of BG-related mood changes presents difficulties. Negative mood changes associated with hypoglycemia, for example, may be misattributed to environmental or interpersonal situations. In fact, our interest in BG–mood relationships was instigated by an episode in which a research subject, unbeknownst to her, experienced very low BG levels during testing. Instead of attributing her symptoms to low BG, the subject became angry, began crying, and accused the staff of "doing something" to upset her. Although research has not addressed the potential negative impact of low BG on social relationships, marital conflict related to hypoglycemia is not uncommon in clinical settings (Cox, Gonder-Federick, & Saunders, in press).

Some of the most important determinants of BG perception and inferences are individual beliefs about symptoms that covery with hypoglycemia and hyperglycemia. After diagnosis of almost any disease, people appear to develop relatively "rigid" beliefs about symptoms (Nerenz & Leventhal, 1983). These beliefs guide and direct attention to symptom feedback, often biasing attention toward instances that confirm symptom beliefs. We evaluated the accuracy of BG symptom beliefs by asking IDDM patients what symptoms best indicated their own BG. This interview was conducted after these patients had completed at least 40 trials of concurrent symptom ratings and BG measurements in order to identify empirically those symptoms that idiosyncratically covaried with glucose.

Patients' symptom beliefs were then compared to those symptoms that were actually related to low and high BG using a signal detection approach (Swets, 1973) to yield measures of accurate symptom beliefs (hits and correct rejections) and inaccurate symptom beliefs (false alarms and misses). Across subjects, the majority of symptom beliefs were accurate, meaning that most were either hits or correct rejections. However, there was also a disturbingly high rate of false alarm belief (mean = 3.0), suggesting a tendency to believe symptoms to be related to BG when, in fact, the symptoms do not reliably co-occur with hypoglycemia or hyperglycemia. Females had a higher rate of false alarm symptom beliefs than males. However, males had a higher rate of missed symptoms, indicating they were unaware of symptoms that did reliably co-occur with BG levels. Similar symptom belief errors have been found in non–insulin-dependent diabetic patients (O'Connell et al., 1990) and in hypertensive patients (Pennebaker and Watson, 1988). Importantly, O'Connell et al. also found that symptom belief inaccuracy was related to diabetes control.

It is not all that surprising that false alarm symptom beliefs occur in chronic illnesses that require patients to focus vigilantly on some physiological parameter, such as diabetes and hypertension. Certainly, for the IDDM patient, the most salient, available, and plausible cause for any perceived symptom is BG level. Once formed, false alarm beliefs do appear to be maintained by perceptual and cognitive biases and are highly resistant to change (Nerenz & Leventhal, 1983). We have frequently observed such resistance in clinical work with IDDM patients. For example, a female patient was convinced that her afternoon headaches indicated hyperglycemia. A diary of her daily headaches and BG measurements showed, however, that the headaches co-occurred with high BG only 50% of the time. This objective, disconfirming evidence had little impact, and the patient continued to believe her headaches were reliable BG cues.

IDDM patients can also be unaware of symptoms that do reliably co-occur with hypoglycemia and hyperglycemia. This may happen most often with the milder, early warning symptoms usually associated with moderately low or high BG. Beliefs about symptoms associated with very extreme BG levels tend to be more accurate. The higher frequency of missed symptoms in males may reflect the general tendency to report and/or attend to somatic and affective changes to a lesser degree than females (Pennebaker, 1982).

Accuracy of Subjective BG Discrimination

Although highly suggestive, symptom belief errors do not necessarily demonstrate that errors in subjective BG detection occur. The potential negative impact of inaccurate symptom beliefs on BG detection may be moderated, or even eliminated, by accurate beliefs. In addition, in the real world symptoms and other internal cues are not the only source of

BG-relevant information available to the patient. External cues, such as information about the time of day, insulin, food, and recent activities, also provide relevant cues. For these reasons, we tested the accuracy of subjective BG detection directly in a series of studies using variations of a repeated-measures design in which subjects are asked to estimate their current BG level just prior to measurement of actual BG.

The first study is described in some detail because it involved separate assessments of BG estimation based only upon internal cues and upon both internal and external cues (Cox et al., 1985). Ability to estimate BG was tested under two conditions: in a controlled hospital setting and at home. For hospital testing, IDDM patients were connected to the Biostator and estimated their BG level every 10 minutes over a 9-hour period (for a total of 54 trials) as their glucose levels were manipulated from 300 to 55 mg/dl. Patients were kept blind to actual BG levels and instructed to base their estimations on symptoms and other internal cues. This procedure allowed us to assess BG perception in a unique setting in which external cues, such as time of day and food intake, did not provide relevant information. After hospital testing, patients estimated their BG just prior to home SMBG, four times each day over a 10-day period.[1] In making home estimates, they were encouraged to consider any and all relevant BG information, including external cues.

Before summarizing the results of this and subsequent BG estimation studies, the issue of accuracy in subjective BG estimates needs to be briefly discussed. Traditionally, comparisons of BG estmates and a reference value have employed correlations or computation of deviation scores. The statistical problems associated with these techniques have been discussed previously (Clarke, Cox, Gonder-Frederick, Carter, & Pohl, 1987; Koschinsky, Dannehl, & Gries, 1988). From an applied perspective, however, their most serious flaw is failure to measure the clinical significance of BG estimations. For example, an estimated BG of 150 mg/dl when actual BG is 300 mg/dl, a 100% deviation, represents a clinically significant error because the person believes BG to be euglycemic when, in reality, it needs to be lowered. On the other hand, an estimated BG of 25 mg/dl when actual BG is 50 mg/dl, another 100% deviation, represents a clinically accurate estimate because in both cases BG needs to be raised.

---

[1] The primary flaw with this home protocol is that some subjects might be tempted to measure BG levels prior to recording estimates in order to appear more accurate. For this reason, we incorporated use of a hand-held computer containing a program which prompts subjects to enter their symptom ratings, BG estimates, and actual BG measurements—in that order. These computers also contain an internal clock programmed to record the time interval between entries of BG estimations and entries of actual BG measurements. Because SMBG requires a 1-minute development period, entries showing that actual BG was recorded in less time indicate that BG was measured before estimation entry. We have employed this procedure in subgroups of subjects in all BG estimation studies and have repeatedly found such "cheating" to be extremely rare.

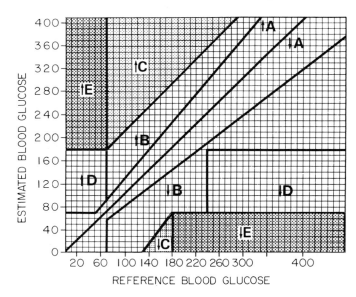

Figure 10-1. Error Grid Analysis. (From C. S. Holmes [Ed.], *Neuropsychology and Behavioral Aspects of Diabetes*, Springer-Verlag, 1990. Reprinted by permission.)

To obtain a clinically relevant measure of BG estimation accuracy, we developed the Error Grid Analysis (EGA), which is seen in Figure 10-1. The EGA provides a measure of the frequency of clinically accurate estimates and different types of clinically negative errors. As shown in Figure 10-1, EGA involves plotting estimated against actual BG so that each estimate falls into one of 10 logically symmetrical EGA zones. The diagonal line represents perfect agreement. Estimates falling above the diagonal are overestimates of BG and estimates falling below are underestimates.

Upper and lower A zones are clinically accurate estimates that are either (1) within 20% of actual BG or (2) below 70 mg/dl when actual BG is hypoglycemic. B zone estimates are not clinically accurate but in most cases are clinically benign in the sense that potentially dangerous consequences are unlikely whether or not action is taken.

Zones C, D, and E represent errors in BG estimation that could have negative clinical implications. Estimates falling into C zones describe instances in which BG is believed to be either hypoglycemic (lower C) or hyperglycemic (upper C) when it is actually euglycemic. Any action to raise or lower glucose based on C zone errors could drive BG from an acceptable to an unacceptable range. D zone errors are potentially dangerous failures to detect hypoglycemia (upper D) and hyperglycemia (lower D). In these instances, BG is believed to be at an acceptable level when it is not, and a patient may fail to take needed action. Finally, E zone errors are those in which BG is believed to be too high when it is actually too low, and vice

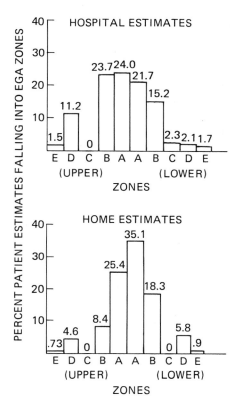

Figure 10-2. EGA results. (From C. S. Holmes [Ed.], *Neuropsychological and Behavioral Aspects of Diabetes*, Springer-Verlag, 1990. Reprinted by permission.)

versa. Obviously, taking action to lower BG level when it is already hypoglycemic, and vice versa, could have very serious consequences.

The first step of EGA involves measuring the frequency of estimates in each zone. A summary statistic, the accuracy index (AI), is then computed by subtracting the summed percentage of estimates in the C, D, and E zones from the summed percentage of estimates in A zones. Thus positive AI scores a higher frequency of clinically accurate estimates as compared to potentially serious errors, while negative AI scores indicate more errors than accurate estimates.

Figure 10-2 summarizes the EGA results from the study described above. BG estimates were clinically accurate 46% of the time in the hospital condition, where patients had access to internal cues only. Home estimates were clinically accurate significantly more often than hospital estimates— 60% of the time—demonstrating that availability of external cues enhanced accuracy. This finding is not surprising because there are many instances in which external information alone can lead to accurate estimates. For example, patients estimating high BG levels 2 hours after eating a meal are likely to be accurate.

Figure 10-2 also shows that patients made a surprisingly high rate of clinically serious errors in both conditions. Almost 19% of hospital estimates and 12% of home estimates fell in zones C, D, and E. The most common type of error was failure to detect hypoglycemia and hyperglycemia (D zones). Other types of errors (C and E zones) were less common, but they did occur. To put these findings in clinical perspective, this means that serious errors in BG discrimination were made an average of four times over a 10-day period.

This pattern of results has been replicated in subsequent studies of BG estimation in adult IDDM patients (Cox, Carter, Gonder-Frederick, Clarke, & Pohl, 1988; Cox, Gonder-Frederick, et al., 1989). Because hospital and home estimation procedures did not yield different results, these studies used home estimates (which have more clinical relevance) to assess accuracy. Across studies, failure to detect BG extremes is consistently the most common clinically serious error. The rate of C zone errors is quite low, showing that patients rarely believe BG is too high or low when it is in a normal range. This may reflect the tendency for patients' estimates to normalize BG fluctuations. We repeatedly find that patients underestimate high BG measurements and overestimate low BG measurements. This finding, in patients who use SMBG on a regular basis, suggests that objective data from self-testing are distorted by biases in BG perception and beliefs.

Ability to estimate BG varies greatly across individual patients, with clinically accurate estimates ranging from 42 to 90%. Unfortunately, confidence in ability to detect hypoglycemia and hyperglycemia does not predict accuracy, suggesting that patients who are not able to estimate BG accurately are not aware of their inability. Adult patients' ability to estimate BG is also unrelated to age, duration of IDDM, frequency of SMBG, or educational level.

Although age does not predict accuracy in adults, BG estimations are significantly less accurate in adolescent patient populations whose AIs average 25% (Freund et al., 1986). A recent study at our Pediatric Clinic found even poorer ability in younger diabetic children (ages 5–11). Their mean AI was 0%, indicating that this age group makes clinically significant errors just as frequently as clinically accurate estimates (Gonder-Frederick, Snyder, & Clarke, 1989). Like adults, the most common error for children was failure to detect BG extremes. However, children were more likely than adults to estimate low BG when BG was actually high (lower E zone errors). These errors may reflect children's lack of experience with BG symptoms or a tendency to interpret any unpleasant symptoms as signs of hypoglycemia. Reinforcement contingencies might also contribute, since children are typically fed carbohydrates when they report hypoglycemic symptoms.

Treatment of IDDM in the young child requires both parent and child to recognize and respond to symptoms and other signs of hypoglycemia or hyperglycemia. We therefore also assessed parents' ability to estimate their diabetic child's BG level. Surprisingly, parents' estimates were just as inaccurate as their children's, with a mean AI of 5%. Obviously, parents are at a disadvantage when estimating their child's BG, since they must rely on overt signs or the child's report of perceived symptoms. Nonetheless, we might expect parents to be much better than children at using external cues to predict BG. As in other studies, confidence in ability to discriminate BG levels was unrelated to measured accuracy for both diabetic children and their parents.

Taken together, the accuracy studies lead to the conclusion that diabetic patients in all age groups make potentially serious errors in subjective BG perception and inference-making. These findings have several implications for diabetes self-treatment and education. First, and most important, clinicians should be cautious when instructing or encouraging patients to treat themselves on the basis of perceived BG. Rather, patients should be encouraged to use SMBG to verify perceived symptoms and decrease zone C or zone E errors.

SMBG should also be used more frequently at times when *no* symptoms are perceived to reduce undetected hypoglycemic and hyperglycemic episodes (D zone errors). IDDM patients of all ages tend to be unaware of the frequency and severity of their hyperglycemia. In addition, patients fail to detect nearly half of hypoglycemic episodes. The high rate of D zone errors demonstrates that absence of perceived symptoms plays a role in subjective BG assessment.

These findings do not support traditional assumptions that patients can "feel" BG extremes. Because there is no relationship between confidence and measured accuracy, clinicians should not rely on patients' self-reported ability to discriminate BG levels. Finally, we suspect that these results describe optimal levels of accuracy. The IDDM patients in these studies were educated in diabetes management, relatively healthy, and highly motivated. This is not representative of the general diabetic population in which the majority of patients are inadequately educated and have numerous health problems due to long-term complications. For these reasons, we would expect to find even more errors in other patient groups.

Clinical Intervention to Improve BG Estimation

Regardless of actual ability, IDDM patients will continue to rely on symptoms and other subjective cues to regulate their illness. Even the most dedicated self-regulator will not always have a reflectance meter available and, if signs of possible hypoglycemia occur, will have to decide whether or not to take action. For this reason, we have developed and tested a clinical intervention designed to improve patients' ability to recognize BG symptoms and estimate glucose levels.

Several studies have shown that provision of BG feedback via SMBG alone does not improve ability to estimate glucose (Moses & Bradley, 1985; Wing et al., 1984). Our intervention, Blood Glucose Awareness Training (BGAT), provides systematic feedback concerning the accuracy of BG estimations and inferences. BGAT is designed to (1) increase awareness of idiosyncratic symptoms and other internal cues that reliably covary with hypoglycemia and hyperglycemia; (2) increase awareness of inaccurate symptom beliefs and other misleading information that causes errors; and (3) increase knowledge about the effects of external factors (food, insulin, stress, etc.) on individual BG patterns.

BGAT is a seven-week training program, with weekly sessions conducted in a group setting. These weekly sessions follow a seven-chapter manual with each chapter containing a didactic section, a self-test of information mastery, and homework exercises.[2] Patients also keep a Blood Glucose Estimation Diary throughout BGAT, requiring at least four entries each day. Diary entries record all internal and external cues believed to be relevant to current BG, record estimated BG based on these cues, test and record actual BG, and plot estimated and actual BG on the error grid for evaluation.

Diaries are reviewed by the group during weekly meetings in order to identify those cues that appear to provide reliable information (i.e., result in A zone estimates) and those cues that appear to be misleading (i.e., result in C, D, and E zone estimates). Participants also try to identify idiosyncratic error patterns such as consistent underestimation of hyperglycemia or failure to detect hypoglycemia.

The clinical utility of BGAT has been tested in three separate studies, using a pre–post design comparing trained patients with untrained control patients (Cox et al., 1988; Cox, Gonder-Frederick, et al., 1989; Cox et al., 1990). Control subjects met in weekly group sessions to discuss the effects of psychological stress on diabetes control and other diabetes-related topics. Control patients also kept stress and BG diaries but did not estimate BG levels during group participation. Figure 10-3 shows that BGAT has consistently improved estimation accuracy, measured by pretraining and posttraining AIs. Improvements in AI among BGAT patients have ranged from 14 to 22%, whereas control groups have shown no significant change.

BGAT also results in a consistent pattern of improvement. The frequency of clinically accurate estimates (A zones) increases and the frequency of errors involving failure to detect BG extremes (D zones) decreases. The number of undetected hypoglycemic and hyperglycemic episodes has been reduced by 50% or more across studies. Even more important from a pragmatic perspective, BGAT appears to have positive effects on metabolic control, as shown by reduced glycosylated hemoglobin measurements after training.

Many questions remain concerning the mechanisms contributing to BGAT's efficacy; the most important questions concern the contributions of

---

[2] Copies of the Blood Glucose Awareness Training Manual are available upon request.

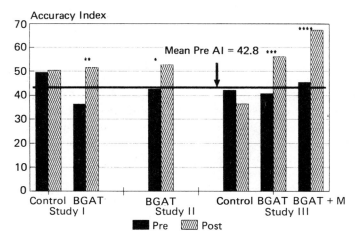

Figure 10-3. Pre- and post-BGAT results. *p = .058; **p < .05; ***p < .005; ****p < .001. (From C. S. Holmes [Ed.], *Neuropsychological and Behavioral Aspects of Diabetes*, Springer-Verlag, 1990. Reprinted by permission.)

internal versus external cue training. The first attempt at BGAT intervention (Study I in Figure 10-3) focused primarily on internal cue training, which resulted in significant improvements in accuracy (Cox et al., 1988). Study II added information about external cues to BGAT, resulting in greater improvement and suggesting that external cue training might enhance the benefits of BGAT. A recent pilot study in Spain found that training in the use of external cues alone resulted in improved BG estimation and glucose control (Raoles-Nieto, 1988).

In our most recent study (study III), we tested the possibility that a procedure designed to enhance internal cue training would increase the effectiveness of BGAT (Cox et al., 1990). Half of the treatment subjects in this study underwent a procedure called *massed practice* prior to BGAT. These subjects were hospitalized and connected to the Biostator, which manipulated BG to low, normal, and high levels. During this procedure, subjects completed approximately 25 practice trials in which they (1) scanned their bodies for symptoms and other internal cues, (2) estimated current BG, (3) received immediate feedback about actual BG, and (4) were instructed to scan their bodies again for internal cues covarying with actual BG level. Massed practice thus provided an opportunity for subjects to form accurate mental representations of subjective sensations that accompany different BG levels.

Figure 10-3 compares the pretraining and posttraining AI scores for control, standard BGAT, and massed practice groups (BGAT + M). Compared to subjects receiving standard BGAT, massed practice subjects showed almost twice as much improvement in AI and better detection of both hypoglycemia and hyperglycemia, but these differences were not statistically significant. However, massed practice subjects did show a significant improvement in glucose control; standard BGAT subjects did not. Although somewhat mixed, these findings suggest that BGAT may be enhanced by similar in vivo procedures involving structured focus on internal cues during hypoglycemia and hyperglycemia. We are currently integrating these findings into BGAT by holding weekly sessions at a time of day when BG levels are likely to be low (just before dinner) then increase dramatically (after eating dinner). Preliminary data show some promise, with these subjects exhibiting larger improvements in AI scores (22%) compared to previous groups.

Other questions remain concerning the effects of BGAT. Compared to control subjects, treatment subjects do not show a reduction in anxiety or depression or an increase in diabetes knowledge, indicating that BGAT has highly specific effects. Following a self-regulatory model, we assume that improvements in glucose control are due to more timely and appropriate self-treatment, made possible by improved detection of extreme BG fluctuations. This model is supported by patient surveys, but it is difficult to measure self-treatment behaviors objectively. However, we have measured pre- and post-BGAT SMBG use by having patients record self-test results with reflectance meters containing memory chips (Gonder-Frederick, Julian, Cox, Clarke, & Carter, 1988). There was no change in the frequency of SMBG after BGAT, indicating that patients do not become overconfident after treatment and rely even more on subjective estimation. On the less positive side, we might hope that patients would use SMBG more frequently as they become more aware of errors in BG estimation.

Conclusion

We have reviewed findings from an in-depth investigation of symptom representations and BG inferences in IDDM patients. These results can be summarized as follows:

1. IDDM BG fluctuations are associated with physical symptoms. In contrast to expectations, however, subjective BG symptoms are highly idiosyncratic.
2. This idiosyncrasy is a result of individual differences in both physiological (e.g., hormonal) and psychological (e.g., attribution) processes.
3. Symptom representations play a central role in self-treatment. Patients trust their ability to recognize symptoms and base self-treatment decisions on perceived BG levels.
4. IDDM patients make errors in their beliefs, attributions, and judgments about BG symptoms. Errors in symptom beliefs and BG estimation are related to diabetes control.

5. Ability to detect symptoms and estimate BG can be improved with systematic training. Improvements in BG estimation have positive effects on clinical outcome.

Throughout this chapter, we have emphasized the clinical implications of symptom representations and BG inferences. However, these studies also provide interesting insight into how IDDM patients process subjective symptom and BG information. A closer look at the types of errors IDDM patients make in BG symptom beliefs and estimation is particularly revealing. The two most common errors are (1) failure to detect low and high BG levels and (2) false alarm symptom beliefs. From an information-processing perspective, both are errors in judgment of covariation (Fiske & Taylor, 1984). As such, they illustrate some of the perceptual and cognitive biases that can distort BG information processing and inference-making in IDDM patients.

Failure to detect BG extremes, for example, is often a failure to make an accurate judgment of covariation between a symptom and glucose levels. This occurs when BG-related symptoms are either not perceived or, if noticed, not attributed to glucose levels. Selective attention can contribute to failures to perceive very mild or subtle symptoms, such as a slight shakiness indicating mild hypoglycemia. In addition, symptoms experienced frequently and in many different contexts (e.g., nervousness or hunger) may not be perceived as related to BG levels. Failure to detect symptoms may also occur because of cognitive expectations. Symptomatic information that does not match expectations and beliefs is more likely to be ignored, rejected, or attributed to other causes.

The frequency of failure to detect BG extremes also highlights the importance of perceived absence of symptoms. Much previous work on symptom representations has focused on the pervasive tendency to seek out, identify, and utilize physical symptoms, even when actual covariations are dubious. We suggest that in some patients there is an equally pervasive bias toward assuming that symptoms are not occurring, indicating physical well-being. Certainly, absence of unusual or aversive symptoms is often a reliable indicator of physical health. However, in patients with chronic illnesses, these assumptions can result in failure to attend to or recognize symptom–BG covariations. The tendency to infer diabetes control is also seen in the frequent "normalization" of subjective BG estimations.

These findings point out that emotional as well as cognitive and perceptual processes influence symptom representations. Inferences that symptoms are absent and BG is regulated have obvious positive implications for feelings of self-esteem and self-efficacy. Health care practitioners and scientists tend to dismiss such perceptual biases and erroneous conclusions as signs of psychological denial. From a self-regulatory perspective, however, such tendencies demonstrate that symptom representations are also important factors in the regulation of emotional distress (Nerenz & Leventhal, 1983).

Human information processors are often willing to sacrifice accurate data in order to reduce anxiety and improve affective well-being.

IDDM patients also tend to have false alarm symptom beliefs. This means that patients are monitoring symptoms for BG information even though those symptoms are, in fact, unrelated to glucose fluctuations. This type of error is analogous to what Fiske and Taylor (1984) term the illusory correlation phenomenon—judgments of covariation when there is no actual relationship. Like failure to recognize covariations, false alarm symptom beliefs illustrate some of the perceptual and cognitive biases that distort BG information processing and inference-making.

Biased beliefs and expectations about BG symptoms arise from a variety of sources, including diabetes education ("Watch for these low blood sugar symptoms."), clinical folklore ("My diabetes makes me crave sweets."), and past experiences with BG extremes ("Just before passing out, I had a horrible headache.") Pennebaker (1982) points out that a single highly salient instance in which a symptom covaries with an illness experience can result in a long-lasting belief in that symptom's informative value. Once beliefs are formed, they result in selective attention to symptom and BG information. Thus patients attend to, process, and remember those instances that confirm expectations and ignore or reject instances that do not.

Our research and clinical observations support the previous conclusion that errors in symptom covariation judgment are resistant to change. The positive effects of BGAT, however, provide encouraging evidence that symptom beliefs and inferences can be altered, resulting in more accurate BG estimation. From an information-processing perspective, BGAT can be viewed as systematic training in making covariation judgments about symptoms and BG. According to Fiske and Taylor (1984), one effective method for improving judgments of covariation is to increase awareness of noncontingencies through repeated exposure to summarized data. In BGAT, the BG Diary provides this learning experience.

By requiring patients to record and evaluate all information relevant to BG inferences at every self-measurement, the BG Diary reduces selective attention to instances that confirm expectations, beliefs, and wishes. The patient must consider instances in which symptoms (and other cues) do not confirm expectations as well as instances which do. This identification of misleading symptoms and cues that contribute to erroneous inferences leads to elimination of false alarm beliefs. The BG Diary is equally effective in reducing failure to recognize symptom and BG covariations. When patients fail to detect extreme BG (make D zone errors), they repeat the procedure of "scanning" their bodies and environment for cues they tend to miss. Tendencies to normalize BG fluctuations also become obvious through plotting estimated and actual glucose levels on the EGA.

We are currently entering a five-year project to investigate BGAT further. Some of the questions to be addressed include whether improvements in BG estimates and diabetes control after BGAT are maintained over time; what aspects of BGAT contribute to improvements; and if BGAT will also be effective of IDDM populations who are not well educated and relatively healthy. In addition, hospital studies using the Biostator will continue investigating patient awareness of BG extremes and the physiological and psychological processes mediating that awareness. The basic goals of these future studies—understanding how IDDM patients process subjective BG information, how these processes affect self-treatment, and how to reduce errors in BG detection—are parallel to the goals of our past studies.

In closing, the question of generalizability of these findings should be addressed. Knowledge about symptom and BG representations in IDDM treatment may not be applicable to other diseases, although evidence suggests that hypertensive patients make similar errors in symptom detection and beliefs, and that patients may reduce these errors with systematic training (Pennebaker & Watson, 1988). In a broader sense, however, the most important conclusion from our research is that these abstract constructs called mental representations have concrete effects on health care behavior and clinical outcome. Therefore, it is not enough to demonstrate that self-treatment is guided by subjective representations or that patients often make errors in these representations. In our opinion, the perceptual and cognitive biases that distort illness information processing should be viewed as potential targets for psychological and behavioral intervention. This conclusion reflects our belief that psychologists can make a unique and viable contribution in the task of providing patients with the tools they need to achieve optimal self-regulation. It may be that this conclusion has relevance for other illnesses and patient populations.

References

Baumann, L. J., & Leventhal, H. (1985). "I can tell when my blood pressure is up, can't I?" *Health Psychology*, *4*, 203–218.

Bradley, C. (1982) Psychophysiological aspects of the management of diabetes mellitus. *International Journal of Mental Health*, *11*, 117–132.

Carney, R. M., Schechter, K., & Davis, T. (1983). Improving adherence to blood glucose testing in insulin-dependent diabetic children. *Behavior Therapy*, *14*, 247–254.

Clarke, W. L., Carter, W. R., Moll, M., Cox, D. J., Gonder-Frederick, L. A., & Cryer, P. E. (1988). Metabolic and cutaneous events associated with hypoglycemia detected by Sleep Sentry. *Diabetes CARE*, *11*, 630–635.

Clarke, W. L., Cox, D. J., Gonder-Frederick, L. A., & Carter, W., & Pohl, S. L. (1987). Evaluating the clinical accuracy of self-blood glucose monitoring systems. *Diabetes CARE*, *10*, 622–628.

Cox, D., Antoun, B., Gonder-Frederick, L. A., Schroeder, D., Cryer, P., & Clarke, W. (1991). A descriptive study of perceived hypoglycemic symptoms. Submitted for publication.

Cox, D. J., Carter, W. R., Gonder-Frederick, L. A., Clarke, W., & Pohl, S. (1988). Blood glucose awareness training in IDDM patients. *Biofeedback and Self-Regulation*, *13*., 201–217.

Cox, D. J., Clarke, W. L., Gonder-Frederick, L. A., Pohl, S., Hoover, C., Snyder, A., Zimbelman, L., Carter, W. R., Bobbitt, S., & Pennebaker, J. W. (1985). Accuracy of perceiving blood glucose in IDDM. *Diabetes CARE, 8,* 529–536.

Cox, D. J., Gonder-Frederick, L. A., Conway, B., Bolton, K., Julian, D., Cryer, P., Lee, J., & Clarke, W. (1991.) Training insulin-dependent diabetic patients to estimate their blood glucose levels. Submitted for publication.

Cox, D. J., Gonder-Frederick, L. A., Lee, J. H., Julian, D. M., Carter, W. R., & Clarke, W. L. (1989). Blood glucose awareness training among patients with IDDM: Effects and correlates. *Diabetes CARE, 12,* 313–318.

Cox, D. J., Gonder-Frederick, L. A., Pohl, S., & Pennebaker, J. W. (1983). Reliability of symptom–blood glucose relationships among insulin-dependent adult diabetics. *Psychosomatic Medicine, 45,* 357–360.

Cox, D. J., Gonder-Frederick, L., Pohl, S., & Pennebaker, J. W. (1986). Diabetes. In K. Holroyd and T. Creer (Eds.), *Self-management of chronic disease: Handbook of clinical intervention and research* (pp. 305–346). Orlando, FL: Academic Press.

Cox, D. J., Gonder-Frederick, L. A., & Saunders, J. T. (in press). Diabetes and its management. In J. J. Sweet, R. H. Rozensky, & S. M. Tovian (Eds.), *Handbook of clinical psychology in medical settings.* New York: Plenum Press.

Cox, D. J., Irvine, A., Gonder-Frederick, L. A., & Nowacek, G. (1987). Fear of hypoglycemia: Quantification, validation, and utilization. *Diabetes Care, 10,* 617–621.

Cryer, P. E., & Gerich, J. E. (1985). Glucose counterregulation, hypoglycemia, and intensive insulin therapy in diabetes mellitus. *New England Journal of Medicine, 313,* 232–241.

Dunn, S. M., & Turtle, J. R. (1981). The myth of the diabetic personality. *Diabetes CARE, 4,* 640–646.

Epstein, L. H., Beck, S., Figueroa, J., Farkas, G., Kazdin, A. E., Daneman, D., & Becker, D. (1981). The effects of targeting improvements in urine glucose on metabolic control. *Journal of Applied Behavior Analysis, 14,* 365–375.

Epstein, L. H., & Cluss, P. A. (1982). A behavioral medicine perspective on adherence to long-term medical regimens. *Journal of Consulting and Clinical Psychology, 50,* 950–971.

Fiske, S. T., & Taylor, S. E. (1984). *Social cognition.* Reading, MA: Addison-Wesley.

Freund, A., Bennett-Johnson, S., Rosenbloom, A., Alexander, B., & Hansen, C. (1986). Subjective symptoms, blood glucose estimation, and blood glucose concentrations in adolescents with diabetes. *Diabetes CARE, 9,* 236–243.

Gerich, J. E. (1988). Glucose counterregulation and its impact on diabetes mellitus. *Diabetes, 37,* 1608–1617.

Gjedde, A., & Crone, C. (1981). Blood-brain glucose transfer: Repression in chronic hyperglycemia. *Science, 214,* 456–457.

Glasgow, R. E., McCaul, K. D., & Schafer, L. C. (1986). Barriers to regimen adherence among persons with insulin-dependent diabetes. *Journal of Behavioral Medicine, 9,* 65–77.

Gonder-Frederick, L. A., & Cox, D. J. (1986). Behavioral responses to perceived hypoglycemic symptoms: A report and some suggestions. *Diabetes Educator, 12,* 105–109.

Gonder-Frederick, L. A., & Cox, D. J. (1990). Symptom perception and blood glucose feedback in the self-treatment of IDDM. In C. Holmes (Ed.), *Neuropsychological and behavioral aspects of insulin- and non-insulin-dependent diabetes* (pp. 155–173). New York: Springer-Verlag.

Gonder-Frederick, L. A., Cox, D. J., Bobbitt, S. A., & Pennebaker, J. W. (1989). Changes in mood state associated with blood glucose fluctuations in insulin-dependent diabetes mellitus. *Health Psychology, 8*, 45–59.

Gonder-Frederick, L. A., Cox, D. J., Pennebaker, J. W., & Bobbitt, S. A. (1986). Blood glucose symptom beliefs in Type I diabetic adults: Accuracy and implications. *Health Psychology, 3*, 327–341.

Gonder-Frederick, L. A., Cox, D. J., Pohl, S. L., & Carter, W. (1984). Patient blood glucose monitoring: Use, accuracy, adherence, and impact. *Behavioral Medicine Update, 6*, 12–16.

Gonder-Frederick, L. A., Julian, D. M., Cox, D. J., Clarke, W. L., & Carter, W. R. (1988). Self-measurement of blood glucose: Accuracy of self-reported data and adherence to recommended regimen. *Diabetes CARE, 11*, 579–585.

Gonder-Frederick, L. A., Snyder, A. L., & Clarke, W. L. (in press). Accuracy of detection of hypo- and hyperglycemia by children with Type I diabetes and their parents. Diabetes *CARE*.

Hamera, E., Cassmeyer, V., O'Connell, K. A., Weldon, G., Knapp, T. M., & Kyner, J. L. (1988). Self-regulation in individuals with Type II diabetes. *Nursing Research, 37*, 363–367.

Hayford, J. T., Weydert, F. A., & Thompson, R. G. (1983). Validity of urine glucose measurements for estimating plasma glucose concentration. *Diabetes CARE, 6*, 40–44.

Haynes, R. B., Taylor, D. W., & Sackett, D. L. (1979). *Compliance in Health Care*. Baltimore: Johns Hopkins University Press.

Koch, M. F., & Molnar, G. P. (1979). Psychiatric aspects of patients with unstable diabetes mellitus. *Psychosomatic Medicine, 36*, 57–117.

Koschinsky, T., Dannehl, K., & Gries, F. A. (1988). New approach to technical and clinical evaluation of devices for self-monitoring of blood glucose. *Diabetes CARE, 11*, 619–629.

Leventhal, H., Meyer, D., & Nerenz, D. (1980). The common sense representation of illness danger. In S. Rachman (Ed.), *Medical psychology* (Vol. 2, pp. 7–30). New York: Pergamon Press.

Manstead, A. S. R., & Wagner, H. L. (1981). Arousal, cognition and emotion: An appraisal of two factor theory. *Current Psychological Reviews, 1*, 35–54.

Mazzuca, S. A., Moorman, N. H., Wheeler, M. L., Norton, J. A., Fineberg, N. S., Vinicor, F., Cohen, S. J., & Clark, C. M. (1986). The diabetes education study: A controlled trial of the effects of diabetic patient education. *Diabetes Care, 9*, 1–10.

Miller, L. V., Goldstein, J., & Nicholaison, G. (1978) Evaluation of patient's knowledge of diabetes self-care. *Diabetes CARE, 1*, 275–280.

Moses, J. L., & Bradley, C. (1985). Accuracy of subjective blood glucose estimation by patients with insulin-dependent diabetes. *Biofeedback and Self-Regulation, 10*, 301–314.

Murawski, B. J., Chazan, M. B., Balodimos, M. C., & Ryan, J. R. (1979). Personality patterns in patients with diabetes mellitus of long duration. *Diabetes, 19*, 259–263.

Nerenz, D. R., & Leventhal, H. (1983). Self-regulation theory in chronic illness. In T. G. Burish & L. A. Bradley (Eds.), *Coping with chronic disease: Research and applications* (pp. 13–37). New York: Academic Press.

Newbrough, J. R., Simpkins, C. G., & Maurer, H. (1985). A family development approach to studying factors in the management and control of childhood diabetes. *Diabetes CARE, 8*, 83–92.

O'Connell, K. A., Hamera, E. K., Knapp, T. M., Cassmeyer, V. L., Eaks, G. A., &

Fox, M. A. (1984). Symptom use and self-regulation in Type II diabetes. *Advances in Nursing Science*, 6, 19–28.

O'Connell, K. A., Hamera, E. K., Schorfheide, A., & Guthrie, D. (1990). Symptom beliefs and actual blood glucose in Type II diabetes. *Research in Nursing and Health*, 13, 145–151.

Pennebaker, J. W. (1982). *The psychology of physical symptoms*. New York: Springer-Verlag.

Pennebaker, J. W., Cox, D. J., Gonder-Frederick, L. A., Wunsch, M. G., Evans, W. S., & Pohl, S. (1981). Physical symptoms related to blood glucose in insulin-dependent diabetics. *Psychosomatic Medicine*, 43, 489–500.

Pennebaker, J. W., & Watson, D. (1988). Blood pressure estimation and beliefs among normotensives and hypertensives. *Health Psychology*, 7, 309–328.

Roales-Nieto, J. G. (1988). Blood glucose discrimination in IDDP: Training in external cues. *Behavior Modification*, 12, 116–132.

Rosenstock, I. M. (1985). Understanding and enhancing patient compliance with diabetic regimens. *Diabetes CARE*, 8, 610–616.

Sanazaro, P. J. (1985). A survey of patient satisfaction, knowledge, and compliance. *Western Journal of Medicine*, 142, 703–705.

Schafer, L. C., Glasgow, R. E., & McCaul, K. D. (1982). Increasing the adherence of diabetic adolescents. *Journal of Behavioral Medicine*, 5, 353–362.

Schafer, L. C., Glasgow, R. E., & McCaul, K. D. (1983). Adherence to IDDM regimens: Relationship to psychosocial variables and metabolic control. *Diabetes CARE*, 6, 493–498.

Schiffrin, A., & Belmonte, M. (1982). Multiple daily self-glucose monitoring: Its essential role in longterm glucose control in insulin-dependent diabetic patients treated with pumps and multiple subcutaneous injections. *Diabetes CARE*, 5, 479–484.

Simonds, J. (1976–1977). Psychiatric status of diabetic youth in good and poor control. *International Journal of Psychiatry in Medicine*, 7, 133–151.

Stone, D. B. (1964). A study of the incidence and causes of poor control in patients with diabetes mellitus. *American Journal of the Medical Sciences*, 241, 436–469.

Surwit, R. S., Feinglos, M. N., & Scovern, A. W. (1983). Diabetes and behavior: A paradigm for health psychology. *American Psychologist*, 83, 255–262.

Surwit, R. S., Scovern, A. W., & Feinglos, M. N. (1982). The role of behavior in diabetes care. *Diabetes CARE*, 5, 337–342.

Swets, J. A. (1973). The relative operating characteristic in psychology. *Science*, 82, 990–1000.

Weiner, M. F., & Skipper, F. P. (1979). Euglycemia: A psychological study. *International Journal of Psychiatry in Medicine*, 9, 281–287.

Williams, T. F., Martin, D. A., Hogan, M. D., Watkins, J. D., & Ellis, E. V. (1967). The clinical picture of diabetic control, studied in four settings. *American Journal of Public Health*, 57, 441–451.

Wing, R. R., Epstein, L. H., Lamparski, D. M., Hagg, S. A., Nowalk, M. P., & Scott, N. (1984). Accuracy in estimating fasting blood glucose levels by patients with diabetes. *Diabetes CARE*, 7, 474–478.

Wing, R. R., Epstein, L. H., Nowalk, M. P., & Lamparski, D. M. (1986). Behavioral self-regulation in the treatment of patients with diabetes mellitus. *Psychological Bulletin*, 99, 78–89.

11
The Active Side of Illness Cognition

Howard Leventhal and Michael Diefenbach

This chapter has three objectives. The first is to provide a few historical details respecting the development of illness cognition research in our laboratory. As these activities extended over three decades, our brief comments may help the interested reader to integrate several lines of research that are frequently viewed as separate. The second, primary objective is to advance a constructivist view of behavioral processes. We believe people are active problem solvers and work in illness cognition must identify the procedures that people use to elaborate and test their illness models. If taken seriously, this theme can generate new directions for conceptual and empirical development. Our third, final objective is to highlight a few of the points made in prior chapters suggesting how they relate to the directions we now envision.

Why Study Illness Cognition?

There are both practical and conceptual reasons for studying illness cognition, many of which are illustrated in the contributions to this volume. Among the practical reasons, one stands in sharp relief: Illness is intrinsic to the life cycle. Every culture, contemporary and remote, has had its institutions, its expert and lay roles, and its rituals for the entry to and exit from life and for the management of illness episodes. Schober and Lacroix's fascinating tour of Western history (this volume) provides evidence of the continuity of everyday, common sense illness thinking dating from Hippocrates through the Enlightenment to the present. Indeed, the continuity in

Research was supported by grant AG 03501 from the National Institute On Aging.

writings from each of these three widely separated epochs is sufficient to allow them to identify each of the six basic attributes of illness representations: symptoms, labels, causes, timelines, consequences, and controllability or cure. We believe this continuity reflects both biological and cultural constraints on the way we construe our bodies and our world. Indeed, there should be no surprise that symptoms and signs were the focus of early medicine and remain the cornerstones of lay illness cognition, as many theories of behavior, even models of perception, were grounded in observation of everyday activity. For example, Helmholtz assigned concrete, somesthetic experience a central role in his theory of visual depth perception, and many psychologists believed thought equivalent to concrete, subvocal speech.

The Universality of Health Beliefs

Two specific experiences persuaded the senior author of the merit of studying beliefs, attitudes, and behavior in the health–illness domain rather than in some other area of social behavior. During the early 1960s while conducting studies on attitude change, it soon became clear to me that the participating subjects often had little interest and even less knowledge of the political and social topics that were the focus of the persuasion process. Indeed, the use of such material seemed reminiscent of Ebinghaus's retreat to the nonsense syllable for the study of memory, and the results may have been equally rewarding. Even when there was some interest in the topics, it was clear that the issues of the day became the forgotten issues of tomorrow, and one could not help but wonder whether a science could develop from data based on ephemeral events.

The second occurred while skimming through Whiting and Child's (1953) examination of the effects of child-rearing practices on personality development. Their analysis of the data from the cross-cultural area files yielded chapter after chapter of negative results until they examined the relationship between child-rearing practices and health attitudes. This finding of the universal importance of health beliefs and practice reinforced my nascent belief that these attitudes merited careful study.

The Need to Account for the Impact of Fear Communications

The factor that finally triggered our study of illness cognition was the data we obtained when examining the impact of fear communications on beliefs and behavior. The results of these studies contradicted the widely held hypothesis that attitudes and behavior could be changed by communications that first aroused fear and then presented a specific strategy or recommendation for coping with the threat agent. The idea was that reducing fear would generate persuasion (Leventhal, 1970; Leventhal & Singer, 1966). The data showed, however, that while high fear messages were more effective than low fear messages in changing attitudes in the direction advocated by the communicator (to quit smoking, use seat belts, etc.), these effects endured only for short periods of time, say, 24 to 48 hours (Leventhal & Niles, 1965). Moreover, high fear messages were no more effective than low fear messages in effecting changes in behavior (e.g., taking tetanus shots or quitting smoking). The messages that were effective in changing behavior, and doing so over relatively long periods of time (e.g., 3 months), used either a high or a low fear message in combination with an action plan, that is, a message that specified how, when, and where to fit action into the context of the individual's daily life pattern. These effects were found for actions such as taking tetanus shots (Leventhal, Jones, & Trembly, 1966; Leventhal, Singer, & Jones, 1965) and quitting smoking (Leventhal, Watts, & Pagano, 1967). We concluded that the combination of a threat message, regardless of its level of fear, and an action plan message was necessary for behavioral change and that neither alone was sufficient.

Two specific findings made clear that it was not fear per se that was the essential ingredient which combined with the planning message to effect behavioral change. First, as mentioned, the combination of the low fear message and the action plan aroused less fear than the combination of the high fear message and the action plan, but each combination was equally effective in producing behavioral change. Second, the favorable effect of the combination was often visible a day or more after exposure to the message (Kornzweig, 1967; Leventhal et al., 1967), sufficient time for decay of the fear state (Leventhal & Niles, 1965). Once we recognized that fear was not responsible for the behavioral effect, we inferred that a change must have occurred in the way the threat was represented or understood (Leventhal, 1970, 1975), and that this new representation was the motivating factor that led to overt action when combined with the plan. The research question which emerged, therefore, was to identify the ingredients of the representation of threat that stimulated action, and then to isolate the message components that could affect the representation.

The implications of these questions for research were clear. First, they suggested that it would be necessary to understand how people process information in response to warnings. This meant we had to examine their everyday or common sense beliefs about specific threats, their procedures for coping with objective threats, their emotional reactions to the threat, and we had to look at how people appraised or evaluated the outcomes of these two parallel coping processes (Leventhal, 1970). Second, it was clear that personality factors, which were the focus of much attention at that time, were likely to be of minor importance in pursuing these questions (Janis & Leventhal, 1967). As Janis (1958) had cogently argued, the focus would be on the individual's perception and interpretation of situational factors. Thus to address our question we looked at people's everyday beliefs and procedures for coping with health threats rather than their personalities.

The Construction of Common Sense Models

Our investigative work is now centered on the procedures used to construct common sense models of illness. Procedures vary in complexity from micro events to macro and meta procedures; micro procedures refer to the automatic and nonconscious interaction of somatic sensations with memory schemata to construct perceptual feelings of sickness. Macro procedures are more or less automatic, schema-driven behaviors (thoughts and overt actions) designed to test hypotheses about the meaning of somatic sensations; they are extended in time, over seconds, and may be performed with relatively low levels of awareness. Meta procedures are generic test procedures that are conscious and answer broad questions about somatic sensations, such as taking aspirins and visiting the doctor. But before discussing our most recent findings on the procedures we have identified and those we expect to identify, we will backtrack and describe the earlier, substantive focus of the research, which brought us to the investigation of this constructivist theme.

The Structure/Organization of Illness Cognition

The Focus on Somatic Sensations: Symptoms

In the late 1960s we began to explore the interpretation of somatic sensations, as we suspected this would be central to understanding illness threats. With the able collaboration of Jean Johnson we generated data which showed that providing information about anticipated somatic sensations, and/or focusing attention on these sensations, led to sharp reductions in emotional distress unless these sensations were given threatening interpretations (Johnson, 1973, 1975; Johnson & Leventhal, 1974; Leventhal, Brown, Shacham, & Engquist, 1979). At least three mechanisms appeared to be involved in the reduction of distress by this type of preparatory information: (1) removal of surprise, which reduces activation due to novelty; (2) habituation, which is facilitated by attending to and processing stimuli as they gradually increase in intensity, a critical factor in passive situations (Ahles, Blanchard, & Leventhal, 1983; Foa & Kozak, 1986; Parrott & Sabini, 1989); and (3) the development of an accurate representation of the environmental stressor, which facilitates instrumental coping reactions (Johnson, Lauvier, & Nail, 1989; Johnson & Leventhal, 1974; E.A. Leventhal, Shacham, & Easterling, 1989). Two critical points emerged from the foregoing data:

1. Somatic sensations and their interpretation play a key role in the arousal and the minimization of intense emotional distress.
2. Somatic sensations play a critical role in guiding coping reactions.

The Hierarchical Organization of Illness Cognition

Having clarified the importance of somatic sensations for the evocation of emotional reactions, we proceeded to examine the role of somatic sensations in the representation of physical illness in sick persons (Leventhal, 1976; Leventhal, Meyer, & Nerenz, 1980; Safer, Tharps, Jackson, & Leventhal, 1979). Unknown to us, Jamie Pennebaker and his students were undertaking their imaginative work on symptom interpretation at the same time (Pennebaker, 1982; Pennebaker & Skelton, 1978, 1981).

As the current status of this activity is so exceptionally well summarized by Bishop (this volume), we will simply highlight three key points. First, experience with illness in oneself and others appears to generate a complex hierarchical residue, or memory structure (Bishop, 1987). Representations of specific illness events—for example, symptom clusters and their labels with their associated expectations respecting timelines, causes, consequences, and beliefs about control (Lau & Hartmann, 1983)—define a relatively "low"-level information structure. These representations are both concrete and abstract: An illness episode can be identified by its somatic sensations (running nose, headache, fatigue) and by its label (flu). And as Lau, Bernard, and Hartman (1988) indicate, comparisons between specific illness schemata can generate yet more abstract dimensions (or propositional statements) for scaling illnesses and specific illness experiences. Examples include the acute–chronic dimension (Keller, Leventhal, Prohaska, & Leventhal, 1989; Leventhal, Nerenz, & Steele, 1984), the fatal–nonfatal dimension (Bishop, this volume), and the dimension of diseases caused by one's own actions versus diseases caused by chance (Lau, Bernard, & Hartmann, 1988).

Second, it is clear that the representation of the physical self, that is, the body schema, affects every level of the illness domain. The representation of the body provides a basic pattern against which deviations are measured and somatic sensations and features are defined as "normal" or potential signs of disease (Shontz, 1975; Suls, Maco & Tobin, in press). In addition to defining the illness-relatedness of specific somatic experiences, the self schema may lead the individual to discriminate signs along abstract dimensions such as whether an illness is related to and/or caused by aging (Keller et al., 1989) and whether a somatic sign is due to illness or a normal change in sexual function (E. Leventhal, in press). Other idiosyncratic dimensions may guide individuals to cluster and organize illness knowledge in unique ways.

Third, social and cultural institutions may also organize illness representations. For example, most health-care institutions are structured to treat acute illness: The patient reports symptoms, which are diagnosed, treated with medication, and cured. These socially defined procedures draw attention to a contrast between illnesses that are acute, readily treated, and self-limited and illness that is chronic and never cured. Moreover, doctors and nurses can reinforce acute models of illness when they ask patients about symptoms, suggest diagnoses, and dismiss the patient with a protocol for cure and an occasional gesture to lifestyle modification to avoid more serious, chronic complications.

The basic outlines of an illness taxonomy are emerging from the foregoing data along with (as yet minimal) evidence regarding the multiple sources that contribute to the development of this knowledge structure. Although efforts to develop a conceptually sound illness taxonomy may not seem an exciting task, it is a critical step for the further development of the area. If we expect to deepen our understanding of the processes underlying the construction and updating of representations and the way representations guide behavior, it is essential that we have a taxonomy that adequately defines our domain. To be optimally useful, we will also have to consider ways of describing the various properties of the categories comprising the taxonomy: their abstract versus their concrete properties, whether they are defined by prototypes or specific instances, and if defined by instances, the variance among these instances. The problem is likely to be complicated, however, by the incompleteness and inconsistencies that appear in common-sense constructions.

The Construction Process

Schober and Lacroix (this volume) open their chapter with a brief citation in which Oliver Sacks (1984, p. 56) describes his euphoria upon discovering that his toes were "twiddling . . . pink and lively" in clear disconfirmation of his hypothesis that his inability to move his leg was due to a cerebral stroke. Sacks's story holds several lessons. First, as we emphasized earlier, people are active problem solvers; they enact procedures that construct and define their illness representations. Thus the repetitive wiggling and cycling of Sacks's toes provided critical information that updated the way he represented his condition. Second, Sacks's representation reflected his common sense views both of his body and of physical illness; he believed, inaccurately, that a stroke that would cripple his leg would necessarily leave him unable to move his toes. Third, his procedures or coping behaviors and his interpretation of these behaviors were guided by his common sense representations of his body and of strokes. Thus Sacks's view of anatomy defined a response, "try to move your leg," and an outcome, your leg/toes either move, which is inconsistent with the stroke hypothesis, or they do not move, which is consistent with the stroke hypothesis. Fourth, the procedures involved in updating and changing the representation have a somewhat accidental or random flavor. It seems unlikely that Sacks made a specific and conscious decision to wiggle his toes to test the stroke hypothesis: The wiggling was likely a by-product of efforts to move his foot and the unexpected feedback from the activity produced the information critical for rejecting the stroke hypothesis. The lesson is that common sense representations of illness and the procedures used to construct them are typically less well organized and efficiently performed than the representations and procedures used in domains in which the individual has a history of study and/or practice.

Our very first study on procedures for appraising representations was conducted in 1965 by Donald Quinlan and the first author (unfortunately, a change in university affiliation disrupted an analysis and write-up). We developed a "Symptom TAT," a set of brief scenarios, each of which asked the respondent what he would think, feel, and do if, for example, he "woke one morning and noticed a lump on his neck while shaving." The array of active procedures that our male undergraduate subjects reported to these scenarios was somewhat astonishing. They suggested ways in which they would explore the stability of the event by means of observational or information-collecting procedures such as searching for correlated symptoms (check to see if I had a sore throat) and searching for information to confirm whether the somatic change was simply a part of normal body structure (e.g., see if I had something like it on the other side). They also reported many active, treatment-oriented procedures, such as applying salves and taking pills, to determine if the symptom was controllable. Both Sacks and our respondents were actively engaged in constructing or defining a symptom/illness representation.

Constructions and Meaning

An important point emerges from our discussion of the passive and active procedures used to construct illness representations: Procedures are clearly related to and/or informed by the individual's illness representations. Thus the somatic sensations and the individual's knowledge about disease generate a representation of the illness problem and that in turn stimulates hypothesis-consistent actions. The initial representation of the problem may be little more than a vague hunch or suspicion about what is wrong, the hunch becoming increasingly specific and clear as the individual evaluates the feedback from a series of procedures. It is fair to say that procedures are expressions of the knowledge structure and as such they both define the structure and are defined by it (Andersen, 1983). As procedures generate meaning and are guided by meaning we can rest assured that the investigation of procedures will provide insight into the cognitive content of illness, the cognitive content of the self system, and their interaction.

The Organization of Coping Procedures

As is true for medical tests such as x-rays and hematological analyses, the very same observational or active coping procedure can be used to make a variety of discriminations between various attributes of an illness representation. Moreover, any single procedure that adds to the definition of a health threat is likely to have multiple implications as clarification of the identity of a problem has vast implications regarding its consequences, timeline (chronic rather than acute), cause, and potential for cure. For example, the easing of a severe headache after taking two aspirins is likely to convince one that he or she was suffering from tension and/or fatigue, and little else. On the other hand, if the headache does not prove treatable and no other physical symptoms or signs are present, one may entertain the hypothesis of a cerebral stoke. The multiple functions of procedures suggest that it may prove impossible to represent them as an organized structure. On the other hand, the intimate connection between procedures and illness representations suggests that a taxonomy of procedures may emerge along with a taxonomy of illness representation.

Hierarchy of Illness Knowledge and Procedures

Although several investigators have generated taxonomic views of the illness domain (Linz, Penrod, Siverhaus, & Leventhal, 1982), Bishop (1987) seems to have made the first clear step toward linking a few specific procedures to an illness taxonomy. After his subjects completed the judgments needed to generate a hierarchical representation of symptom–disease clusters, he asked them to indicate the likelihood of engaging in each of eight specific health-maintaining behaviors given the presence of 30 of the 60 symptoms. The behaviors included procedures such as "reduce daily activities," "take prescription/nonprescription medicine," "go to a doctor," and/or "ignore the symptoms altogether." The data, analyzed separately for male and female respondents, showed that some procedures, such as reduce daily activities, fell rather high in the tree structure, whereas others, such as visit a doctor, fell toward the bottom. Thus reduction in daily activities was involved in discriminations among very broad or inclusive sets of symptoms rather than discriminations among specific illness conditions. Seeking expert medical advice, on the other hand, came into play at a lower level—at the point where discriminations would be made about the diagnostic implications of specific symptom subsets.

Relative to male respondents, the females respondents also made differential use of the repertoire of coping behaviors Bishop provided. Females selected different actions at different levels of the tree structure; they reported they would discuss the symptom with friends, see somebody who was not a doctor (e.g., a nurse), take nonprescription medicine, and/or ignore the symptom at different points in the hierarchy of symptoms clusters. Males, on the other hand, reported doing all of these things at a common point in time—namely, when they were faced with making specific diagnoses among the entire set of the smallest symptom clusters. Thus male respondents used all of the behaviors for the same purpose: to pinpoint which problem was at issue. This use of procedures may reflect that males are less threatened by health issues and ignore them until the very last minute or that males fail to perform distinct procedures at different levels of the knowledge structure because they lack the knowledge and coping skills needed for informed responding and problem-based coping. Our most recent data support the second interpretation of gender differences in health and illness behavior.

Important as they are, Bishop's findings provide little more than a first glance at the relationship between knowledge systems and procedures as he used a relatively small set of behavioral items in a simulated setting. People may perform a wide range of automatic acts to test suspicion that a symptomatic swelling is an infection rather than a cancer or that a headache is a sign of stress rather than an indicator of hypertension or a brain tumor, and they may be unable to report on them. Moreover, Bishop's list of procedures was quite brief and it is unlikely that his data exhaust all of the procedures that people use to "test" the broad distinctions between trivial, self-limited conditions and truly "serious" chronic illnesses.

The Temporal Unfolding of Illness Episodes

The pattern of disease is important in providing a changing landscape of sensations that are translated as moods and feelings of illness or well-being. As this somatic landscape shifts, so too will the procedures used for coping and appraisal. Although specific diseases such as hypertension, cancer, or the common cold can take idiosyncratic form in a given individual, the temporal unfolding of many diseases is likely to follow a similar pattern allowing us to define common phases across multiple illnesses. For example, colds and other acute illnesses begin with minor symptoms (e.g., slight stuffiness of the nose, barely perceptible soreness of the throat, tightness about the eyes, build to clear, flaring symptoms, and with time (and or treatment) disappear. Chronic illnesses have a different picture: Some provide early warnings, whereas others, such as heart attacks, introduce themselves in cataclysmic fashion (Matthews, Siegel, Kuller, Thompson, & Vanat, 1983).

To explore the procedures used with the unfolding of different phases of illness, Safer, Tharps, Jackson, and Leventhal (1979) used Suchman's (1965) distinctions to define three phases of illness that precede the individual's contact with the medical care system: (1) an *appraisal* phase, initiated by a change in body sensations and ending with the decision that one is ill; (2) an *illness* phase, beginning with the decision that one is ill and ending with the decision to call for professional care; and (3) a *utilization* phase, beginning with the decision to contact a treatment authority and ending by contact with a provider. (See Caccioppo, Andersen, Turnquist, & Petty, 1985, and Green, 1984, for further elaboration of these and later stages.) These phases of illness are important as they are likely to involve different body sensations, different procedures for coping, and different criteria for appraisals over the course of an illness episode. For example, Safer et al.'s (1979) data showed that the early, appraisal phase was dominated by procedures for collecting information including monitoring symptoms for signs of change (a "wait and see" procedure) and reading about symptoms. Respondents who adopted these procedures had relatively long appraisal delays. During the illness phase, that is, after the decision one was ill, procedures for managing the emotional upset of the illness threat proved to be the most salient factor in delay.

The data suggest, therefore, that a variety of procedures are used to track and update the representation of health problems. Some of these procedures may be used throughout the illness history, whereas others are more frequently used at early stages rather than later ones and vice versa. The selection of a hypothesis-testing procedure varies, therefore, as the underlying questions or discriminations at issue change while the illness episode unfolds. These changes are motivated by the changing biological display of the disease process and the changes in the individual's social context; as the episode evolves, the individual moves from talking with friends to talking to professionals. Thus the psychological system involved in constructing the representation is exposed to different somatic and social information over the illness history.

Procedures to Determine the Identity of Somatic Sensations

As we suggested earlier, a fundamental question to be answered about a somatic sensation is whether it represents an illness and if it represents an illness, its identity. Answers to these identity questions—"Is it illness?" and if so, "What illness is it?"—provide the immediate, "causal" explanation for somatic symptoms and signs. These questions and the procedures used to answer them are fundamental as they focus on the meaning of the somatic change and whether it does or does not pose an immediate or long-term threat and how the threat might be managed.

We have treated the question of identity separately from that of cause, the former concerning the labeling of the disease or illness, the latter concerning the conditions that initiated the threat (e.g., having eaten contaminated food or exposing oneself to stress or adverse climatic conditions). The identity of an illness threat can have important implications for all of its attributes. For example, if a large, soft tissue mass in the shoulder is (accurately) labeled a malignant sarcoma rather than a benign lipoma, the implications are vastly different for the individual's experience of consequences, duration, and controllability of the threat. The degree to which knowledge of identity brings these implications to the fore depends on the individual's prior knowledge; knowing a growth is a sarcoma will have limited cognitive and/or emotional impact if the individual does not understand the implications of having a rapidly growing, untreatable, soft tissue malignancy. Because causal information is often helpful (but only sometimes necessary) to establish the identity of a symptom, similar procedures can be used to elaborate both identity and cause. Some of these procedures appear to involve internal or historical comparison processes (Suls & Wan, 1989), comparing current to prior illness experiences and arriving at common labels for similar symptom patterns, whereas many will be identified that draw upon external information, both social and nonsocial (Sanders, 1982).

Decision Rules and Procedures for Discriminating Between Illness and Nonillness States

We have been able to identify a number of decision rules that people appear to use for discriminating between illness and nonillness states. Decision rules involve a hypothesized contrast, for example, "Am I sick or am I under stress?," relevant data, and procedures for acquiring and using these data to make such decisions. Two such rules have been documented in our research: (1) the stress–illness rule and (2) the aging–illness rule.

The Stress–Illness Rule. Practicing physicians often report that a patient will ask whether he or she is ill or emotionally upset. This stress–illness distinction was also suggested by data in our studies of hypertension. In several different samples, patients in treatment for hypertension made clear that they used somatic sensations as indicators of blood pressure elevation. It was also clear that many of these sensations could be signs of emotional distress—symptoms such as headache, face flushing, and nervousness (Meyer, Leventhal, & Gutmann, 1985). As the very same symptoms are reported by patients new to treatment and patients who have been in treatment for several years, we suspected it might even be the case that these symptoms were suggested by the label, hyper-tension (Blumhagen, 1980). Given that these symptoms are very common and that the majority of people do not think they are hypertensive, it seemed plausible to suspect these symptoms are frequently attributed to stress rather than illness.

We conducted a laboratory study to see whether this stress–illness discrimination guided procedures for self-appraisal. The study was quite simple. College undergraduates who volunteered to participate were asked to consider whether they would think they were ill or would think they were under stress (rated on 7-point scales) if they experienced a set of six symptoms on the following day. This simulation was conducted on two different days: Half the subjects were run on a Friday before an open weekend and the other half the day before their psychology midterm examination. The experimenters gave no special notice to the day. Subjects participating the day before their midterm were very much more likely to judge the symptoms as signs of stress rather than signs of illness (Baumann, Cameron, Zimmerman, & Leventhal, 1989), whereas subjects participating on a Friday before an open weekend were more likely to judge the symptoms as signs of illness rather than signs of stress. The data clearly suggest that subjects use external contextual (environmental) information in appraising symptoms. The effect did not hold, however, for all three of the symptom sets used; one was ambiguous, one representative of diabetes, and one representative of mononucleosis. Because undergraduates are familiar with the signs of mononucleosis, appraisals of that set were not influenced by context. Thus the data also show that prior knowledge constrains the effect of external context.

There is a direct parallel between the data reported above and the findings of Skelton and his colleagues: our subjects discounted their (presumably) own symptoms as signs of illness on a stressful (examination) day, and observers also discounted symptoms as signs of illness for individuals reported to have complex life stresses such as examinations and disrupted love relationships (Skelton, this volume). We should be cautious not to assume that these contextual factors lead subjects to totally discount the reality and illness potential of symptoms. The data suggest the illness potential is minimized, but they do not indicate that the symptoms are ascribed a totally symbolic status and regarded as physically unreal.

It should also be possible to identify other active procedures for making stress–illness decisions. For example, people commonly self-medicate with aspirin and other analgesics to treat headaches; the outcome of treatment defines the identity of the disorder, with stress headaches clearing up with treatment but the complete disappearance of illness-induced headache requiring cure of the underlying illness.

The Age–Illness Rule. Distinguishing pathological changes from the normal changes of age—the age–illness distinction—is an increasingly common task as people grow order. For example, reductions in energy and athletic prowess are common as one moves from the third to the fourth decade of life, and the late middle years (50's and 60's) see reductions in both visual and auditory capacities and a variety of orthopedic changes such as bone loss and arthritis; all occur with normal aging.

Data relevant to the age–illness rule were obtained in two separate studies. One was a simulation, in which respondents ranging in age from 20 to 80+ were randomly assigned to evaluate brief symptom scenarios; in another, respondents (age range 40–94) were interviewed at the point of entry to self-initiated visits to the medical care system (Prohaska, Keller, Leventhal, & Leventhal, 1987). The data show that attribution to age rather than to illness to more common for mild symptoms of gradual onset and somewhat more common, though not strikingly so, in older (over 65 years) than younger respondents. Attribution of symptoms to age had two important effects: It reduced reports of emotional distress and enhanced reports of delay in seeking help in the scenario study, and it was associated with considerably longer delays in seeking medical care in the patient study.

The information and procedures involved in age–illness decisions are not completely known, but it is clear that slow rate of symptom onset is important in biasing judgments toward an aging decision. It appears likely that these evaluations require careful appraisal of one's current state against an existent prototype or memory template of the body, and that slow onset makes such evaluations more difficult. It also seems likely that this discrimination would be especially difficult for individuals who pay relatively little attention to their bodies. The decision that one is ill may also be difficult for individuals who are threatened and defend against the recognition that they are ill. On the other hand, the extensive literature on individual differences in illness behavior (Mechanic, 1980, 1986; Pilowsky, 1986) suggests the presence of a subset of individuals predisposed toward monitoring symptoms and accepting illness labeling (see also, Croyle and Jemmott, this volume)

Establishing the Identity of a Disorder

Having decided that one is suffering from an illness, the typical next step is further diagnostic specification or labeling of the disorder. Past experience teaches us that symptoms vary as a function of the underlying disorder, and the individual compares the changing picture to underlying notions relevant to generic (acute versus chronic) and specific disease categories. Some diseases may be assumed to change rapidly (e.g., with injury and food poisoning), others slowly (e.g., with diabetes and cancer), and others in a monotonic manner. Thus an individual suffering from a painful, swollen lymph node that suddenly declines in severity may conclude that the pain does not reflect an underlying disease such as cancer, because he assumes that cancer symptoms increase monotonically, always getting worse over time.

Clustering and Labeling. The pattern, or *clustering*, of symptoms will usually suggest an initial, provisional diagnosis. This was seen in the stress–illness study described previously: The symptom cluster describing mononucleosis was familiar and the subjects recognized the set as an indicator of a specific illness and this recognition clearly played an important role in limiting the impact of context (exam or no exam tomorrow) on judgments. Although there is relatively little research on clustering and labeling, recent data show that people have little difficulty in grouping their symptoms. For example, in a sample of 366 adult respondents 45–90 years of age, the average number of symptoms reported was 7.9 and these symptoms were placed into an average of 5.6 clusters (range 1 to 20), the largest group averaging 3.1 symptoms. When asked which symptom bothered them most, these respondents had no difficulty selecting one from among a set, the typical choice being a rather concrete, physical somatic event.

Additional evidence on clustering appeared in our studies of hypertension. When asked if people "can tell when their blood pressure is up," 80% of a group of patients in treatment believed that "people cannot tell," but in this same group, 88% believed their symptoms reflected changes in their pressure (Meyer et al., 1985). Thus they accepted the medical dogma that hypertension is an asymptomatic illness when it affects *other* people, but not with respect to themselves. While respondents were not asked to cluster symptoms, those who claimed they could use symptoms to monitor changes in blood pressure reported multiple symptoms such as headache, palpitations, face flushing, and nervousness.

The Symmetry Rule. The consistent association of symptom clusters with illness labels (see Lau, Bernard, & Hartman, 1989) was the source of the first rule for self-appraisal that we proposed: the symmetry rule. It states that a person who suffers from a set of symptoms will seek to label the symptoms, and a person who is labeled (i.e., diagnosed) as having an illness will expect to experience specific symptoms. Because the relationship between illness and symptoms is ingrained in people's knowledge structures, the procedures used to establish symmetry and to generate clusters are often automatic micro procedures in which label and symptoms are joined on the basis of existent schemata of illness or of nonconscious, rapidly performed search procedures to form symptom clusters. This interpretation is reinforced by data indicating that clusters from the same set of somatic sensations (e.g., rapid heart beating, headache, tenseness, tiredness, warm face) are used as indicators in widely varied samples of respondents, including adult patients in treatment for hypertension and undergraduates who have been given false feedback that their blood pressure is elevated (Baumann et al., 1989).

Scenarios provided by individuals suggest the linkage between symptoms and labels is not always automatic; elaborate, consciously performed procedures are also involved. For example, on one occasion, a health professional who attended a presentation on illness cognition informed the speaker that she could monitor her blood pressure symptomatically; she took her blood pressure and always observed a high reading whenever she felt tension, headache, and/or face flushing. Unfortunately, her *active testing* was seriously biased as she confirmed the "validity" of her symptoms by taking her blood pressure whenever she had the relevant symptoms, but she did not take it when asymptomatic.

As the symmetry rule suggests, symptoms are virtually synonymous with illness. It is not surprising, therefore, that subjects report having had symptoms relevant to a specific disorder when given false feedback purported to show that their blood pressure is elevated (Baumann et al., 1989) or that they lack a pancreatic enzyme, as shown in the results of an elegant study by Croyle and Sande (1988). But, although symptoms are clearly powerful guides to belief and behavior, subjects even discount diagnostic information when it is inconsistent with their recall of relevant symptoms (Croyle & Sande, 1988); their beliefs about the cause of an illness limit whether they judge themselves to have experienced the symptoms of that illness. For example, when told their blood pressure was elevated, subjects reported symptoms commonly believed to be indicators of that disorder if their belief about the cause of hypertension (stress or genetic) was consistent with information about the level of stress (high or low) in their own lives (Baumann et al., 1989).

Matching Prototypes and Instances

The various rules and procedures discussed in the preceding sections suggest that procedures for assessing whether one is well or ill and for labeling or specifying the nature of the illness vary as a function of the comparison being made. Thus when a new somatic episode comes into experience, different procedures are used to check the features of this episode and to generate new information about it as a function of the individual's existent knowledge base. If there is a prototype or exemplar in the declarative reservoir and the information is sensory in nature, the individual is likely to utilize intrapersonal procedures for testing, to engage in memory searches in which he or she attempts to compare and contrast the current somatic sensations with these prior touchstones (Suls, et al. in press). For example, imagine a person suffering from intense abdominal cramps who has had such pains in the past and attributed them to food poisoning. It is reasonable to expect that the recurrence of the pain will lead to a similar attribution, that is, food poisoning. Such a description ignores, however, the procedures that are likely to be used to make the attribution. The most likely first step will be to recall the prior incident of cramping and to compare the past condition with the present one. If memory is sufficiently clear and the present *feels* the same as the past, the identical self-diagnosis is likely. The notion of a sufficiently "clear" memory may imply recall of a specific member rather than recall of the "prototype." Efforts to match to a prototype—that is, it feels like "food poisoning would feel"—seem inherently more likely to yield uncertain outcomes than would a match to a specific member—"it feels just like it did when I had food poisoning at that other time." The uncertainty associated with the prototypic match, would probably motivate additional and more active search procedures.

More active search procedures might also be elicited by the severity of the symptoms and the concerns and fears they elicit respecting possible consequences. Thus severe gastrointestinal distress might elicit a range of automatic and deliberate coping reactions ranging on the automatic side from writhing, massaging, and probing of the abdomen to more deliberate procedures such as drinking water or taking a household remedy. These procedures may be motivated to contain the pain and distress, but they can also have important appraisal value as their consequences serve further to define the identity or immediate meaning of the distressing symptoms.

Accessing the Social Environment

When uncertainty continues because the symptoms change their pattern or fail to ameliorate, or the comparison to prior episodes raises questions about cause or control, or simply because the sensations become too severe to tolerate, the individual is likely to turn to others for support. An initial step might be to seek informational support; for example, if he had eaten with friends or family members, he might ask if they experienced similar pains and if so, whether they suspect the same foods that he had eaten (Sanders, 1982). If the information indicates similar problems and sources, further search will be unnecessary. If, however, the information is nonconfirmatory, the search for other explanations will continue and at some point there may be a felt need and decision to seek expert medical care. The expert practitioner has the medical background, the epidemiological information, and the diagnostic tools to remove the uncertainty and give meaning to the symptom state.

In their excellent review of their carefully executed research program, Croyle and Jemmott (this volume) make a strong case for the reduction of perceived danger and threat via social comparison. Subjects informed of an alleged enzyme deficiency are far more upset by this information if they are the only person in a set of individuals so diagnosed. When a majority of those present receive a similar diagnosis, the threat is appraised as less life-threatening; prevalence reduces perceived threat to self. It is unclear whether this reduction is a consequence of prevalence per se: Merely sharing a noxious fate may reduce its emotional impact. Instead, it may be a consequence of the implications for prevalence on severity: If most people have a problem with their pancreas and few people are dying if it, it cannot be very serious. Whatever its source, it is clear that prevalence information alters the meaning of diagnostic information. Because it is often difficult or impossible to generate prevalence information on one's own, it is frequently obtained when seeking medical care.

Procedures to Regulate Threat, Uncertainty, and Affect

We have said little about the interaction of illness cognitions—the representations, coping procedures, and appraisals involved in generating adaptive responses to health threats—with the fear, anger, and distress that accompany these adaptive efforts. We will mention just two aspects of these interactions here: illness cognition and the elicitation of emotion, and procedures that serve to regulate both emotion and illness threats.

Provocation to Fear and Worry

There is virtually no limit to the evidence that health threats are a source of worry, fear, distress, and anger. Fear and anger of the intensity of a "blow on the head" are commonly reported reactions at the point that symptoms are diagnosed as cancer (Jamison, Wellisch, & Pasnau, 1978; Myerowitz, 1980) and intense anger is especially common upon discovery of recurrence (Andersen et al., 1984; Silberfarb, Maurer, & Crouthamel, 1980). Emotional reactions of fear and distress can be provoked, therefore, at virtually every step of information processing, from the initial detection and labeling of somatic changes through the distress generated by the noxious effects of treatment to the severe distress and dejection evoked by treatment failure.

Fear and worry can be stimulated, however, by more subtle processes of illness cognition. Easterling and Leventhal (1989) examined worry about breast cancer as a function of three factors: women's belief in their vulnerability to cancer, their generic (noncancer) symptomatic complaints, such as headache and tiredness, and the cross-product of these two factors, that is, vulnerability times symptom complaints. Neither vulnerability feelings nor generic complaints were strongly related to worry about cancer either in a sample of women who had been treated for breast cancer four to five years earlier and were now disease-free or in a sample of their close friends who had not had cancer. The cross-product did, however, predict worry. Thus women who felt vulnerable to cancer (believed their chances of contracting it were 7 in 10 or better) reported increasing levels of worry as their level of generic symptoms increased. But if these vulnerable women were asymptomatic, they did not report more worry than women who felt invulnerable. In addition, visits to the doctors, a cue to worry for the ex-patients, were reported to stimulate worry by these women but not for their friends who had never had cancer. Finally, the ex-patients reported a higher level of worry about cancer than did their close friends. Thus cues such as symptoms and doctor visits provoke worry about cancer if interpreted within a framework of perceived vulnerability. These factors did not, however, predict general level of negative mood: The effects are specific to worry about cancer.

Little use has been made to date of the role of somatic sensations as reminders of vulnerability, elicitors of worry, and potential motivators of preventive and treatment behaviors. It is likely they have been ignored because of their double-edged character: Somatic reminders can instill motivation to control or regulate threat and they can instill loss of hope and passivity. The interpretation of somatic sensations and the responses to them are key; that is, are they interpreted as signs of disease and an uncontrollable and dire fate or are they seen as cues to necessary preventive or treatment actions where failure to act, and not the somatic signs, elicit the perception of threat and loss?

In contrast to the ambiguity regarding symptom interpretation and threat, data on the impact of diagnostic labels strongly suggest that positive diagnoses elicit a defensive process which reduces the judged severity of the diagnosed disorder (Croyle & Sande, 1988; Jemmott, Ditto, & Croyle, 1986). Interestingly, this dynamic seems partially independent of symptom perception; it appears to reflect coping with threat-elicited fear rather than a distortion of the perception of the presence of the illness itself (Croyle & Sande, 1988).

Procedures to Limit Threat and Emotion

Defensive Style. Both the psychoanalytic (Freud, 1957/1915) and psychological (Byrne, 1961) literatures describe various defenses or modes of limiting the impact of threat and/or negative emotions. Recent descriptions focus on mechanisms and personality types such as repression and repressors, that is, individuals who report low levels of anxiety and high levels of socially appropriate behaviors (Crowne & Marlowe, 1960; Weinberger, Schwartz, & Davidson, 1979), vigilance and sensitizers (Byrne, 1961), monitoring and distraction (Ahles et al., 1983), and monitoring and blunting (Miller, 1980). It is clear that individual differences of this type affect emotional reactions to illness and medical treatment. For example, compared to sensitizers, repressors report fewer somatic complaints (Byrne, 1961), and among patients in chemotherapy treatment for cancer, repressors report less intense and sometimes fewer somatic effects from treatment than nonrepressors (Ward, Leventhal, & Love, 1988). Avoiding somatic sensations is a plausible way of avoiding emotional upset, but it is not precisely clear how the avoidance is managed: Do repressors distract by engaging in alternative, positive thought, do they "grit their teeth" and ignore the distressing sensations of treatment, do they forget or refuse to report what they feel, or do they have fewer somatic sensations? The reduced symptom awareness of repressors does not seem to require an interval of time for "forgetting," at least not for cancer patients in chemotherapy treatment (Ward, Leventhal, & Gilderson-Duwe, in preparation).

The way that individuals reduce distress in health-threatening situations is clearly in need of further exploration given the evidence that both avoidance/repression and monitoring can be equally effective in reducing distress under different treatment conditions (E. A. Leventhal et al., 1989; Leventhal & Johnson, 1983; Suls & Fletcher, 1985; Suls & Wan, 1989). We can predict outcomes from "personality" scales, but doing so clearly fails to uncover the processes underlying the correlation, and the existent data clearly suggest these processes can vary from what appear to be relatively "passive" and covert mental events—for example, just don't think about it—to active monitoring and coping.

Limiting Threat Through Vigilant Coping. We have uncovered an interesting example where vigilance and confrontation appear to be used to reduce emotional distress. In two studies designed to examine delay in seeking health care, we compared the duration of total delay and delay at each of two key phases, *appraisal delay*, time from first noticing sensory changes till deciding one was ill, and *illness delay*, time from deciding one was ill to calling for care. The participants spanned a considerable age range. Both data sets revealed, as expected, swifter seeking of health care for severe than for mild symptoms and shorter delay at each phase for older (over 65) than for middle-aged respondents. What was most startling, however, was an interaction between the respondents' appraised severity of the symptoms and illness delay. When a symptom was of unknown or uncertain quality and appraised at onset as neither clearly mild nor severe, older people were very quick to seek care and middle-aged persons very slow. This difference was particularly pronounced for illness delay (the second stage) and the lengthy delays among the middle-aged appeared to be due to active efforts at denial (admissions of delay, fear it may be serious, not wanting to know what it is) while brief delays among the older and oldest subjects appeared to be due to unwillingness or inability to tolerate uncertainty and its associated dysphoria. There were no clear differences between the age groups in the type of complaint, reports of difficulty in getting to the doctor, or being urged to seek care by family and friends. Indeed, where differences appear (e.g., being advised to seek care), they are in a direction opposite to the foregoing effects: The younger persons were more likely than the older to receive such advice.

Evidence that health care can be used to reduce distress is not new. Prior data tend to emphasize, however, the use of care to reduce distress due to nonmedical factors, for example, non-European immigrants to Israel used the health-care system to reduce anxiety, form new relationships, and obtain advice about resettlement (Shuval, 1970). Similar functions have been emphasized in the primary care literature. We do not know whether our data reflect an age-related change (learning an efficient way to manage health threats with increasing illness experience), a reduction in perceived threat due to higher prevalence of disease in the elderly (Croyle & Sande, 1988; Jemmott et al. 1986), or a survivor effect (the efficient users are the ones who make it to old age). It seems clear, however, that it does reflect the use of a common coping response, seeking health care, to manage two objectives: the threat of illness and the emotional distress associated with uncertainty. It may be that the elderly "conserve" more energy by acting promptly and that adopting a "wait and see" attitude, common in the middle-aged participants, is too costly for the oldest subjects. The data also highlight the difference between a process-oriented approach characteristic of the investigations of illness cognition and the more traditional approach, which presents correlations between variables such as age, anxiety (Watson, 1988) or proclivity toward illness behavior (Pilowsky, 1986) and outcome measures. Traditional approaches would not reveal such interaction effects nor would they provide an account for their underlying dynamics.

Conclusion

Our intention in writing this chapter was to provide readers with an overview of our research program that would allow them to see the relationships between current work on illness cognition and earlier work on fear communications and control of emotional distress in both laboratory and medical settings. Thus we began with a flashback to our early work on fear communications, which served as the basis for our model of the effects of affect and cognition on beliefs and behavior. The impact of fear messages on beliefs, attitudes, and intentions seemed fairly direct (for contradictory view here, see Rogers, 1983) but of relatively short duration. More important were data showing the conditions under which a fear message would result in behavioral change: the combination of a threat message with a detailed action plan, that is, a suggestion stimulating subjects to think over and integrate the desired behavior into their daily life schedule. This combination affected behavior both in the immediate postcommunication setting and for up to three months later. The level of fear, however, was irrelevant for long-term effects, and both strong and weak fear messages resulted in behavior change when combined with a plan message that bridged the threat-induced motivation to the action system.

Studies of patients facing stressful medical procedures (e.g., gastritis intubation) made clear that somatic sensations play a critical role in the arousal of emotional reactions and that prior preparation identifying these experiences and action plans are valuable for controlling (reducing) these emotional reactions. These studies led us to the strong hypothesis that the representation of an illness will include both abstract (disease label) and concrete components, the two elements defining the identity (what it is) of an illness. We also hypothesized that the concrete or lower level of the information structure would play a powerful role in motivating (energizing and directing) behavior. At a still higher level of cognitive organization—that is, when comparing illness representations to one another (Lau et al., 1989)—representations appear to be organized about an acute–chronic or fatal–nonfatal dimension (see also Keller et al., 1989). Finally, contextual factors—for example, the self system including body schema as influenced by gender and age and the institutional organization and roles involved in health care—play an important role in the interpretation and organization of information within the illness domain. We have termed these representations and the processes involved in their construction "common sense models of illness."

Sacks's description of his exploratory "toe-wiggling" is a prime example of the use of procedures in the construction of illness representations. In this context it is important to realize that procedures are both a reflection of the knowledge structure they emerge from and operations which add to and create these knowledge structures. The virtually limitless number of cognitive and behavioral procedures poses some problems for an organized presentation and exploration of their functioning. A possible solution to this obstacle is to define the rules, decisions, or choices that guide the use of procedures. Data from recent field and laboratory studies identified at least two rules important for distinguishing illness from nonillness conditions: the stress–illness rule and the aging–illness rule. Studies involving the stress–illness relationship underscore the individual's use of situational and contextual cues in addition to personal history and symptoms in evaluating somatic sensations. For example, undergraduate students judged a potential set of symptoms as a likely reflection of stress if they were asked to evaluate these symptoms on the day prior to their midterm exam in psychology but did not evaluate them that way on the day before a free Saturday.

Studies with elderly patients revealed changes in the attributional rules applied to somatic sensations. Thus, compared to younger people, older people were more likely to attribute somatic changes to age rather than to illness, and this attribution was more common for mild symptoms with gradual onset. Although the age attribution is more frequent among the elderly, its effects are the same in both older and younger subjects: It appears to reduce emotional distress and to increase delay in seeking health care. But even though age attributions delay care and are somewhat more common for older than younger persons, compared to younger persons the elderly delay less in seeking care. This effect is most pronounced, however, for symptoms of intermediate severity; both groups delay substantially, and about equally so, for very mild symptoms, and they are both very swift to seek care for very severe symptoms. The older subjects appear to seek care rapidly for moderately severe symptoms, both to reduce the threat of illness and to reduce the distress and emotional upset contingent upon uncertainty regarding the symptoms diagnosis. Concern about the potential seriousness of the symptoms and fear of diagnosis seem, however, to enhance delay in the middle-aged respondent. The data provide an example of a procedure used to control both the objective threat and the affective component of an illness experience.

The literature on personality variables and their effects on symptom experience is vast, descriptive rather than analytic, and consequently inconclusive in outcome. Two aspects of the personality–health relationship need careful analysis: (1) the role of personality as direct and indirect contributor to the complex processes involved in the initiation and promotion of acute and chronic illnesses; and (2) the role of personality factors in the construction of illness representations and the appraisal of strategies for coping with health threats. A reader familiar with research on coping will quickly notice the contrast between our approach that advocates the identification of a host of rules and procedures for constructing illness representations, in contrast to traditional approaches that focus on one or two broad personality dimensions related to coping, such as repression and sensitization (Byrne, 1961; Lazarus & Launier, 1978; Miller, 1980). We accept the hypothesis that higher order "traits" or personality dispositions may influence lower level rules and procedures, but we do not believe that traits and dispositions can directly predict and/or account for the underlying dynamic processes which make up the appraisal and coping mechanisms (Contrada, Leventhal, & O'Leary, 1990). Similarly, we take a dim view of recent attempts to interpret negative affect as an all-encompassing disposition that is a major source of symptom generation and the factor responsible for significant relationships between stress and illness and stress and use of health care. The descriptive finding ought not be confused with the analysis of the mechanism by which negative affect may or may not influence symptom generation and the development of illness representations. Ignoring these process questions uses personality variables in ways reminiscent of the "good old times" of personality research where factor-analytically derived concepts were presented as the answer to all questions of personality.

We hope these concluding remarks will help to more sharply delineate our viewpoint and assume that in their general form they are agreeable to most of the contributors to this volume. The area of illness cognition has become increasingly important both for health psychology and for deepening our understanding of the complex processes involved in the representation, coping, appraisal, and updating of problem situations. In addition, research on illness cognition offers multiple possibilities for studying the interaction of cognition and emotion and of the interaction of the physiological processes underlying both. While some may find health psychology "too applied" or too far from the "mainstream" of social psychology, we believe it provides a unique opportunity to work at a critical interface that will generate important contributions to psychology. We hope that the intellectual excitement stimulated by the excellent contributions in this volume will lead aspiring social psychologists to pursue further the study of illness cognition.

References

Ahles, T. A., Blanchard, E. B., & Leventhal, H. (1983). Cognitive control of pain: Attention to the sensory aspects of the cold pressor stimulus. *Cognitive Therapy and Research, 7*, 159–177.

Anderson, J. (1983). *The architecture of cognition.* Cambridge, MA: Harvard University Press.

Baumann, L., Cameron, L. D., Zimmerman, R., & Leventhal, H. (1989). Illness representations and matching labels with symptoms. *Health Psychology, 8*, 449–469.

Bishop, G. D. (1987). Lay conceptions of physical symptoms. *Journal of Applied Social Psychology, 17*(2), 127–146.

Blumhagen, D. (1980). Hyper-tension: A folk illness with a medical name. *Culture, Medicine, and Psychiatry, 4*, 197–227.

Byrne, D. (1961). The repression–sensitization scale: Rationale, reliability and validity. *Journal of Personality, 29*, 344–349.

Cacioppo, J. T., Andersen, B. L., Turnquist, D. C., & Petty, R. E. (1985). Psychophysiological comparison processes: Interpreting cancer symptoms. In B. L. Andersen (Ed.), *Women with cancer: Psychological perspectives* (pp. 141–171). New York: Springer-Verlag.

Contrada, R., Leventhal, H., & O'Leary, A. (1990). Personality and health. In L. Pervin (Ed.), *Handbook of personality: Theory and research* (pp. 638–669). New York: Guilford.

Crowne, D. P., & Marlowe, D. (1960). A new scale of social desirability independent of psychopathology. *Journal of Counselling Psychology, 24*, 349–354.

Croyle, R. T., & Sande, G. N. (1988). Denial and confirmatory search: Paradoxical consequences of medical diagnosis. *Journal of Applied Social Psychology, 18*(6), 473–490.

Easterling, D., & Leventhal, H. (1989). The contribution of concrete cognition to emotion: Neutral symptoms as elicitors of worry about cancer. *Journal of Applied Psychology, 74*, 787–796.

Foa, E. B., & Kozak, M. J. (1986). Emotional processing of fear: Exposure to corrective information. *Psychological Bulletin*, *99*, 20–35.

Freud, S. (1957). Instincts and their vicissitudes. In J. Strachey (Ed. and Trans.), *The standard edition of the complete psychological works of Sigmund Freud* (pp. 111–142). London: Hogarth Press. (Original work published 1915)

Green, L. W. (1984). Modifying and developing health behavior. *Annual Reviews of Public Health*, *5*, 215–236.

Jamison, K. R., Wellisch, D. K., & Pasnau, R. O. (1978). Psychosocial aspects of mastectomy. I. The woman's perspective. *American Journal of Psychiatry*, *135*, 432–436.

Janis, I. L. (1958). *Psychological stress*. New York: Wiley.

Janis, I. L., & Leventhal, H. (1967). Human reactions to stress. In E. Borgatta & W. Lambert (Eds.), *Handbook of personality theory and research* (pp. 1041–1085). Chicago: Rand McNally.

Jemmott, J. B., III, Ditto, P. H., & Croyle, R. T. (1986). Judging health status: Effects of perceived prevalence and personal relevance. *Journal of Personality and Social Psychology*, *50*, 899–905.

Johnson, J. E. (1973). Effects of accurate expectations about sensations on the sensory and distress components of pain. *Journal of Personality and Social Psychology*, *27*, 261–275.

Johnson, J. E. (1975). Stress reduction through sensation information. In I. G. Sarason & C. D. Spielberger (Eds.), *Stress and anxiety* (Vol. 2, pp. 361–373). Washington, DC: Hemisphere Publishing.

Johnson, J. E., Lauvier, D. R., & Nail, L. M. (1989). Process of coping with radiation therapy. *Journal of Consulting and Clinical Psychology*, *57*, 358–364.

Johnson, J. E., & Leventhal, H. (1974). The effects of accurate expectations and behavioral instructions on reactions during a noxious medical examination. *Journal of Personality and Social Psychology*, *29*, 710–718.

Keller, M. L., Leventhal, H., Prohaska, T. R., & Leventhal, E. A. (1989). Beliefs about aging and illness in a community sample. *Research in Nursing and Health*, *12*, 247–255.

Kornzweig, N. D. (1967). *Behavior change as a function of fear arousal and personality*. Unpublished doctoral dissertation, Yale University, New Haven, CT.

Lau, R. R., Bernard, T. M., & Hartman, K. A. (1989). Further explorations of common sense representations of common illnesses. *Health Psychology*, *8*, 195–219.

Lau, R. R., & Hartman, K. A. (1983). Common sense representations of common illnesses. *Health Psychology*, *2*, 167–185.

Lazarus, R. S. (1966). *Psychological stress and the coping process*. New York: McGraw-Hill.

Lazarus, R. S., & Launier, R. (1978). Stress related transactions between person and environment. In L. A. Pervin & M. Lewis (Eds.), *Perspectives in interactional psychology*. New York: Academic Press.

Leventhal, E. A. (in press). Gender and their aging: Women and *their* aging. In D. M. Reddy, V. J. Adesso, & R. Fleming (Eds.), *Psychological perspectives on womens's health*. New York: Hemisphere.

Leventhal, E. A., Leventhal H., Shacham, S., & Easterling, D. V. (1989). Active coping reduces reports of pain from childbirth. *Journal of Consulting and Clinical Psychology*, *57*, 365–371.

Leventhal, H. (1970). Findings and theory in the study of fear communications. *Advances in Experimental Social Psychology*, *5*, 119–186.

Leventhal, H. (1975). The consequences of depersonalization during illness and treatment: An information processing model. In J. Howard & A. Strauss (Eds.), *Humanizing health care* (pp. 119–161). New York: Wiley.

Leventhal, H. (1976). Comments on the study of smoking and the study of special subcultures and cancer. In J. W. Cullen, B. H. Fox, & R. N. Isom (Eds.), *Cancer, the behavioral dimensions* (pp. 111–115). New York: Raven Press.

Leventhal, H. (1979). A perceptual-motor processing model of emotion. In P. Pliner, K. Blankstein, & I. M. Spigel (Eds.), *Advances in the study of communication and affect: Perception of emotion in self and others* (Vol 5, pp. 1–46). New York: Plenum Press.

Leventhal, H., Brown, D., Shacham, S., & Engquist, G. (1979). Effects of preparatory information about sensations, threat of pain, and attention on cold pressor distress. *Journal of Personality and Social Psychology, 37,* 688–714.

Leventhal, H., & Johnson, J. E. (1983). Laboratory and field experimentation: Development of a theory of self-regulation. In P. J. Wooldridge, M. H. Schmitt, J. K. Skipper, & R. C. Leonard (Eds.), *Behavioral science and nursing theory* (pp. 189–262). St. Louis: Mosby.

Leventhal, H., Jones, S., & Trembly, G. (1966). Sex differences in attitude and behavior change under conditions of fear and specific instructions. *Journal of Experimental Social Psychology, 2,* 387–399.

Leventhal, H., Meyer, D., & Nerenz, D. (1980). The common sense representation of illness danger. In S. Rachman (Ed.), *Contributions to medical psychology* (Vol. 2, pp. 17–30). New York: Pergamon Press.

Leventhal, H., Nerenz, D., & Steele, D. (1984). Illness representations and coping with health threats. In A. Baum & J. Singer (Eds.), *A Handbook of Psychology and Health* (Vol. 4, pp. 219–252). Hillsdale, NJ: Lawrence Erlbaum Associates.

Leventhal, H., & Niles, P. (1965). Persistence of influence for varying durations of exposure to threat stimuli. *Psychological Reports, 16,* 223–233.

Leventhal, H., Singer, R., & Jones, S. (1965). Effects of fear and specificity of recommendations upon attitudes and behavior. *Journal of Personality and Social Psychology, 2,* 20–29.

Leventhal, H., & Singer, R. P. (1966). Affect arousal and positioning of recommendations in persuasive communications. *Journal of Personality and Social Psychology, 4,* 137–146.

Leventhal, H., Watts, J. C., & Pagano, F. (1967). Effects of fear and instructions on how to cope with danger. *Journal of Personality and Social Psychology, 6,* 313–321.

Linz, D., Penrod, S., Siverhus, S., & Leventhal, H. (1982). *The cognitive organization of disease and illness among lay persons.* Unpublished manuscript, University of Wisconsin, Madison.

Matthews, K. A., Siegel, J. M., Kuller, L. H., Thompson, M., & Vanat, M. (1983). Determinants of decision to seek medical treatment by patients with acute myocardial infarction symptoms. *Journal of Personality and Social Psychology, 44,* 1144–1156.

Mechanic, D. (1972). Social psychological factors affecting the presentation of bodily complaints. *New England Journal of Medicine, 286,* 1132–1139.

Mechanic, D. (1980). The experience and reporting of common physical complaints. *Journal of Health and Social Behavior, 21,* 146–155.

Mechanic, D. (1986). Illness behavior: An overview. In S. McHugh & T. M. Vallis (Eds.), *Illness behavior: A multi-disciplinary model.* New York: Plenum Press.

Meyer, D., Leventhal, H., & Gutmann, M. (1985). Commonsense models of illness: The example of hypertension. *Health Psychology, 4,* 115–135.

Miller, S. (1980). When is a little information a dangerous thing? Coping with stressful events by monitoring versus blunting. In S. Levine & H. Ursin (Eds.), *Coping and health: Proceedings of a NATO conference* (pp. 145–169). New York: Plenum Press.

Myerowitz, B. E. (1980). Psychosocial correlates of breast cancer and its treatments. *Psychological Bulletin, 87*, 108–131.

Parrott, G. W., & Sabini, J. (1989). On the "emotional" qualities of certain types of cognition: A reply to arguments for the independence of cognition and affect. *Cognitive Therapy and Research, 13*, 49–65.

Pennebaker, J. W. (1982). *The psychology of physical symptoms.* New York: Springer-Verlag.

Pennebaker, J. W., & Skelton, J. A. (1978). Psychological parameters of physical symptoms. *Personality and Social Psychology Bulletin, 4*, 524–530.

Pennebaker, J. W., & Skelton, J. A. (1981). Selective monitoring of bodily sensations. *Journal of Personality and Social Psychology, 41*, 213–223.

Pilowsky, I. (1986). Abnormal illness behavior: A review of the concept and its implications. In S. McHugh & T. M. Vallis (Eds.), *Illness behavior: A multidisciplinary model* (pp. 391–408). New York: Plenum Press.

Prohaska, T. R., Keller, M. L., Leventhal, E. A., & Leventhal, H. (1987). Impact of symptoms and aging attribution on emotions and coping. *Health Psychology, 6*, 495–514.

Rogers, R. W. (1983). Cognitive and physiological processes in fear appeals and attitude change: A revised theory of protection motivation. In J. T. Caccioppo & R. E. Petty (Eds.), *Social psychophysiology* (pp. 153–176). New York: Guilford Press.

Sacks, O. (1984). *A leg to stand on.* London: Duckworth.

Safer, M. A., Tharps, Q. J., Jackson, T. C., & Leventhal, H. (1979). Determinants of three stages of delay in seeking care at a medical clinic. *Medical Care, 12*(1), 11–29.

Sanders, G. S. (1982). Social comparison and perceptions of health and illness. In G. S. Sanders & J. Suls (Eds.), *Social psychology of health and illness* (pp. 129–157). Hillsdale, NJ: Lawrence Erlbaum Associates.

Shontz, F. C. (1975). *The psychological aspects of physical illness and disability.* New York: Macmillan.

Shuval, J. T. (1970). *Social functions of medical practice: Doctor–patient relationships in Israel.* San Fransisco: Jossey-Bass.

Silberfarb, P. M., Maurer, L. H., & Crouthamel, C. S. (1980). Psychosocial aspects of neoplastic disease. I. Functional status of breast cancer patients during different treatment regimens. *American Journal of Psychiatry, 137*, 450–455.

Suchman, E. A. (1965). Stages of illness and medical care. *Journal of Health Social Behavior, 6*, 114.

Suls, J., & Fletcher, B. (1985). The relative efficacy of avoidant and non-avoidant coping strategies: A meta-analysis. *Health Psychology, 4*, 249–288.

Suls, J., Maco, C. A., & Tobin, S. (in press). *The role of temporal comparison, social comparison, and direct appraisal in the elderly's self-evaluations of health. Journal of Applied Social Psychology.*

Suls, J., & Wan, C. K. (1989). Effects of sensory and procedural information on coping with stressful medical procedures and pain: A meta-analysis. *Journal of Consulting and Clinical Psychology, 57*, 372–379.

Suls, J. Wan, C. K., & Sanders, G. S. (1988). False consensus and false uniqueness in the perception of health-promotive behaviors. *Journal of Applied Psychology, 18*, 66–79.

Tulving, E. (1972). Episodic and semantic memory. In E. Tulving & W. Donaldson (Eds.), *Organization of memory*. New York: Academic Press.

Ward, S., Leventhal, H., & Gilderson-Duwe, C. *Repression and the experience of chemotherapy: A self-regulation perspective*. Manuscript in preparation.

Ward, S., Leventhal, H., & Love, R. (1988). Repression revisited: Tactics used in coping with a severe health threat. *Personality and Social Psychology Bulletin, 14*, 735–746.

Watson, D. (1988). Intraindividual and interindividual analyses of positive and negative affect: Their relation to health complaints, perceived stress, and daily activities. *Journal of Personality and Social Psychology, 54*, 1020–1030.

Watson, D., & Pennebaker, J. W. (1989). Health complaints, stress, and distress: Exploring the central role of negative affectivity. *Psychological Review, 96*, 234–254.

Weinberger, A. D., Schwartz, G. E., & Davidson, R. J. D. (1979). Low-anxious, high-anxious, and repressive coping styles: Psychometric patterns and behavioral and physiological responses to stress. *Journal of Abnormal Psychology, 88*, 369–380.

Whiting, J. W. M., & Child, I. L. (1953). *Child training and personality* (pp. 119–128). New Haven, CT: Yale University Press.

Index

Within-subject research design, 77–78,
    100, 228
Wong, S., 156
Work, return to, predictors of, 203–207
Workers' Compensation Board, 194,
    202–203, 209

Worry, and generic symptoms, 263

Zimmerman, R., 97
Zola, I. K., 90